Principles
of
Obstetrics

Principles
of
Obstetrics

Edited by

Ronald M. Caplan, M.D.

Clinical Associate Professor
Obstetrics and Gynecology
Cornell University Medical College
New York, New York

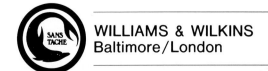

WILLIAMS & WILKINS
Baltimore/London

Library of Congress Cataloging in Publication Data

Main entry under title:

Principles of obstetrics.

  Includes index.
  1. Obstetrics. I. Caplan, Ronald M. [DNLM: 1. Obstetrics. WQ 100 P9572]
RG524.P825   618.2   81-14794
ISBN 0-683-01436-6   AACR2

Composed and printed at the
Waverly Press, Inc.
Mt. Royal and Guilford Aves.
Baltimore, MD 21202, U.S.A.

TO WILLIAM J. SWEENEY III, M.D.

superb clinician, confidant, friend.

PREFACE

We no longer can expect a medical student to be totally competent in the practice of obstetrics for several reasons. Among these are lack of sufficient curriculum time and lack of sufficient numbers of pregnant patients "available" at many schools of medicine for the medical student to deliver. The rapid expansion of knowledge in the field and the goal of giving each mother an infant in optimal condition make it mandatory for the person caring for the pregnant patient to be knowledgeable and experienced and to have access to immediately available expert help and sophisticated equipment in case of complications.

In this setting, we assume that anyone desirous of caring for the pregnant patient and her forming child will avail themselves of appropriate postgraduate training.

It is essential, however, for every medical student to have a thorough grounding in reproductive physiology as part of the greater understanding of the functioning of the human body. The student should be aware of the new physiologic demands of pregnancy and of how these may alter various disease states. The diagnosis of pregnancy should be learned: this should be kept in mind when dealing with any female patient in her reproductive years. It is important to understand the mechanisms of labor and delivery as part of the physiologic interaction between mother and child.

It is with this philosophy in mind that this textbook was written.

ACKNOWLEDGMENTS

I wish to acknowledge the contribution of Dr. Graham Hawks, who has been instrumental in providing statistical and clinical data. I appreciate the enthusiasm of Dr. William Ledger, who has been most supportive. Most importantly, I wish to thank the contributors, whose unselfish hard work and expertise were instrumental in the creation of this text.

Ms. Diane Abeloff and Mr. Michael Budowick are superb professionals: they are the creators of the original drawings in the book.

I thank Ms. Charlene Varnis for her help with the statistics and Ms. Randy Sue Caplan for many hours of library research. My gratitude is extended to Dr. Joseph F. Artusio, Jr., and Dr. Fritz Fuchs for their constructive suggestions.

I wish to convey my sincere gratitude to Ms. Susan Vitale of the Williams & Wilkins Company for her innovative thought, support and understanding, without which this text would not have been written. I also thank the many others in the Williams & Wilkins organization who have done so much to bring this book to fruition.

CONTRIBUTORS

Lucien I. Arditi, M.D.
Clinical Associate Professor of Medicine,
Cornell University Medical College
New York, New York

Alan Berkeley, M.D.
Assistant Professor,
Obstetrics and Gynecology
Cornell University Medical College
New York, New York

Ronald M. Caplan, M.D.
Clinical Associate Professor,
Obstetrics and Gynecology
Cornell University Medical College
New York, New York

Lars L. Cederqvist, M.D.
Associate Professor of Clinical Obstetrics
and Gynecology
Cornell University Medical College
New York, New York

Yves Clermont, Ph.D.
Professor and Chairman,
Department of Anatomy
McGill University
Montreal, Quebec, Canada

M. Yusoff Dawood, M.D., M.Med.
Professor of Obstetrics and Gynecology
Abraham Lincoln School of Medicine
University of Illinois
Chicago, Illinois

Maurice L. Druzin, M.B., B.Chir.
Assistant Professor,
Obstetrics and Gynecology
Cornell University Medical College
New York, New York

John F. Dwyer, M.D.
Associate Clinical Professor,
Obstetrics and Gynecology
Columbia University College of
Physicians and Surgeons
New York, New York

Joseph Finkelstein, M.D.
Clinical Instructor,
Obstetrics and Gynecology
Cornell University Medical College
New York, New York

Anna-Riitta Fuchs, D.Sc.
Associate Professor of Reproductive
Biology
Cornell University Medical College
New York, New York

Fritz Fuchs, M.D.
Professor of Obstetrics and Gynecology
Cornell University Medical College
New York, New York

Philip Grimley, M.D.
Pathologist
Suburban Hospital
Bethesda, Maryland

Donald E. Henson, M.D.
Chief, Diagnostic Section
Breast Cancer Program Coordinating
Branch
Division of Cancer Biology and Diagnosis
National Cancer Institute
Bethesda, Maryland

Lois Jovanovic, M.D.
Assistant Professor of Medicine and
Obstetrics and Gynecology
Cornell University Medical College
New York, New York

Elmer E. Kramer, M.D.
Professor of Obsterics and Gynecology
and Pathology
Cornell University Medical College
New York, New York

Robert Landesman, M.D.
Clinical Professor of Obstetrics and
Gynecology
Cornell University Medical College
New York, New York

Niels H. Lauersen, M.D.
Associate Professor,
Department of Obstetrics and
Gynecology
Division of Perinatology
The Mount Sinai School of Medicine
New York, New York

William Ledger, M.D.
Given Foundation Professor
of Obstetrics and Gynecology
Chairman, Department of
Obstetrics and Gynecology
Cornell University Medical College
New York, New York

Norton M. Luger, M.D.
Clinical Associate Professor of Medicine
and Clinical Associate Professor of
Medicine in Obstetrics
Cornell University Medical College
New York, New York

Paul S. Milley, M.D.
Associate Director of Laboratories
Sisters of Charity Hospital
Buffalo, New York

Charles M. Peterson, M.D.
Associate Professor
Laboratory of Medical Biochemistry
The Rockefeller University
New York, New York

Richard A. Ruskin, M.D.
Clinical Professor,
Obstetrics and Gynecology
Cornell University Medical College
New York, New York

Zoltan Saary, M.D.
Assistant Professor of Clinical Obstetrics
and Gynecology
Cornell University Medical College
New York, New York

Brij B. Saxena, Ph.D., D.Sc.
Professor of Biochemistry and
Endocrinology
Cornell University Medical College
New York, New York

Edwina Sia-Kho, M.D.
Instructor of Anesthesiology
Cornell University Medical College
New York, New York

Frederick Silverman, M.D.
Clinical Associate Professor,
Obstetrics and Gynecology
Cornell University Medical College
New York, New York

Joe Leigh Simpson, M.D.
Professor of Obstetrics and Gynecology
Section of Human Genetics
Department of Obstetrics and
Gynecology
Northwestern University Medical School
Chicago, Illinois

William J. Sweeney III, M.D.
Clinical Professor,
Obstetrics and Gynecology
Cornell University Medical College
New York, New York

Marion S. Verp, M.D.
Fellow, Section of Human Genetics
Department of Obstetrics and
Gynecology
Prentice Women's Hospital
Chicago, Illinois

Robert E. Wieche, M.D.
Clinical Associate Professor,
Obstetrics and Gynecology
Cornell University Medical College
New York, New York

Olavi Ylikorkala, M.D.
Professor of Obstetrics and Gynecology
University of Helsinki
Helsinki, Finland

Luciano Zamboni, M.D.
Professor of Pathology
University of California at Los Angeles
School of Medicine
Chairman, Department of Pathology
Harbor-UCLA Medical Center
Torrance, California

CONTENTS

Reproductive Physiology

Perinatology

Labor and Delivery

Postpartum

Section 1

Reproductive Physiology

CHAPTER 1

The Menstrual Cycle

BRIJ B. SAXENA, Ph.D., D.Sc.

The measurement and the study of the interaction of the hormones secreted by the central nervous system (CNS)-hypothalamic-hypophyseal-gonadal axis have provided insight into the sequence of events in the regulation of the menstrual cycle. This has been done by the application of sensitive, specific radioimmunoassays in the determination, in the same individuals, of daily or more frequent levels of endocrine and neuroendocrine components which circulate in low concentrations in the body fluids.

In the human, the menstrual cycle is the result of a precise coordination of the functional characteristics of the central nervous system, the hypothalamus, the pituitary, the ovary and the endometrium, which regulate the cyclic release of the gonadotropin releasing factors (luteinizing hormone-releasing hormone: LH-RH), gonadotropins (follicle stimulating hormone: FSH, and luteinizing hormone: LH) and ovarian steroids (estradiol: E_2, and progesterone). Prolactin and prostaglandins play a facilitatory role in the regulation of the menstrual cycle. In general, ovulation does not occur prior to menarche. The menstrual cycle is timed from the onset of blood flow to the similar onset with the next cycle. During the normal reproductive years this period is of an average of 28 days. However, an increase in the intermenstrual interval occurs at adolescence and at the menopausal transition due to the frequent occurrence of anovulatory cycles. Due to variability in the length of the menstrual cycle from 28 to 35 days, the day of maximum preovulatory LH surge

has been used as a marker for the midcycle or the "O" day (Fig. 1.1). The period from the day of menses until 1 day prior to the LH surge is designated as the *follicular* or *preovulatory* phase, which can be functionally subdivided into the first half as "early" and the late second half as "late" follicular phases, each of 7 days' duration. The late follicular phase is followed by an "ovulatory" phase. During this period, there is a rapid rise in the plasma LH level which leads to ovulation, which is the final maturation of the Graafian follicle in the ovary; the follicle ruptures approximately 24 hours following the LH surge, resulting in the formation of the corpus luteum. The interval between the beginning of the maturation of a follicle and ovulation is as yet unknown. The period between 1 day following the LH peak and the day of the onset of the next menses is designated as the *luteal* or *postovulatory* phase. The first half of the luteal phase can be considered as the "early luteal phase" and the second half as the "late luteal phase."

MORPHOLOGICAL CHANGES

From the seventh month of fetal life until the menopause, follicular maturation is continuous in the ovary. After the menarche, atresia, a follicular degenerative process which continues until the last oocyte is removed from the ovary, persists.[12, 21] Ovulation of one follicle gives rise to a corpus luteum during each menstrual cycle. Ovulation begins with rapid enlargement of a follicle and is followed by its protrusion from the surface of the

3

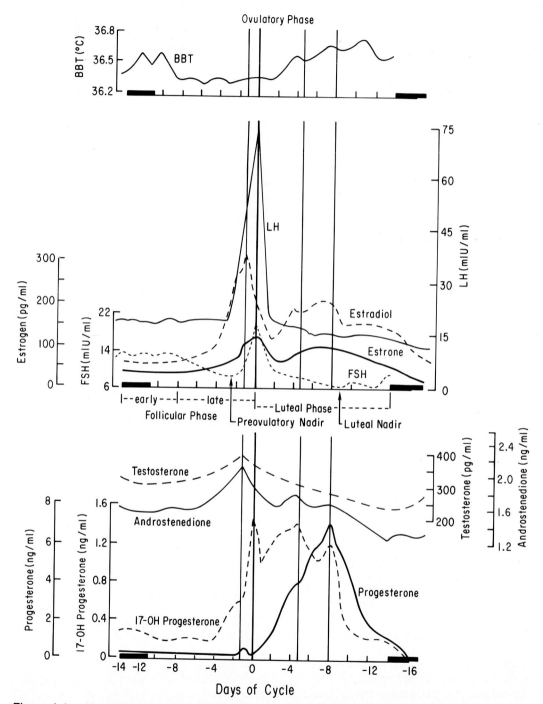

Figure 1.1.   Hormonal levels in the menstrual cycle. The basal body temperature curve shown in the top figure is biphasic, rising after ovulation. The dramatic preovulatory LH surge is shown.

ovarian cortex and rupture, with an extrusion of an oocyte and adhering cumulus oophorus.[4] In the human ovary, this sequence occurs over a 5–6 day period prior to the preovulatory LH surge which precedes actual rupture by as much as 16 hours.[30] Following rupture of the follicle, capillaries and fibroblasts from the theca cells proliferate and penetrate the basal lamina. The mural granulosa cells undergo "luteinization," and these cells, surrounding theca cells, capillaries and blood vessels intermingle to give rise to the corpus luteum.[10] The corpus luteum is the major source of steroid hormones secreted by the ovary during the postovulatory phase of the cycle.[15] Endometrial development is necessary for implantation: in unfertilized cycles, regression of the endometrium occurs in the form of menstrual bleeding. The corpus luteum functions for about 14 ± 2 days, after which it spontaneously regresses and is replaced by an avascular scar called a *corpus albicans*, unless pregnancy occurs.[28] The endometrial changes and their correlation with the menstrual cycle are presented in Figure 1.2. In an ideal 28-day cycle in a normal woman, after ovulation the progestational or secretory phase lasts 14 days and is followed by 3 days of menstruation which is succeeded by 11 days of the proliferative phase during which the repair of the endometrium takes place. Prior to the onset of menses, there is withdrawal of estrogen and progesterone and desquamation of the endometrium. Bleeding is preceded by intense spasmodic constrictions (vasospasm) of the spiral arteries of the uterus and ischemic necrosis. Vasospasm and increased uterine contraction are thought to be initiated by local production of prostaglandins, which are found in high concentrations in the menstrual blood.[29] The estrogen and progesterone withdrawal causes a decrease in lysosomal stability and a release of phospholipase which stimulates prostaglandin synthesis. Aspirin and indomethacin increase the stability of lysosomal membranes and inhibit the prostaglandin synthesis. The menstrual flow is also facilitated by the noncoagulability of the blood due to the fibrinolytic activity of the endometrium, which is maximum at the time of menstruation.

GONADOTROPIN-OVARIAN INTERACTIONS IN THE REGULATION OF THE MENSTRUAL CYCLE

The human fetal pituitary produces FSH and prolactin preferentially, even prior to the establishment of the hypothalamic-hy-

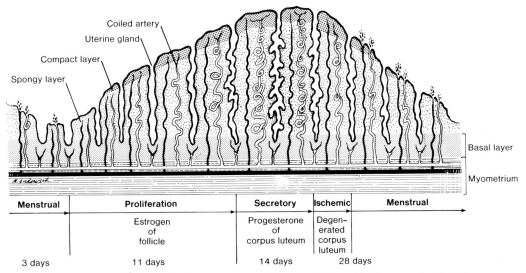

Figure 1.2. Endometrial changes and their correlation with the menstrual cycle.

pophyseal portal system, and the ratio of FSH to LH is greater than 1. The androgens present in the ovary potentiate FSH release by the pituitary, independent of the aromatizing step.[1] The progressive appearance of estrogen in circulation and of follicular "inhibin" which selectively inhibits FSH release decreases the ratio of FSH to LH to less than 1 during sexual maturation and induces the initiation of the menstrual cycle.[6]

HORMONAL LEVELS IN A NORMAL CYCLE (Fig. 1.1)[7, 27, 29]

The metabolic clearance rate (MCR) of LH is greater than FSH.[24] The MCR of FSH and LH are not affected by large differences in the concentrations of the hormone; hence the variations in the plasma concentrations of FSH and LH are considered equivalent to the pituitary secretions.

FOLLICULAR PHASE

The level of FSH is relatively high in plasma in the early follicular phase and reaches a maximum prior to the onset of menstruation. Due to the low levels of steroids at the end of the preceding postovulatory luteal phase, FSH stimulates follicular growth with minimal secretion of the estrogens estrone (E_1) and estradiol (E_2). Ovarian secretion of estrogens, androgens and progestins is at a relatively constant level during the early follicular phase. The late follicular phase begins approximately 7 or 8 days prior to the preovulatory LH surge and is characterized by an increase in ovarian secretion of E_1 and E_2. The rise of E_1 is not as great as but parallels that of E_2. The rate of secretion of the estrogens is dependent upon the blood levels of gonadotropins and, more importantly, on the intraovarian levels of estrogens and androgens. The rise of the plasma estrogen level results in a decreased FSH level during the late follicular phase that reaches a low point called the *preovulatory nadir*. This is accompanied by a small but steady increase in basal LH levels. When plasma estrogens reach a threshold value there is an explosive pre-

ovulatory discharge of LH from the pituitary, resulting in ovulation, provided that the morphological changes in the follicle have kept pace with the changes in the hormone levels. In association with the rise of estradiol, the concentrations of prolactin, growth hormone, adrenocorticotrophic hormone (ACTH), cortisol, parathyroid hormone and calcitonin also show a progressive increase toward midcycle, indicating a modulatory role of estrogen on neurohypophyseal and adenohypophyseal function as well as on calcium metabolism. Urinary excretion of catecholestrogens (2-OHE$_1$ or 2-OHE$_2$) is also increased to 50 μg/24 hours at midcycle as compared with 10 μg/24 hours during the early follicular phase.

OVULATORY PHASE

During this period the FSH and LH rise in the plasma and an abrupt midcycle surge of FSH usually occurs on the same day as LH release. This leads to the final maturation of the Graafian follicle and follicular rupture, approximately 16–24 hours following the LH surge. The precise mechanism for the selection of a single follicle for ovulation is not known. The role of the simultaneous midcycle rise of FSH with LH level in ovulation is not clearly understood and is speculated to be a fail-safe support to assure that rupture follows follicular maturation. The level of estradiol drops sharply prior to the midcycle LH surge and prior to ovulation.

There is a minor elevation in plasma progesterone levels prior to the ovulatory phase. Subsequently the plasma progesterone concentration begins to rise on the day of the LH peak and reaches a maximum of 25 mg daily, about 8 days after the midcycle LH peak. The maximum levels of progesterone coincide with the FSH luteal nadir. Increased serum progesterone and urinary pregnanediol derived from progesterone are regarded as an index of ovulation and of adequate corpus luteum function, which may be further confirmed by the biopsy of the endometrium showing secretory phase. The 17-OH progesterone, secreted by the ovary, increases significantly to coincide with the midcycle LH and FSH surges but declines transiently to rise again in a fashion similar to that of progesterone.

LUTEAL PHASE

Following ovulation and adequate maturation of the follicle, a surge of LH is followed by the rupture of the follicle, extrusion of an ovum and formation of a corpus luteum. The follicular cells are luteinized and there is significant increase in progesterone secretion by the corpus luteum. The elevation of the basal body temperature (BBT) is a reflection of the increasing plasma concentrations of progesterone. The mean BBT is elevated during the luteal phase for a period of 9 days.

Maximal luteal phase concentrations of gonadal hormones (17 α-hydroxyprogesterone, progesterone and estrogen) coincide with minimal concentration to FSH and LH. During the luteal phase, the FSH and LH levels decline. The day the mean FSH levels decline to the lowest level is designated as the day of the *luteal nadir*. When the concentration of the steroid hormones begins to decline, pituitary secretion of FSH and LH is resumed and another cycle of follicular maturation is initiated. After ovulation occurs, small amounts of LH are necessary for the normal function of the corpus luteum and, unless there is a secondary luteotropic stimulus to the corpus luteum (presumably by the blastocyst), the steroid levels start to decrease 7 or 8 days after ovulation, accompanied by the regression of the endometrium, and a new cycle starts.

THE INTERACTION OF HORMONES AND RECEPTORS IN THE REGULATION OF THE MENSTRUAL CYCLE

The ovary contains a pool of nonproliferating germ cells which are surrounded by a layer of granulosa cells, a basement lamina and a theca layer outside of the basement membrane. The interaction of FSH and LH with theca and granulosa cells is involved in the regulation of follicular growth and maturation. The target for FSH is exclusively the granulosa cell, while LH acts upon thecal, stromal and luteal as well as granulosa cells.

During the early follicular phase, increasing levels of FSH induce an increase in FSH receptors to allow FSH to influence the proliferation of granulosa cells, follicular growth, and induction of an aromatizing enzyme. This enzyme provides the essential step for estradiol production via conversion of androgens seen during the late follicular phase. Estradiol increases its own receptors, thereby exerting a direct mitogenic action on granulosa cells to cause proliferation.[8, 23] FSH and estradiol induce the production of LH receptors which may be responsible for preovulatory progesterone production.[14] During the luteal phase the theca interna develops specific receptors for LH, leading to the synthesis of androgens which diffuse into the follicular fluid and are aromatized to estrogen by granulosa cells[1] and theca cells. The androgens, especially non-aromatizing androgen dihydrotestosterone, induce follicular atresia[23] and a decrease in E_2 production. The deprivation of E_2 initiates, via the negative feedback mechanism, the synthesis and release of FSH to maintain a tonic level during the later period of the luteal phase, which initiates growth of new follicles for the next cycle.

In the human ovary the binding of prolactin to the ovary[25] may be implicated in follicular maturation and corpus luteum function. Prolactin regulates its own receptors[20] and acts as a permissive hormone to facilitate the optimum action of other hormones.

The functional life of the corpus luteum is transient and can be extended by human chorionic gonadotropin (hCG) only temporarily, which may be due to the downregulation of LH-hCG receptors of the corpus luteum.[5]

FEEDBACK MECHANISM IN THE REGULATION OF THE MENSTRUAL CYCLE

The hypothalamic-pituitary axis can be considered functionally in three components: 1) The CNS-hypothalamic complex is a signal generator and a coordinating element which is under feedback control of the ovary. 2) The pituitary is a transducer, dependent upon cyclic input of the hypothalamus and a cyclic control via long-loop feedback exerted by the ovary. The synthesis and release of pituitary gonadotropins may also be regulated by short-loop feedback of pituitary LH to the hypothalamus via countercurrent blood flow.[3, 18] 3) The ovary is the cyclic feedback control, via estrogen, progesterone and recently described follicular "inhibin" (Fig.

1.3). The target gland hormones, such as estrogen, androgen and progestin, not only provide feedback signals to the hypothalamic-pituitary complex but also operate as a local feedback system within the ovarian unit. Estrogens and progesterone exert a negative feedback and inhibit the release of FSH and LH.[7, 27] Prolonged administration of estrogen results in gonadal atrophy. Similarly, gonadectomy is followed by increased gonadotropin release.[11, 16] In the normal cycle, 2–3 days prior to menstruation the concentration of estradiol and progesterone are at their lowest level, which

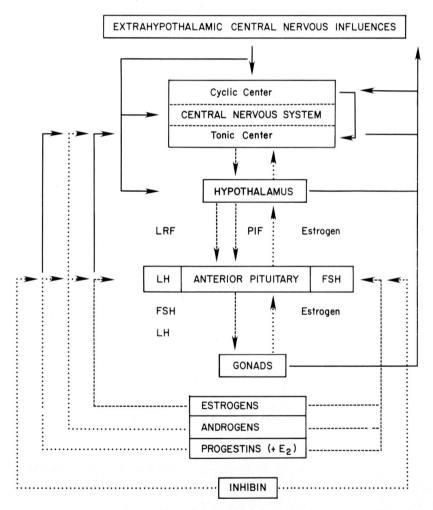

Figure 1.3. Interaction of releasing hormones, pituitary gonadotropins and ovarian steroids in the regulation of the menstrual cycle. PIF: prolactin inhibiting factor.

stimulates, via the negative feedback mechanism, a release of FSH and LH from the pituitary. As the follicle develops and increasing amounts of estradiol are secreted, the secretion of FSH actually falls; when the estradiol secretion reaches approximately 200 μg/day, the preovulatory release of LH and FSH is stimulated by positive feedback.

The interaction of releasing hormones, pituitary gonadotropins and ovarian steroids in the regulation of the menstrual cycle is illustrated in Figure 1.3. An "ovarian clock" and hypothalamic tonic and cyclic centers for the regulation of gonadotropin release are inherent features of the female reproductive system.

Estrogen exerts a profound effect directly on the pituitary and on the CNS-hypothalamic complex. There is a greater binding of estradiol to the pituitary than to the hypothalamus, and the release of gonadotropin by the pituitary is determined by the direct input of luteinizing hormone releasing factor (LRF) modulated by the feedback input of E_2. The LRF causes a biphasic, acute and delayed, release of pituitary gonadotropins.[29] The sum of these two pools is designated as pituitary capacity, which is modulated by E_2 and thus synchronizes with the cyclicity of ovarian steroid levels. The sensitivity of the pituitary to LRF and the consequent release of LH during the early follicular phase are minimal but increase with increasing levels of E_2 toward midfollicular phase and dramatically near the midcycle. The binding of LRF to the pituitary is highest at midcycle.[26] The pituitary may control the midcycle gonadotropic surge. Pituitary sensitivity to LRF and reserve of gonadotropin are reduced progressively during the luteal phase. Experimental evidence for the induction of LH surge by estradiol has been provided (Leyendecker et al., 1976).

The progressive increase in the circulating estradiol augments the responsiveness of gonadotropes to LRF. E_2 augments norepinephrine and inhibits dopamine neuronal activity, contributing to the acute LRF release. The catecholestrogens may serve as biochemical links between estrogens and catecholamines in the modulation of neuronal activity and release of the ovulatory surge of LH.[2, 9, 19] Prostaglandins may participate by promoting LRF neuronal activity directly. The follicular "inhibin," a nonsteroidal factor, has been implicated in the selective inhibition of FSH via an exclusive feedback system of the granulosa-FSH axis.

There is evidence that fetal androgens desensitize the cyclic center in the male and this can be reversed by the administration of antiandrogen to the male fetus *in utero.* Animals treated with antiandrogen *in utero* elicit the pituitary discharge of LH after the administration of E_2. The presence of an androgen-sensitive cyclic center is further validated from the observation that *in utero* androgen-treated females lose the ability of pituitary LH discharge on stimulation with E_2. Preovulatory changes in progesterone may provide a fail-safe or augmentary mechanism by virtue of the ability to elicit acute gonadotropin release in estrogen-primed women. However, progesterone subsequently blocks the cyclic center for further induction by the high circulating levels of E_2, a mechanism which may explain the lack of LH surges in the luteal phase of the cycle when the levels of E_2 are also high.[13, 17, 22]

References

1. Armstrong, D.T., and Papkoff, H. Stimulation of aromatization of exogenous and endogenous androgens in the ovaries of hypophysectomized rats *in vivo* by FSH. *Endocrinology* 99:1144, 1976.
2. Ball, P., Knuppen, R., Haupt, M., and Breuer, H. Interactions between estrogens and catecholamines. *J. Clin. Endocrinol. Metab.* 34:736, 1972.
3. Bergland, R.M., and Page, R.B. Pituitary secretion to the brain (anatomical evidence). *Endocrinology*, in press.
4. Blandau, R.L. Follicular growth, ovulation and egg transport. In *The Ovary*, edited by Mack, H.C. Charles C Thomas, Springfield, IL, 1968.
5. Davies, T.F., Dufau, M.L., and Catt, K.J. Gonadotropin receptors: Characteristics and clinical applications. *Clin. Obstet. Gynaecol.* 5:329–362, 1978.
6. De Jong, F.H., and Sharpe, R.M. Evidence for inhibin-like activity in bovine follicular fluid. *Nature* 263:71, 1976.
7. Dhont, M., et al. Daily concentrations of plasma

LH, FSH, estradiol, estrone, and progesterone throughout the menstrual cycle. In *Ovarian Function*, edited by Eskes, T.K., et al. Excerpta Medica Foundation, Amsterdam, 1974, p. 153.

8. Erickson, G.F., Challis, R.G., and Ryan, K.J. A developmental study of the capacity of rabbit granulosa cells to respond to trophic hormones and secrete progesterone *in vitro*. *Dev. Biol. 40:* 208, 1974.

9. Fishman, J., and Norton, B. Catecholestrogen formation in the central nervous system of the rat. *Endocrinology* 96:1054, 1975.

10. Harrison, R.J. The structure of the ovary. In *The Ovary*, edited by Zuckerman, S., Mandl, A.M., and Eckstein, P. Academic Press, London, 1962, pp. 143–182.

11. Hohlweg, W., and Junkmann, K. Die hormonal-nervose Regulierung der Funktion des Hypophysenvorderlappens. *Klin. Wochenschr.* 11:121, 1932.

12. Ingram, D.L. Atresia. In *The Ovary*, edited by Zuckerman, S., Mandl, A.M., and Eckstein, P. Academic Press, London, 1962, pp. 247–273.

13. Leyendecker, G., Wildt, L., Gips, H., Nocke, W., and Plotz, E.J. Experimental studies on the positive feedback effect of progesterone, 17α-hydroxyprogesterone and 20α-dihydroprogesterone on the pituitary release of LH and FSH in the human female. *Arch. Gynaek.* 221:29, 1976.

14. Makris, A., and Ryan, K.J. Progesterone, androstenedione, testerone, estrone and estradiol synthesis in hamster ovarian follicle cells. *Endocrinology* 96:694, 1975.

15. Mikhail, G. Hormone secreting by the human ovary. *Gynecol. Invest.* 1:5, 1970.

16. Moore, C.R., and Price, D. Gonad hormone function and the reciprocal influence between gonads and hypophysis. *Am. J. Anat.* 50:13, 1932.

17. Odell, W.D., and Swardloff, R.S. Progesterone-induced luteinizing and follicle stimulating hormone surge in post-menopausal women: A simulated ovulatory peak. *Proc. Natl. Acad. Sci. USA* 61:529, 1968.

18. Oliver, C., Mical, R.S., and Porter, J.C. Hypothalamic-pituitary vasculature evidence for retrograde blood flow in the pituitary stalk. *Endocrinology 101*:598, 1977.

19. Paul, S.M., and Axelrod, J. Catecholestrogens: Presence on brian and endocrine tissues. *Science 197*:657, 1977.

20. Posner, B.I., Kelly, P.A., and Friesen, H.G. Prolactin receptors in rat liver: Possible induction by prolactin. *Science 187*:57, 1975.

21. Potter, E.L. *Pathology of the Fetus and the Newborn.* Yearbook Publishers, Chicago, 1952.

22. Rakoff, J.S., Rigg, L.A., and Yen, S.S.C. Assessment of progesterone (P)-induced LH-release as a test for the hypothalamic-gonadotropin function. *Gynecol. Invest.* 8:31(A), 1977.

23. Richards, J.S., Ireland, J.J., Rao, M.C., Bernath, G.A., Midgley, A.R., Jr., and Reichert, I.E., Jr. Ovarian follicular development in the rat: Hormone receptor regulation by estradiol, follicle-stimulating hormone and luteinizing hormone. *Endocrinology* 99:1562, 1976.

24. Ross, G.T., Cargille, C.M., Lipsett, M.B., et al. Pituitary and gonadal hormones in women during spontaneous and induced ovulatory cycles. *Recent Prog. Horm. Res.* 26:1–62, 1970.

25. Saito, T.; and Saxena, B.B. A sensitive, rapid and economical radioimmunoassay of human growth hormone using ethanol-ammonium acetate. *J. Lab. Clin. Med.* 85:487, 1975.

26. Saxena, B.B. Regulation of LH-RH receptor in the pituitary gland of the rat. In *Clinical Psychoneuroendocrinology in Reproduction*, edited by Carenza, L., Pancheri, P., and Zichella, L. 1978, p. 165.

27. Saxena, B.B., Demura, H., Gandy, H.M., and Peterson, R.E. Radioimmunoassay of human follicle stimulating and luteinizing hormones in plasma. *J. CLin. Endocrinol* 28:519, 1968.

28. Valdes-Dapena, M.A. The normal ovary of childhood. *Ann. N.Y. Acad. Sci.* 142:597, 1967.

29. Yen, S.S.C. *Reproductive Endocrinology*, edited by Yen, S.S.C., and Jaffe, R.B. W.B. Saunders, Philadelphia, 1978, p. 126.

30. Yussman, M.A., and Taymor, M.L. Serum levels of FSH and LH and of plasma progesterone related to ovulation by corpus luteum biopsy. *J. Clin. Endocrinol.* 30:396, 1970.

CHAPTER 2

Oogenesis

LUCIANO ZAMBONI, M.D.

The term *oogenesis* refers to the series of complex events which occur in the female gonad and accompany the differentiation of the primordial germ cells at first into oogonia and then into oocytes. The process includes an embryonal and a postembryonal phase. Its duration varies considerably, not only among species but also among individual cells in the same animal. It is shorter in those species in which the gestation period is brief and sexual maturity is attained swiftly than in those in which the gestational and prepubertal periods are long. The oogenetic process is shortest for those oocytes which are ovulated soon after the attainment of sexual maturity and is longest for those released from the ovarian follicles toward the end of the fertile period. In the human female, the life span of individual germ cells and, thus, oogenesis vary from a minimum of about 12 years to a maximum of several decades.

EMBRYONAL PHASE

Upon arriving at the genital ridges at the end of their migration from the yolk-sac, the primordial germinal cells establish close and permanent association with somatic elements which will later differentiate into the definitive granulosa cells (Fig. 2.1). Recent studies performed on fetal ovaries of different species have shown that these somatic cells do not originate from the mesothelial cells lining the surface of the gonad or from the mesenchymal cells of the gonadal stroma as postulated by classic theories (for a review, see Zuckerman and Baker, 1977) but are exclusively mesonephric in origin and derive from the epithelial elements of regressing mesonephric glomeruli and/or tubules.[4]

At first, germinal and somatic cells become associated in small clusters which, in sequential stages of development, undergo progressive enlargement and organization, eventually becoming coalescent and forming the *ovigerous cords*. These are elongated structures demarcated by a basal lamina and extending with radial courses throughout the cortex of the fetal ovary (Fig. 2.2). Within the cords the germ cells multiply, actively giving rise to various generations of *oogonia* which can be distinguished from the somatic cells of the cords (the precursors of the *granulosa cells*) due to their large size, spheroidal shape, a large vesicular nucleus provided with one or more nucleoli, and an expanded cytoplasm. Ultrastructurally, the oogonia display characteristics of highly undifferentiated cells; the organelles consist only of sparse ergastoplasmic reticulum cisternae, a few mitochondria, a modest Golgi complex and numerous free ribosomes. Loose, non-membrane-bound aggregates of a dense, finely granular material are also present in the cytoplasm of oogonia. This component, referred to as *nuage* and probably analogous to the "chromatoid body" which is characteristic of the cytoplasm of spermatocytes and spermatids, may represent a reserve of proteinaceous material earmarked for endogenous utilization. Centrioles are also a part of the organelle population of the oogonium; the presence of these structures

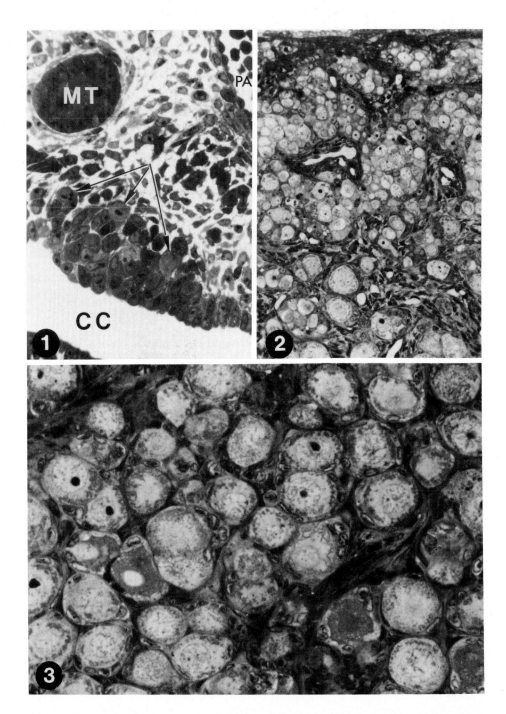

Figure 2.1. Germinal cells (*arrow*) and somatic cells in the genital ridge of an 11-day-old mouse embryo. *MT*, mesonephric tubule; *CC*, coelomic cavity; *PA*, primitive aorta.

Figure 2.2. Ovigerous cords in the ovary of a 162-day-old rhesus macaque fetus. While the most superficial segments of the cords still contain oogonia (upper portion of the micrograph), follicles are forming from the innermost segments (lower portion of the micrograph). The intermediate segments contain oocytes in meiotic prophase.

Figure 2.3. Formation of early follicles from the innermost tips of the ovigerous cords of a 132-day-old rhesus macaque fetus.

is noteworthy since, after the last mitotic division, they normally disappear, being seen in oocytes only in abnormal situations.

At the end of the various waves of mitotic proliferation, the oogonia enter *meiotic prophase* and differentiate into *oocytes.* The meiotic process proceeds through diplotene and then becomes arrested; normally, it resumes in the adult ovary either as preliminary to atretic involution or as part of the maturative process which the oocyte undergoes prior to ovulation (see below). The morphology of oocytes undergoing meiotic prophase in the fetal ovary has been found to be essentially identical in all species. While the general organization of the cytoplasm is essentially identical to that of oogonia, profound modifications occur in the nucleus. At preleptotene and leptotene, there is condensation of the chromatin into discrete chromosomes. At zygotene, the chromosomes become polarized in one nuclear hemisphere with one of their extremities closely associated with the nuclear membrane; at this stage, some chromosomes may appear in pairs, indicating that pairing of homologous chromosomes has begun. At pachytene, the paired chromosomal masses display central, longitudinally oriented tripartite ribbons made up of three linear, parallel structures separated from one another by translucent areas. These structures, which are referred to as *synaptinemal complexes,* represent the core of each bivalent; their presence indicates that at this stage the homologous chromosomes are in fully synaptic condition. At diplotene, the chromosomes become individualized again. At the same time, they become less densely aggregated and less sharply demarcated, remaining in this condition throughout the ensuing long period of meiotic arrest; while in oocytes of some species (primates, for example), their evanescent outlines can still be made out, in those of others (rodents, lagomorpha), chromosomes can no longer be distinguished and the chromatin becomes dispersed in a "dictyate" form not undifferent

from that of interphase nuclei. The proliferation of oogonia and the meiotic differentiation of the oocytes occur concomitantly with successive waves of extensive cell degeneration which result in a drastic reduction of the original number of the germinal elements.

In many species, the main phenomena which occur during the embryonal phase of oogenesis are characterized by a high degree of synchronization; not only is there correspondence between stages of development and predominant stage (mitotic, meiotic, degenerative) of cellular activity but also the germinal elements mature in groups, each of which consists of elements at an identical stage (mitotic, meiotic, degenerative) of differentiation. It was established that the structures responsible for such synchronization of cell maturation are *cytoplasmic bridges* (Fig. 2.4) connecting variable numbers of germinal cells which thus remain associated in clusters having a syncytial organization.[3] These bridges, which probably form in the course of successive mitotic divisions characterized by incomplete cytokinesis, consist of cylindrical portions of cytoplasm containing conventional organelles (mitochondria, ribosomes) that are freely exchanged from one cell to the other; it is very probable that this exchange of material and, thus, of information is the main factor responsible for the synchronous pattern of cell differentiation.

The development of *follicles* from the ovigerous cords usually occurs toward the end of ovarian development (Figs. 2.2 and 2.3). Follicle formation is a gradual process which initiates at the innermost extremities of the ovigerous cords and extends toward more superficial segments; the first follicles may form when the outermost portions of the ovigerous cords still contain mitotic oogonia, or oocytes just entering meiosis (Fig. 2.2). The development of follicles from the ovigerous cords results from the interaction of several factors which include, among others, the disappearance of the intercellular bridges, with consequent individualization of the oo-

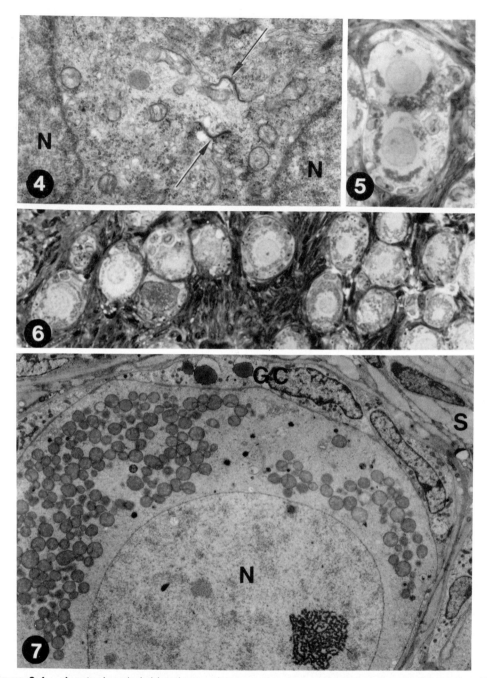

Figure 2.4.   A cytoplasmic bridge (*arrows*) connecting two oogonia in a human fetal ovary. The bridge contains organelles being exchanged between the connected cells. *N*, nucleus.
Figure 2.5.   Polyovular follicle in a human fetal ovary.
Figure 2.6.   Unilaminar follicles in the ovarian cortex of a young adult woman.
Figure 2.7.   Electron micrograph of a portion of a unilaminar follicle in the ovarian cortex of a young adult woman. *N*, oocyte nucleus; *GC*, granulosa cells; *S*, stroma.

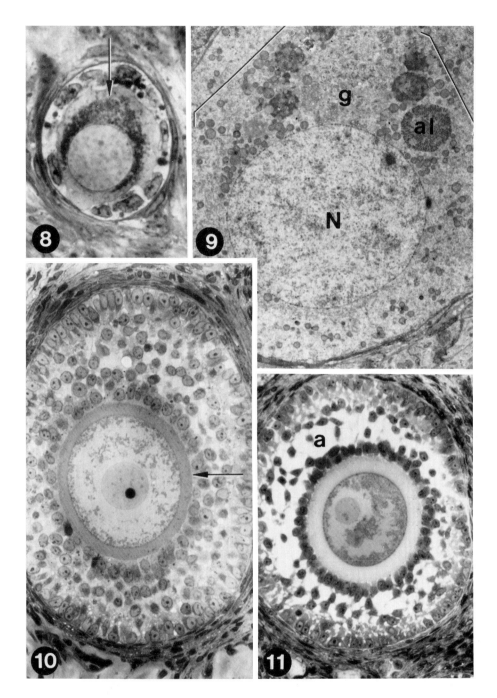

Figure 2.8. Unilaminar follicle in human ovary. The oocyte displays a prominent Balbiani's vitelline body (*arrow*; for explanation, see text and the following micrograph).

Figure 2.9. Electron micrograph of oocyte in a human unilaminar follicle. The bars demarcate a large Balbiani's vitelline body consisting of a prominent Golgi complex (*g*), mitochondria, lysosomes, and annulate lamellae (*al*). *N*, oocyte nucleus.

Figure 2.10. Incipient stage of maturation of a human follicle. Due to mitotic activity, the granulosa cells have increased in number and are now arranged in concentric layers around the oocyte. *Arrow* points to a continuous zona pellucida.

Figure 2.11. Early stage of antrum (a) formation in maturing human follicle.

cytes, and the rapid development of the ovarian stroma, whose cellular and extracellular components encroach upon the cords and eventually bring about their fragmentation. Any deviation of these phenomena from normalcy may result in anomalies of follicle development; for example, persistence of the intercellular bridges may result in the formation of polyovular follicles in which two or more oocytes which failed to become individualized are surrounded by a single layer of granulosa cells (Fig. 2.5). Should the oocytes within these follicles undergo cytoplasmic fusion, polynucleated forms may result.

POSTEMBRYONAL PHASE

The postembryonal phase of oogenesis includes the interval separating birth from the attainment of sexual maturity and the postpubertal period. During the first period, follicles either remain quiescent or undergo *atresia*. During the second period, the follicles enter maturation in preparation for either *ovulation* or atresia. Oogenesis ends at the close of the fertile period with complete or nearly complete exhaustion of the follicle population, due either to ovulation or to atresia.

Albeit a physiological event in the life history of the majority of mammalian follicles, atresia does not constitute an integral part of oogenesis; on the contrary, it represents a derangement, followed by cessation, of the normal event of oogenesis.

The changes which the maturing oocyte undergoes prior to its release from the follicle at ovulation occur concomitantly with and depend upon modifications of the surrounding granulosa cells and other follicle changes.

At any given time, small follicles consisting of a miniscule, immature oocyte arrested in the prophase of the first meiotic division (see above) and of a single layer of granulosa cells resting on a thin basal lamina represent the predominant elements of the follicle population of the sexually mature ovary (Fig. 2.6). These *unilaminar follicles*, which are preferentially situated in the most superficial layers of the cortex, are frequently referred to as "resting" or "quiescent" to distinguish them from those which are progressing through maturation. These terms, however, should not be taken as an indication that they are in a state of metabolic quiescence or inertia since the occurrence of intense protein and RNA synthesis, as well as an avidity for exogenous substances, has been amply and unquestionably demonstrated by biochemical, autoradiographic and tracer studies.

In follicles of this type, the oocyte ranges from 50 to 70 microns in diameter. Its outline is regular (Fig. 2.7), its shape is spheroidal (Figs. 2.6–2.9) and its surface is usually smooth and closely apposed against the plasma membranes of the encircling granulosa cells (Fig. 2.7). The nucleus is prominent, spheroidal and provided with a large nucleolus (Fig. 2.7); the characteristics of the chromatin are identical to those of oocytes which have reached the diplotene stage of the meiotic prophase in the fetal ovary (see above). The cytoplasmic organelles are usually concentrated in the perinuclear region (Figs. 2.7–2.9) where they form a crescentic aggregate which includes one or more large Golgi complexes, mitochondria, elements of the ergastoplasmic reticulum, lysosomes and annulate lamellae (Fig. 2.9). While their functional significance remains to be established with certainty, it is possible that these organelle aggregates, also referred to as *Balbiani's vitelline bodies* or *yolk nucleus complexes*, have important metabolic functions; thus, their localization in the perinuclear area would indicate that the oocyte metabolic activities at this stage are concentrated in and around the nucleus. On the other hand, the occurrence within these aggregates of lysosomes and annulate lamellae, elements which are often an expression of cell sufferance, may also indicate that the oocytes in which these crescents are found may be in early stages of atretic involution. This possibility underlines the extreme difficulty of distinguishing, on the basis of morphologic evidence exclusively, oocytes earmarked for atretic regression from those which are destined to complete maturation. The possibility that oocytes not showing obvious signs of regression still may be embarked toward atresia should always be kept in mind, especially considering that oocytes earmarked for atresia represent the vast majority of the entire oocyte population.

The thickness of the granulosa cells forming the wall of the unilaminar follicles varies markedly not only among different follicles but also in different areas of the wall of individual follicles, and ranges from extremely attenuated sheets of cytoplasm less than 1 μ in thickness to the whole thickness of the cell (Figs. 2.6–2.9). The granulosa cell investment around the oocyte may also be discontinuous, adjacent granulosa cells being separated by gaps which are normally occupied by "naked" portions of the oocyte surface. These fluctuations in the structural organization of the follicle wall are very probably related to the metabolic requirements of the follicle as a whole and especially to those of the oocyte. It is entirely possible, in fact, that through modifications of their thickness, the granulosa cells may monitor the access of extrafollicular substances entering into the follicle by means of transcellular transport mechanisms.

Profound changes occur in the oocyte and surrounding granulosa cells at the time the follicle leaves the stage of "quiescence" and enters the maturative phase. These changes are heralded by vigorous mitotic activity of the granulosa cells which increase considerably in number and become arranged in multiple concentric layers (Fig. 2.10); at the same time, the granulosa cells change their shape from attenuated to cuboidal. These phenomena obviously result in a marked increase in the thickness of the follicle wall and are responsible for the structural and functional isolation of the oocyte in the maturing follicle from the extrafollicular compartment.

The *zona pellucida* becomes formed concomitantly with these early changes (Fig. 2.10). At first, there is focal deposition of mucopolysaccharide-rich material in the narrow intercellular slits separating the granulosa cells from the oocyte; these areas then become confluent, resulting in the formation of a continuous zona layer around the oocyte which, when fully developed, ranges from 10 to 15 μ in thickness.

The formation of the follicular *antrum* (Fig. 2.11) is another change which takes place in the early stages of maturation. Antrum formation is the result of the secretion of *liquor folliculi* by the granulosa cells and its accumulation in the interstices between the cells which are situated midway in the thickness of the follicle wall. Due to progressive accumulation of the liquor, irregular lacunae appear which, isolated at first, become confluent and result in the development of a cavity separating the oocyte and the innermost layers of granulosa cells from the granulosa cells situated more peripherally (Fig. 2.11). Secretion and accumulation of liquor and concomitant expansion of the antrum continue throughout maturation of the follicle, being, in fact, the most important factors in the progressive enlargement of the latter and, probably, playing a determining role also in its dehiscence. The progressive distention of the antrum is also responsible for the eccentric position that the oocyte and its surrounding mantle of granulosa cells, the *cornea radiata*, usually occupy within the follicle cavity (Fig. 2.13).

While the origin of the liquor as a product of the secretory activity of the granulosa cells is well established, little is known of the origin of the zona pellucida, some authors claiming that it is synthesized by the oocyte, others by the granulosa cells, and others by both. It is possible that a role in the synthesis and deposition of both zona pellucida precursor material and liquor folliculi may be played by the *Call-Exner bodies* (Fig. 2.12); these are spheroidal, cystic formations that are delimited by a single layer of concentrically arranged granulosa cells, the basal surfaces of which rest on a basal lamina and constitute the wall of the structure. The nature and identity of the content of the Call-Exner bodies is unknown; it displays in-

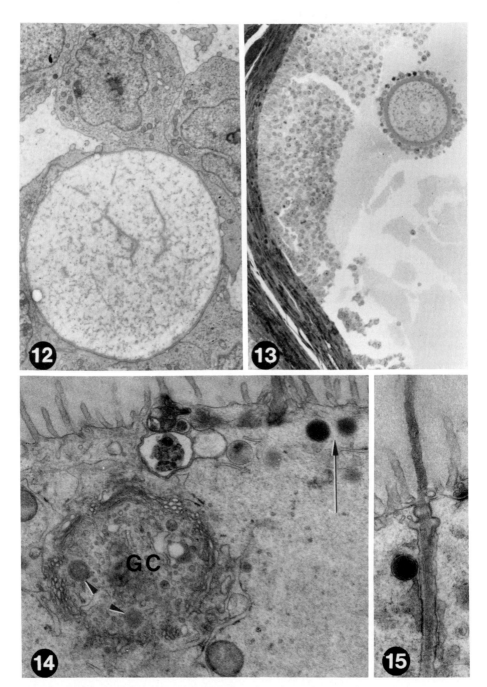

Figure 2.12. Electron micrograph of a Call-Exner body in a human ovary.

Figure 2.13. Oocyte and its corona radiata in a distended antral follicle. Notice the uniform distribution of the organelles throughout the oocyte cytoplasm.

Figure 2.14. Golgi complex (*GC*) near the surface of a human oocyte in antral follicle. The Golgi complex is involved in formation of cortical granules (*arrowheads*). *Arrow* points to two mature cortical granules situated just below the oocyte plasma membrane.

Figure 2.15. A slender cytoplasmic process of a corona radiata cell penetrating into the cytoplasm of a human oocyte in a large antral follicle. Notice the presence of microvilli on the oocyte surface (shown also in the previous micrograph).

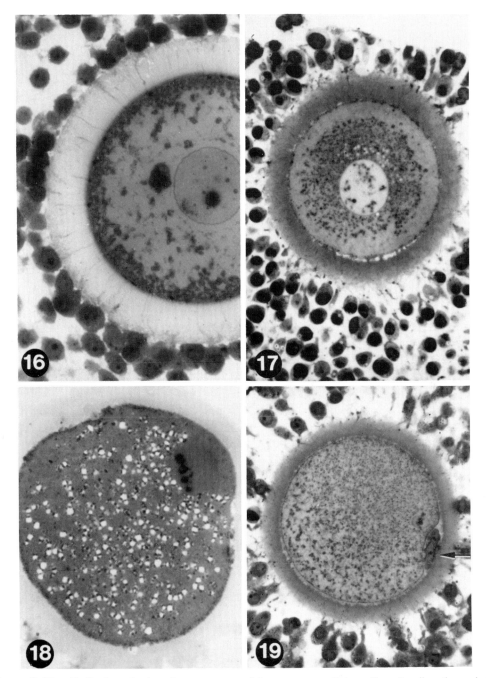

Figure 2.16. Delicate cytoplasmic processes of the corona radiata cells extending through the zona pellucida of an oocyte in antral follicle.

Figure 2.17. Human oocyte in early stage of resumption of the first meiotic division. The oocyte chromatin is undergoing condensation into chromosomes.

Figure 2.18. Human oocyte in anaphase of the first meiotic division; chromosomes and meiotic spindle are clearly visible. The deformation of the oocyte profile from 12 to 2 o'clock indicates that the asymmetric cleavage leading to the extrusion of the first polar body is underway.

Figure 2.19. Mature oocyte in human follicle. The first meiotic division has been completed and the first polar body has been extruded (*arrow*); the haploid oocyte chromosomes are aligned on the equatorial plate of the second metaphase spindle. They will remain in this condition until and unless the ovulated oocyte is penetrated by the spermatozoon.

19

tense PAS-positivity and, ultrastructurally, it appears as filamentous material forming a delicate network, the threads of which may be occasionally continuous with the basal lamina subjacent to the basal surfaces of the granulosa cells delimiting the cyst. The presence of this structure is also surprising since granulosa cells are not provided with a basal lamina, with the exception of those situated at the extreme periphery of the follicle wall which rest on the basal lamina of the follicle. The hypothesis that the Call-Exner bodies may be involved in the deposition of the zona pellucida and liquor folliculi rests on the observation of Call-Exner bodies with interrupted walls in the apparent process of liberating their content at the outer aspect of the developing zona pellucida and on the absence of these structures in large follicles with fully distended antra.[2]

The above-described follicle changes are accompanied by profound modifications of the oocyte. The cell enlarges progressively, attaining a diameter of 150–180 μ by the end of maturation. The organelles cease to be polarized in the perinuclear region and become uniformly distributed throughout the ooplasm (Fig. 2.13). The mitochondria increase in number concomitantly with a marked development of the ergastoplasmic reticulum, a phenomenon which is obviously related to the increased rate of protein synthesis during the maturative period. The Golgi complex becomes subdivided into multiple aggregates of vesicular and tubular elements which are prevalently localized at the periphery of the cell where they become involved in the formation of *cortical granules* and in the synthesis of their constituent material (Fig. 2.14). It is known that these granules, which are liberated outside the ovum at the time of its penetration by the spermatozoon, play an instrumental role in rendering the zona pellucida and/or the oolemma impermeable to supernumerary spermatozoa.[1] They are spheroidal structures averaging 0.5–0.8 μ in diameter, lined by single membrane and entirely occupied by a PAS-positive matrix which ultrastructurally displays a homogeneous texture and a medium to high electron opacity

(Fig. 2.14). In nearly mature or fully mature oocytes, they are distributed in a single layer all around the cell perimeter just below the surface.

Another modification undergone by the oocyte during the maturative stage is the development of vegetations of *microvilli* which protrude for variable distances into the thickness of the zona pellucida (Figs. 2.14 and 2.15). Their presence seems to be related to the metabolic functions of the cell. This is evident especially in consideration of the fact that the zona pellucida is traversed by numerous, long cytoplasmic projections of the corona radiata cells (Figs. 2.15 and 2.16) which either end with bulbous terminations at the oolemma, where they are closely surrounded by the oocyte microvilli, or penetrate deeply into the ooplasm (Fig. 2.15). In addition to conventional organelles, these cytoplasmic extensions also contain numerous fat droplets and aggregates of glycogen, substances which are likely provided to the oocyte for its metabolic requirements. It is evident, thus, that the presence of microvilli, which markedly increase the oocyte surface, facilitates absorption processes.

A few hours prior to its liberation from the cavity of the fully distended, *preovulatory follicle*, the oocyte undergoes the last of the important processes associated with its maturation, i.e., *completion of the first meiotic division*. Resumption of meiotic prophase is heralded by dispersion of the nucleolar material and condensation of the chromatin into discrete chromosomes (Fig. 2.17). These phenomena are soon followed by fragmentation and then disappearance of the nuclear envelope, and spindle microtubules may be seen inside the nucleus at the time its envelope is still intact or only minimally interrupted. Just how the microtubules become organized in the oocyte in the absence of centrioles, which in other cell types are responsible for the synthesis and the organization in microtubular form of the contractile proteins needed for spindle assembly and function, has not yet been established. At metaphase, the chromosomes become arranged on the equatorial plate of the spindle. At anaphase, there is incipient and asymmetric cleavage of the oocyte cytoplasm (Fig. 2.18) which becomes complete at telophase, with the liberation of a small portion of the oocyte and one half of the original chromosome complement as first polar body (Fig. 2.19). These phenomena represent the culmination of the oogenetic process and signal the transformation of the oocyte into a mature ovum which is now ready to undergo fertilization and postfertilization development.

References

1. Szollosi, D. Development of cortical granules and the cortical reaction in rat and hamster eggs. *Anat. Rec. 159*:431–446, 1967.

2. Zamboni, L. *Fine Morphology of Mammalian Fertilization.* Harper & Row, New York, 1971.

3. Zamboni, L., and Gondos, B. Intercellular bridges and synchronization of germ cell differentiation during oogenesis in the rabbit. *J. Cell Biol. 36*:276–282, 1968.

4. Zamboni, L., Upadhyay S., Bézard, J., Luciani, J.M., and Mauléon, P. The role of the mesonephros in the development of the mammalian ovary. In *Endocrine Physiopathology of the Ovary,* edited by Tozzini, R.I., Reeves G., and Pineda, R.L. Elsevier/North-Holland Biomedical Press, Amsterdam, 1980, pp. 3–42.

5. Zuckerman, S., and Baker, T.G. The development of the ovary and the process of oogenesis. In *The Ovary,* edited by Zuckerman, S., and Weir, B. Academic Press, New York, 1977, vol. 1, pp. 41–67.

CHAPTER 3

Spermatogenesis

YVES CLERMONT, Ph.D.

The male gametes or spermatozoa are produced by the testis as a result of a complex series of cytological changes which involve three distinct classes of germinal cells—the spermatogonia, the spermatocytes and the spermatids. The spermatozoa themselves are highly differentiated cells which have a haploid nucleus attached to a structurally complex and motile tail. These germinal cells together with the somatic cells, called *Sertoli cells*, form the seminiferous epithelium. The latter epithelium lines a limiting membrane delineating the seminiferous tubules, which have a diameter of 300 to 400 μm (Fig. 3.1). In the center of the tubules there is a narrow lumen in which the spermatozoa are released and migrate, carried by the flow of a luminal fluid, toward the rete testis which connects with the epididymis. Thus the seminiferous epithelium shows spermatogonia close to the limiting membrane, spermatocytes which form a second layer of cells, and the spermatids which form the innermost layer and border the lumen (see Figs. 3.1, 3.3, 3.4, and 3.6).

Spermatogenesis is usually divided into three phases: the first phase concerns the spermatogonia which proliferate to give rise to spermatocytes and to new spermatogonia that serve as stem cells for future generations of germ cells; the second phase involves the spermatocytes that go through the meiotic divisions leading to the formation of spermatids; the third phase concerns the spermatids which differentiate into spermatozoa, a process usually referred to as spermiogenesis.

SPERMATOGONIA

In man and other primates, three classes of spermatogonia can be identified on the basis of the morphological appearance of the nucleus, i.e., the dark type A spermatogonia (Ad), the pale type A spermatogonia (Ap) and the type B spermatogonia (Figs. 3.2–3.4). The two classes of type A cells show ovoid nuclei containing a fine dustlike chromatin which is uniformly distributed throughout the nucleus except in the area occupied by the nucleoli which are attached to the nuclear envelope. While in the dark type A spermatogonia the chromatin is deeply and uniformly stained with basophilic dyes (hematoxylin or toluidine blue), in the pale type A spermatogonia the chromatin is much less chromophylic and assumes a ground glass texture (Figs. 3.3 and 3.4). The dark type A spermatogonia in man also show a central spherical zone, referred to as a vacuole, free from deeply stained chromatin. The type B spermatogonia show a spherical nucleus containing granules of heavily stained chromatin attached to the nuclear envelope or suspended in the nucleoplasm (Figs. 3.2 and 3.4). A centrally located nucleolus is also associated with chromatin. The exact behavior of these three classes of spermatogonia in man is not fully elucidated as yet, but a number of investigations on monkeys suggest that both the Ap and the Ad spermatogonia may be considered as stem cells.[2] The Ad spermatogonia is a class of cells with a low proliferative rate in normal animals and could thus be

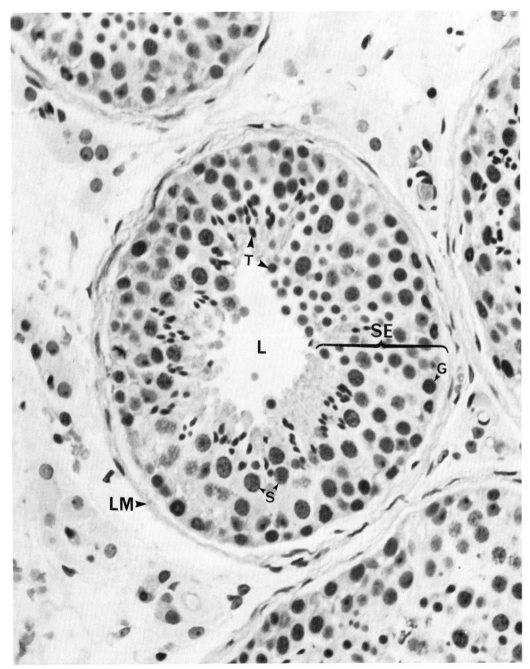

Figure 3.1.   Cross section of a human seminiferous tubule showing the limiting membrane (*LM*), the seminiferous epithelium (*SE*) and the tubular lumen (*L*). The seminiferous epithelium is composed of three main classes of germinal cells, i.e., the spermatogonia (*G*) close to the limiting membrane, the spermatocytes (*S*) and the spermatids along the tubular lumen (*T*).

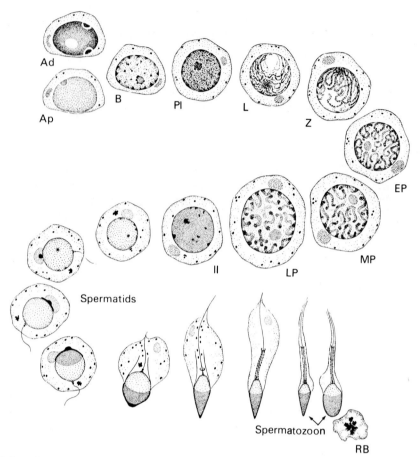

Figure 3.2. Steps of human spermatogenesis. *Ad*, dark type A spermatogonium; *Ap*, pale type A spermatogonium; *B*, type B spermatogonium. Spermatocytes; *Pl*, preleptotene; *L*, leptotene; *Z*, zygotene; *EP*, early pachytene; *MP*, mid pachytene; *LP*, late pachytene; *II*, secondary spermatocytes; *RB*, residual bodies. Description in the text.

considered as a "reverse stem cell." These cells may reconstitute the spermatogonial population if some of the spermatogonia are destroyed. The Ap spermatogonia are cells which at regular intervals undergo one or more successive mitoses, which result in the formation of both new Ap spermatogonia and of type B spermatogonia. The Ap spermatogonia could thus be considered as "renewing stem cells" which actively proliferate to yield new cells of their own kind that are set aside for the production of future generations of germ cells and to yield a new category of cells, the type B spermatogonia. The latter group of cells divide mitotically to yield spermatocytes; since all type B spermatogonia

are destined to produce spermatocytes, they may be considered as "committed" or "differentiated" spermatogonia. While in man the number of successive mitoses of type B cells leading to the production of spermatocytes is not yet known, in monkeys there are four successive generations of type B spermatogonia, referred to as types B_1, B_2, B_3 and B_4, respectively, the type B_4 being the one which in a last wave of mitoses yields a generation of spermatocytes.[2]

SPERMATOCYTES

The spermatocytes undergo meiosis, i.e., the two successive divisions leading to the

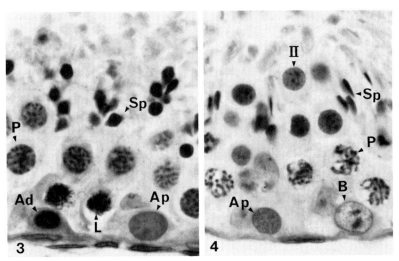

Figures 3.3. and 3.4.   Photographs of small segments of the seminiferous tubules of the monkey showing, along the limiting membrane, dark (*Ad*), pale (*Ap*) type A spermatogonia, type B (*B*) spermatogonia; leptotene spermatocytes (*L*). Closer to the lumen of the tubule, pachytene (*P*) primary spermatocytes, secondary (*II*) spermatocytes and spermatids (*Sp*) at various steps of spermiogenesis are visible.

production of haploid spermatids (Fig. 3.2). The morphological appearance of the chromatin in meiotic cells is different from that of the divisions of somatic cells, and the terms used to refer to the various steps of the prophase of the first divisions reflect this fact. Thus, soon after their formation by the type B spermatogonia, the spermatocytes enter a long phase referred to as a *preleptotene stage* during which DNA-synthesis takes place and the chromosomal filaments replicate. During this stage the nucleus of the spermatocytes resemble the nuclei of type B spermatogonia, i.e., they show granules of heterochromatin either attached to the nuclear envelope and nucleolus or suspended in the nucleoplasm (Fig. 3.2). Following this preleptotene stage, the spermatocytes enter the first step of the prophase of the first meiotic division, called the *leptotene stage*. The chromatin then takes on a fine filamentous texture which is the early sign of the formation of chromosomes. This is followed by the *zygotene stage* during which the homologous chromosomes undergo pairing. The paired chromosomes assume the shape of loops attached by their extremities to the nuclear envelope. Electron

microscope studies of such paired chromosomes revealed the presence, along the facing chromosomes, of an electron dense tripartite structure made up of two bands separated by a space in which a thin and dense line is visible. This structure, called the *synaptinemal complex*, is obviously the site where the homologous chromosomes bind together and keep them face to face. During the next or *pachytene stage* of the prophase of the first maturation division, the paired chromosomes shorten and thicken. Since this stage of meiosis is particularly long in all mammals (e.g., it lasts close to 16 days in man), these pachytene spermatocytes are seen in all tubular cross sections and form a major component of the seminiferous epithelium (Figs. 3.3, 3.4, and 3.6). During the pachytene stage, not only the nucleus but also the cytoplasm increases in volume. This cytoplasm contains, in addition to a juxtanuclear spherical Golgi apparatus, numerous interconnected cisternae of endoplasmic reticulum and spherical mitochondria. Following the pachytene stage, the two homologous chromosomes separate from each other slightly but remain attached at certain points (chiasmata) along the facing

chromosomes. This stage of short duration, called the *diplotene stage*, is followed
by the metaphase of the first maturation
division. During the following anaphase,
the homologous chromosomes (made up of
replicated DNA-filaments or chromatids)
move to the two poles of the achromatic
spindle; after telophase, the condensed
chromosomes despiralize, the nuclear envelope reappears and the nuclei of the
daughter cells, called *secondary spermatocytes*, assume an interphasic appearance.
Such nuclei are small and spherical and
contain a few dense heterochromatin granules and a small nucleolus (Figs. 3.2 and
3.4). The cytoplasm of these cells contains
a spherical juxtanuclear Golgi apparatus,
a sparse endoplasmic reticulum and spherical mitochondria. The life span of interphasic secondary spermatocytes is short
and, therefore, these cells are rarely seen
in the seminiferous epithelium. In contrast
to primary spermatocytes, no DNA repli-
cation takes place in the nuclei of secondary spermatocytes before these cells enter
prophase of the second maturation division. During this division the chromosomes split in half and the chromatids
move to the opposite poles of the spindle,
where they form the haploid nuclei of a
new class of cells, the spermatids. While
meiosis is a rather complex mechanism
that nature has invented to reduce the
number of chromosomes of germ cells by
half, other elaborate processes also take
place within these cells. Thus, for example,
genetic recombination (crossing-over) at
the level of the paired chromosomes during the zygotene stage, or the long pachytene stage, results in a rearrangement or
redistribution of the genes in the two sets
of homologous chromosomes. RNA synthesis takes place in the nucleolus of the
prophasic nucleus, and the RNA (messen-
ger) produced is carried through the two
meiotic divisions into the spermatids
where it is said to play a role in the differentiation of these cells into spermatozoa.
Chromosomal anomalies also occur as a
result of a defective meiosis and may be
carried to the spermatozoa and the off-
springs with rather tragic pathological
consequences.

SPERMATIDS AND SPERMIOGENESIS

The newly formed spermatid is a small
cell with a centrally located spherical nucleus, a juxtanuclear spheroidal Golgi apparatus, a pair of centrioles located outside
the Golgi apparatus next to the plasma
membrane, dispersed small spherical mitochondria, a system of interconnected cisternae of endoplasmic reticulum, and some
ribosomes either attached to the ER or free
in the hyaloplasm. There is also a small
chromophilic mass made up of a granulo-
filamentous material called the *chromatid
body*. This cell undergoes an extremely
complex series of structural modifications
that results in the production of the free
motile cell, the spermatozoon (Figs. 3.2 and
3.5). The major features of this metamor-
phosis, called *spermiogenesis*, involve the
condensation of the nucleus which takes
a shape specific for each species, the elab-
oration of the acrosome by the Golgi apparatus, the formation of the flagellum and
the shedding of most of the cytoplasm not
utilized in the formation of the flagellum.[2, 4]

During an early phase of spermiogenesis, the Golgi apparatus elaborates a number of secretory-like granules, called
proacrosomic granules, which are rich in
glycoproteins and contain a number of
substances, some lysosomal in nature (e.g.,
acid phosphatases).[1] These granules, like
any other secretory granules, are membrane delimited. These granules coalesce
to form a single acrosomic granule which
becomes closely associated to the nuclear
envelope. Concurrently, the pair of centrioles migrate toward the nucleus and one
of the two centrioles, called *proximal centriole*, becomes closely bound to the nuclear envelope in the so-called implantation fossa located opposite the acrosomic
granule (Figs. 3.2 and 3.5). The other centriole, called *distal centriole*, oriented at a
right angle to the proximal centriole initiates the formation of the axoneme of the
future sperm-tail. This axoneme is a collection of microtubules arranged in nine
peripheral doublets plus one central pair,
which characterizes cilia.

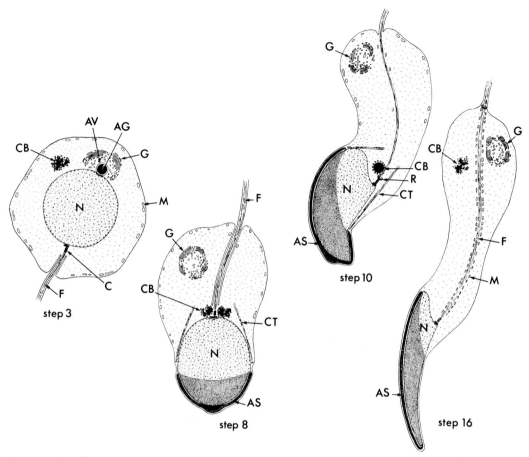

Figure 3.5. Four steps, respectively labeled steps 3, 8, 10 and 16, of spermiogenesis of the rat as seen with the electron microscope. *N*, nucleus; *C*, centrioles; *F*, flagellum; *M*, mitochondria; *CB*, chromatoid body; *G*, Golgi apparatus; *AV*, acrosomic vesicle; *AG*, acrosomic granule; *AS*, acrosomic system; *CT*, caudal tube; *R*, ring or annulus. Description in the text. (From F.R. Susi and Y. Clermont (9).)

Subsequently the Golgi apparatus actively continues to add material to the acrosomic granule, which increases in volume and then spreads over the surface of the nucleus. This acrosomal apparatus or system then assumes the shape of a cap over the nucleus. At the top of this membrane-delimited head cap there is a hemispherical swelling, referred to as the *acrosome*, which under the electron microscope is seen to be made up of a dense material (Figs. 3.2 and 3.5).

Once the acrosomic system is fully developed, the nucleus which up to this stage was centrally located now displaces toward the periphery of the cell, with the acrosomic system adhering to the plasma membrane. The cell then becomes elongated, with the bulk of the cytoplasm forming a lobule along the growing flagellum. The Golgi apparatus also detaches from the acrosomic system and migrates caudally. The chromatoid body displaces toward the centrioles and contributes material to a minute ringlike structure,[9] called the *annulus*, which surrounds the proximal portion of the flagellum (Figs. 3.2 and 3.5). A caudal tube or manchette made up of microtubules also appears at the caudal pole of the nucleus and surrounds, as a veil, the proximal portion of the flagellum (this transitory structure probably regulates the streaming of cytoplasm along the flagellum). Meanwhile, the nuclear chromatin initiates its condensation and the nucleus assumes an elongated shape (pyriform in man). Some material is also added to the surface of the centrioles, which are solidly attached to the nuclear envelope; this part of the tail is referred to as the neck or connecting piece.

Then the spermatids undertake a final series of structural modifications initiated by the migration of the annulus along a predetermined length of the flagellum (short in man); this is immediately followed by a rapid migration of the mitochondria toward the segment of the flagellum extending from the centrioles to the annulus. There they attach to the flagellum, condense and take an elongated shape, and arrange themselves side by side and circularly around the flagellum to form the so-called mitochondrial sheath which demarcates the middle piece of the flagellum. Soon after this migration of mitochondria, the caudal tube undergoes dissolution (Figs. 3.2 and 3.5). Simultaneous to this peculiar behavior of mitochondria, a lot of protein material is deposited along the axoneme in the form of coarse outer dense fibers and in the form of a fibrous sheath of circumferential fibers along the principal piece (beyond the annulus and over the rest of the flagellum). Thus the flagellum of spermatozoa is markedly different structurally from an ordinary cilium. The functions of the outer dense fibers and the fibrous sheath are still unclear. During these changes the nucleus and the acrosomic system undergo a final condensation and give the head of the future spermatozoon its definitive shape (Figs. 3.2 and 3.5). Lastly, the lobule of cytoplasm which throughout this series of modifications was seen along the proximal portion of the flagellum flows toward the nucleus, and the surplus of cytoplasm which has not been utilized in the formation of the flagellum separates from the spermatid and is discarded as a residual body (Fig. 3.2). Then the spermatid detaches from the seminiferous epithelium and could be considered as a free spermatozoon. The complexity of the changes taking place during spermiogenesis are such that errors in the program of the cells differentiation are frequent, in man in particular, and in such cases structural anomalies appear in the degenerating spermatids.

SPECIAL FEATURES OF SPERMATOGENESIS

One main characteristic of spermatogenesis is that its duration and the duration of each one of its phases or steps are fixed and constant for a given species of animal. For example spermatogenesis lasts approximately 60 days in man.[7] External physical factors such as temperature and internal factors such as hormones have no influence on the duration of this process. Renewing spermatogonial stem cells enter spermatogenesis at regular intervals (in man every 16 days). Furthermore, such stem cells undertake spermatogenesis in groups or clusters, the various cells of a group being connected by open intercellular bridges.[2] The daughter cells arising from dividing spermatogonial stem cells, i.e., type B spermatogonia, and spermatocytes remain connected to each other by intercellular bridges. Similarly the spermatids arising from spermatocytes remain connected by these bridges until the end of spermiogenesis, when the spermatids cast off their residual cytoplasm. It is believed that such open intercellular bridges serve in part to synchronize the differentiation of groups or generations of germinal cells. Lastly, as a result of the above features, germ cells at various steps of spermatogenesis are not arranged at random within the seminiferous epithelium but tend to form cellular associations of fixed composition. Thus, owing to the precise and regular timing of the steps of spermatogenesis, spermatids at given steps of spermiogenesis are associated with spermatocytes and spermatogonia at given steps of their respective development. These characteristic cellular groupings, which reappear at regular intervals in segments of seminiferous tubules, represent stages of a cycle of the seminiferous epithelium that may be defined as "a complete series of successive cellular associations appearing in any one area of the seminiferous tubules."[3, 8] The duration of such a cycle in the human is 16 days.

SERTOLI CELLS AND SPERMATOGENESIS

The transformation, described above, of a spermatogonial stem cell into a spermatozoon requires a suitable environment; this environment is provided by the somatic cell, the Sertoli cell, which serves as a support or sustentacular element of the whole epithelium. This large, stellate, nondividing cell is attached to the basement membrane and extends between germ cells to reach the tubular lumen (Fig. 3.6). It shows a large polymorphous nucleus and an abundant cytoplasm rich in organelles, i.e., mitochondria, a large Golgi apparatus, a profuse endoplasmic reticulum, lysosomes, as well as cytoplasmic filaments and microtubules but no secretory granules. The lateral cell membrane of the Sertoli cells forms numerous veil-like processes which extend between spermatocytes and spermatids and attach to these cells by means of various types of junctional devices. The Sertoli cells are phagocytes, eliminating from the seminiferous epithelium residual bodies and degenerat-

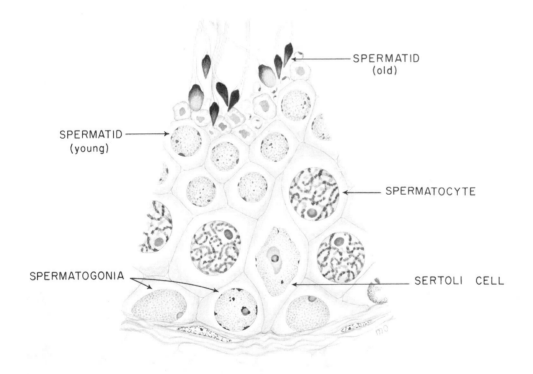

SPERMATID (old)

SPERMATID (young)

SPERMATOCYTE

SPERMATOGONIA

SERTOLI CELL

Figure 3.6.   Drawing of a small portion of a seminiferous tubule showing the main types of germ cells forming the seminiferous epithelium and their relations to the Sertoli cells.

ing germ cells; they also play an active role in the release of spermatozoa in the tubular lumen. On the luminal side of the layer of spermatogonia, lateral veil-like extensions of adjacent Sertoli cells come in contact and attach to each other by means of tight junctions (*zonula occludens*). These tight junctions, fusing the membranes of Sertoli cells, constitute the structural component of the "blood-testis barrier" which separates the seminiferous epithelium into two compartments, namely the "basal" compartment containing spermatogonia and preleptotene spermatocytes and the "adluminal" compartment containing meiotic spermatocytes and spermatids.[5, 6] The blood-testis barrier regulates the molecular composition of the intercellular fluid present in the adluminal compartment and creates a favorable milieu for the differentiation of the more advanced germ cells into spermatozoa. Stimulated by FSH and androgens, the Sertoli cell thus plays a most important role in the maintenance of spermatogenesis.[6]

References

1. Allison, A.C., and Hartree, E.F. Lysosomal enzymes in the acrosome and their possible role in fertilization. *J. Reprod. Fertil.* 21:501, 1970.
2. Clermont, Y. Kinetics of spermatogenesis in mammals: Seminiferous epithelium cycle and spermatogonial renewal. *Physiol. Rev.* 52:198, 1972.
3. Clermont, Y. Cycle of the seminiferous epithelium in man. *Am. J. Anat.* 112:35, 1963.
4. de Kretser, D.M. Ultrastructural features of human spermiogenesis. *Z. Zellforsch.* 98:477, 1969.
5. Dym, M., and Fawcett, D.W. Observations on the blood-testis barrier of the rat on the physiological compartmentation of the seminiferous epithelium. *Biol. Reprod.* 3:308, 1970.
6. Fawcett, D.W. The ultrastructure and functions of the Sertoli cells. In *Handbook of Physiology, Sec. 7, Endocrinology.* Edited by Hamilton, D.W., and Greep, R.O. Physiological Society, Washington, D.C. pp. 21–55.
7. Heller, C.G., and Clermont, Y. Kinetics of the germinal epithelium in man. *Recent Prog. Horm. Res.* 20:545, 1964.
8. Leblond, C.P., and Clermont, Y. Definition of the stages of the cycle of the seminiferous epithelium in the rat. *Ann. N.Y. Acad. Sci.* 55:548, 1952.
9. Susi, F.R., and Clermont, Y. Fine structural modifications of the rat chromatoid body during spermiogenesis. *Am. J. Anat.* 129:177, 1970.

CHAPTER 4

Fertilization and Implantation

WILLIAM J. SWEENEY III, M.D.
JOSEPH FINKELSTEIN, M.D.

Fertilization is that process by which the spermatozoon successfully penetrates the barriers surrounding the ovum. This is followed by the fusion of the chromosomes of the spermatozoon and the oocyte, with the formation of a zygote. Following formation of the zygote, various stages of segmentation and maturation occur in the process of the formation of a blastocyst. Implantation of this blastocyst will then occur; in normal situations, this implantation takes place within the uterine cavity approximately 6 days after fertilization. The zona pellucida, the antrum, and the cumulus oophorus are the protective layers that must be penetrated by the capacitated sperm.

During the development of the primary oocyte, maturation halts at the completion of the first meiotic division a few hours prior to ovulation, so that all primary oocytes prior to fertilization are found at metaphase of the second meiotic division. The further maturation of the primary oocyte will proceed only if fertilization takes place. Fertilization can take place only if ovulation has occurred. If the spermatozoa are unsuccessful in penetration of the protective barrier of the oocyte within 24 to 36 hours after ovulation, the oocyte degenerates. If, however, fertilization is successful the oocyte will enter the second maturation division of meiosis, and the chro-

mosomal changes necessary for the formation of the zygote are initiated.

In order that the spermatozoon can be successful in the process of fertilizing the primary oocyte, several conditions must be present. Sperm capacitation must occur. The spermatozoa must be motile and aided in their motility. The spermatozoa have to penetrate the protective barriers surrounding the oocyte, and the successful fusion of the chromosomal components of the sperm and the oocyte must take place.

Sperm capacitation involves changes in the stability of the membrane of the sperm head, resulting in the release of specific enzymes needed to break down the protective barrier created by the zona pellucida of the ovum.

These enzymes are hyaluronidase and trypsin-like substances. The midpiece connects the sperm head to the flagellum or tail, which is partly responsible for sperm motility. The actual movement of the sperm toward the ovum in the ampullary portion of the fallopian tube involves sperm motility related to the flagellum of the sperm, uterine contractile forces, and ciliary motion within the fallopian tube.

The flagellum of the sperm generates movement of the spermatozoon through the mucus plug of the cervix and it is also important in the immediate environment of the egg in the ampulla of the oviduct where fertilization takes place. Once the spermatozoon passes through the mucus plug, which acts as a favorable environment for the spermatozoa as well as a reservoir of sperm, rhythmic contractions of the myometrium propels it toward the cornual insertion of the oviduct. After the sperm has reached the oviduct, the ciliary action within the fallopian tube helps propel it and the egg that awaits fertilization together in the ampullary portion of the fallopian tube (Fig. 4.1).

At the time of ovulation the fimbriae of the fallopian tube surround the ovulation site, and the contents of the follicle containing the egg are engulfed by the fimbriae. The egg then lies freely within the ampullary portion of the oviduct until fertilization occurs. If fertilization does not occur within 24–36 hours after ovulation, the ovum will degenerate. If fertilization does occur, then the ovum that is fertilized will migrate down the fallopian tube to-

ward the uterine cavity. This migration is aided by the ciliary action of the oviduct. The migration of the fertilized ovum to the cavity of the uterus takes 3 or 4 days. Once in the uterus, the process of implantation occurs.

Although the average volume of male ejaculate is 2–4 ml, with an average concentration of 40–80 million sperm per milliliter, only 20–50 spermatozoa are successful in reaching the ovum. As soon as one spermatozoon penetrates the zona pellucida, all other sperm entry is inhibited.

The passage of sperm through the zona pellucida is aided by the alteration in the stability of the plasma membrane of the sperm head, allowing the release of enzymes. These enzymes allow the breakdown of the zona pellucida, with passage of the spermatozoon into the vitelline space. Once the spermatozoon penetrates this barrier, swelling of the sperm head can be seen. The midpiece of the sperma-

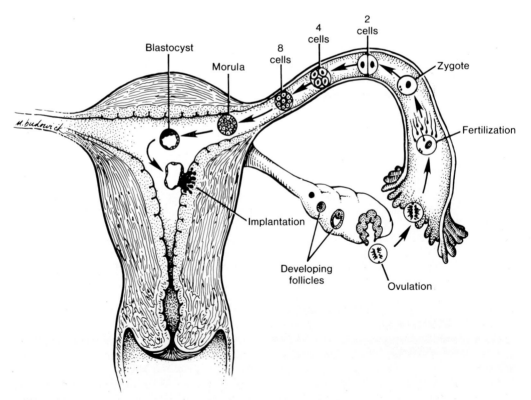

Figure 4.1.   Progression of the ovum through the fallopian tube to implantation in the uterus.

tozoon as well as the flagellum are then engulfed and incorporated within the oocyte. The swelling of the sperm head is one of the major signs that fertilization has taken place. The nuclear change that occurs concomitant with the swelling of the sperm head is the process of the second meiotic division. The chromosomes of the spermatozoon go through anaphase and telophase of the second meiotic division. At the same time the primary oocyte, which had remained at the metaphase of the second meiotic division, resumes the completion of the second stage of meiosis. The aggregation and condensation of both the sperm and the egg chromosomal components then occurs, with the formation of a zygote which is now ready for cleavage.

The entire process of fertilization takes place in the ampullary portion of the fallopian tube (Fig. 4.1). Once fertilization is completed with the successful formation of a zygote, the process of cleavage or segmentation with differentiation begins. Division of the zygote into cells called *blastomeres* takes place. The blastomeres continue to divide until a mass of cells, called the *morula* , develops. Following the development of the morula, fluid accumulates between the cells, leading to the differentiation and formation of the blastocyst. This entire process takes 3 days and includes not only differentiation but also transport of the morula and then blastocyst into the uterine cavity. The blastocyst which at this point lies freely within the uterine cavity is now ready for implantation which occurs 6 or 7 days after ovulation.

In preparation for this event the endometrium undergoes various anatomical changes (see Chapter 5). If fertilization does not occur, then the secretory endometrium formed following ovulation undergoes fragmentation and necrosis with the end result of menstruation. If, however, fertilization occurs the blastocyst implants into the endometrium which undergoes changes resulting in the formation of the decidua. The decidua represents that endometrium whose secretory activity is maintained and increased by the progesterone secretion of the corpus luteum of pregnancy. The blastocyst readily adheres to this decidual lining and becomes embedded within it.

References

1. Austin, C.R. Scientific and clinical aspects of fertilization and implantation. *Proc. R. Soc. Med.* 67:925–927, 1974.
2. Brackett, B.G., Seitz, H.M., Jr., Rocha, G., and Mastroianni, L., Jr. The mammalian fertilization process. In *Biology of Mammalian Fertilization and Implantation*, edited by Moghissi, K.S., and Nafez E.S.E. Charles C Thomas, Springfield, IL, 1972, pp. 165–184.
3. Edwards, R.G., and Steptoe, P.C., Control of human ovulation, fertilization and implantation. *Proc. R. Soc. Med.* 67:932–936, 1974.
4. Park, W.W. Abnormalities of human implantation. *J. Reprod. Fertil.* 25 (suppl.):105–116, 1976.
5. Wimsatt, W.A. Some comparative aspects of implantation. *Biol. Reprod.* 12:1–40, 1975.

CHAPTER 5

Development and Endocrine Physiology of the Placenta

ELMER E. KRAMER, M.D.
M. YUSOFF DAWOOD, M.D.

There are three components which go into the development of the placenta. One of the components is of maternal origin and the other two are of fetal origin. At the time of fertilization, neither the egg nor the maternal component, the endometrium, is ready for implantation so that during the subsequent 6 days certain developments take place to prepare them.

MATERNAL COMPONENT— ENDOMETRIUM

The endometrium consists of glands and stroma. The glands are tubular and extend through the entire thickness of the endometrium. Around the glands is the compact type of connective tissue known as the endometrial stromal cells. The endometrium is divided into the *functional portion*, which makes up the upper two thirds approximately, and the *nonfunctional portion* which makes up the basilar portion of the endometrium (Fig. 5.1). The endometrium does not have a limiting membrane and the nonfunctional portion of the endometrium does not undergo any change throughout the 28 days of the menstrual cycle nor during pregnancy. Each *gland* is divided into 1) the *neck*, which empties on the surface, 2) the *body* and 3) the *basilar tip*. Around the neck of the gland is a compact layer of stromal cells. This is important in pregnancy. It is known as the

stratum compacta in the nonpregnant state and beneath it is the stratum spongiosa. Under the effect of the ovarian hormones, the endometrium is pushed rapidly in 4–6 days into a 1-cm thick lining referred to as the *decidua*. Thus the thin stratum compacta becomes a thick compacta. The body of the gland undergoes tremendous changes also and this is particularly noted in the nuclei in the various cells lining the glands, which become quite bizarre. The change is known as the *Arias-Stella reaction*. It is a sign of pregnancy and is used to diagnose ectopic pregnancy. The compacta is the maternal component which goes into the formation of the placenta.

FETAL COMPONENTS
Trophoblast

Meanwhile, in the fallopian tube, the egg has divided into a strawberry-like mass, the *morula phase*, and finally reaches the blastodermic vesical phase, or *blastocyst*, which consists of a batch of cells that become the *formative cells* off to one side and a single layer of cells that is referred to as the *auxiliary cells* (Fig. 5.2). The fertilized egg must reach this phase prior to implantation. The dividing ovum is nourished by the granulosa cells during its journey in the fallopian tube. The cumulus oophorus is cast out with the egg and nour-

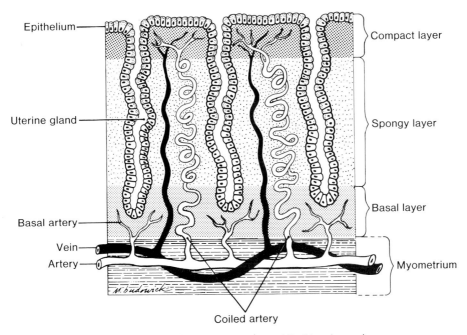

Figure 5.1.   The endometrium and its blood supply.

ishes it down the fallopian tube. It reaches the uterus on about the fourth day after fertilization and wanders a little before finally selecting a site to implant, which is usually high up in the fundus anteriorly or posteriorly. The outer ring of *auxiliary cells* has a sticky substance that allows it to adhere to the endometrium and has catalytic properties which allow it to burrow into the compacta. Usually when the blastocyst implants, the formative pole goes into the endometrium first. Shortly after implantation, the auxiliary cells have become two-layered. These are the first fetal component and they are the primitive chorion, the so-called trophoblast from which the villi will gradually begin to grow. The villi sprout all the way around the circumference. Their objective is to form an attachment and then a circulation.

Amniotic Vesicle

On the dorsal surface of the growing ovum, the amniotic vesicle is formed. This vesicle will come to completely surround the cavity and rest up against the chorion, which will house the amniotic fluid eventually.

For the first 3 weeks, the fertilized egg is generally referred to as an *ovum*, from 3 to 6 weeks it is called an *embryo* and thereafter it is a *fetus* until birth. It is an infant only after delivery.

CHANGES IN THE ENDOMETRIUM

In the normal ovulatory menstrual cycle, ovarian follicles develop during the first 14 days and the corpus luteum develops in the second 14 days. When the woman becomes pregnant, the corpus luteum undergoes further growth and triples in size. This gradual enlargement of the corpus luteum does not by any means explain the marked changes that occur in the endometrium in the 4–6 days after conception. These changes are more striking than those normally seen in the 14 days of the secretory phase. Details on the endocrine changes responsible for this are discussed in Chapter 7. With radioimmunoassay, it is now possible to detect human chorionic gonadotropin (hCG) as early as 3 days after fertilization. It is possible that hCG production accounts for the marked changes that occur in the endometrium.

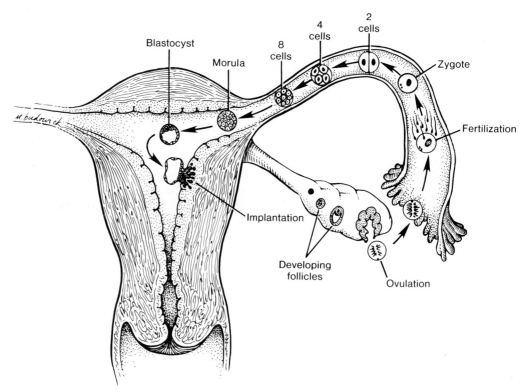

Figure 5.2. Progression of the ovum through the fallopian tube to implantation in the uterus.

The villi have more tissue to grow into in the basal area and the placenta eventually forms in this area. Villi on the outer rim of the implanted ovum gradually undergo atrophy and disappear.

DECIDUA

The portion of the decidua where the placenta forms is the *decidua basalis* (Fig. 5.3). That portion which covers the implanted ovum is called the *decidua capsularis*. That portion which has no direct relationship to the implantation on the opposite side of the cavity is known as the *decidua vera*, or *decidua parietalis*. It takes 4 to 4½ months for the pregnancy to fill the entire uterine cavity; at that time the decidua capsularis fuses with the decidua vera so that they become indistinguishable.

The *amniotic vesicle* continues to enlarge and surrounds the entire pregnancy but why it does not cover the whole fetus is unclear. Hertig feels that the growing embryo herniates into the sac and therefore does not become covered over by the amnion. Both are derived from the ectoderm. The body stalk becomes the umbilical cord. Small blood lakes form in the villi and subsequently connect to form longer lakes. The yolk sac apparently participates in the formation of the circulation. The blood cells are produced in the stroma of the villi and migrate into the capillaries. Thus, the circulation gradually becomes established and eventually connects the capillaries with the embryo. The placenta normally begins to function at 17–21 days. After implantation and in the early period of development, the ovum is nourished by osmosis. At this stage, the embryo is in a bloodless state. Only after the placenta has formed, by 17–21 days, is the circulation between the embryo and the placenta established. The placental circulation then accounts for fetal nourishment.

DIFFERENTIATION OF EMBRYONIC PLATE

The embryonic plate divides into the *ectoderm, mesoderm* and *endoderm* and gives rise to the structures listed in Table 5.1. The mesoderm gives rise to bone, muscle, and the circulatory and urogenital systems. Mixed mesodermal tumors in the uterus are thought to arise from the mesoderm and the various tissues that arise from the mesoderm such as muscle and bone can be present.

Figure 5.4A shows a very early implantation. There are formative cells, the embryonic pole and the trophoblast. The ovum has not been covered over as yet. A 12-day implantation ovum is covered by endometrium (the decidua capsularis) but is still in the previllous stage (Fig. 5.4B). No villi have sprouted from the trophoblast. The ovum is in the compacta and spongiosa. The actual embryo and fetus will eventually develop in the formative plate (Fig. 5.5).

CHANGES IN THE VILLI

An immature villus is very large, cellular, avascular and lined by a double layer

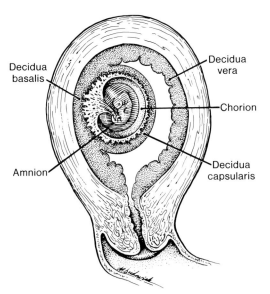

Figure 5.3. The decidua. Eventually, the decidua capsularis and decidua vera fuse as the pregnancy fills the uterine cavity.

Table 5.1.   Structures Derived from the Embryonic Plate

Ectoderm	Mesoderm	Endoderm
Skin	Bone	Respiratory system
Brain	Muscle	Digestive system
Nervous system	Circulatory system	
	Urogenital system	

of cells, the trophoblast (Fig. 5.6). As pregnancy progresses, the vessels develop and the placenta begins to function at day 17–21. There are various developmental landmarks that can be used to decide on the period of pregnancy. The red blood cells are nucleated in the early part of pregnancy. At about 6 weeks, the red blood cells are very immature erythroblasts and are dominated by strikingly large nuclei. At 8 weeks the fetal hemoglobin surrounds the nucleus, and the red blood cells are 100% nucleated. By 10 weeks, only 10% of the red blood cells are nucleated.

The trophoblast consists of two layers of cells which are present up to the 20th week of pregnancy. The outer layer is called the syncytial cells or the syncytiotrophoblast. The inner layer is called Langhans' layer or cytotrophoblast. Presumably Langhans' layer produces the chorionic gonadotrophic hormone which the pregnancy test depends on. At 20 weeks, the two layers of cells become progressively indistinct and the Langhans' layer disappears completely. A small amount of hCG continues to be produced by the trophoblast all through pregnancy but, in general, after 20 weeks there is only one layer of trophoblastic cells. By term, approximately 4 villi occupy the space of one that was present in early pregnancy. The villi consist primarily of blood vessels which have progressed to the surface and hence protrude from it so as to bring about a better interchange between the maternal and the fetal blood. However, the two circulations are completely separate. Prior to the division of the villi, there is poor maternal-fetal interchange. The villi are large,

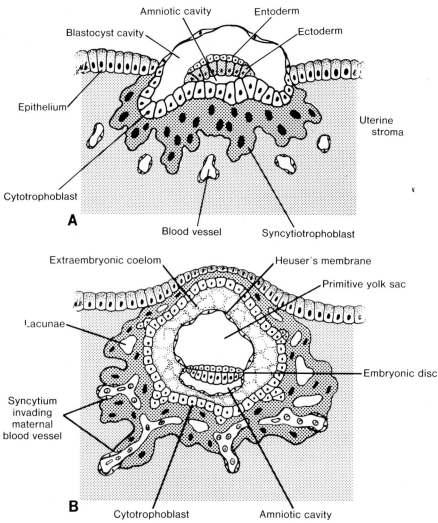

Figure 5.4A.　Early implantation. The ovum is not yet covered over.

Figure 5.4B.　Twelve-day implantation.

lined by a double layer of cells, with tiny vessels that are located centrally. After 20 weeks, the villi gradually divide and become smaller, and the vessels become more prominent and approach the surface.

At term, under the scanning electron microscope the vessels are seen to balloon out from the terminal villi. Under the ordinary microscope, it would appear that the only thing separating the mother's blood from the fetal blood is the endothelium. Under the electron microscope, it is clear that there is a definite cell wall, which rings the entire villus, inside of which endothelium is present. As term approaches, the single layer of syncytial cells lining the villi are frequently pushed together to form syncytial knots. This brings the fetal vessels closer to the intervillous pool, effecting a better interchange.

The membranes of the placenta consist of a single layer of cells, the amnion, which is attached to the thicker chorion by means of connective tissue.

A section of a term placenta that has been fixed shows a rather solid structure but in vivo it is quite different and is spread out over a large area. On the fetal side, there is a single layer of cells, the amnion and the chorionic plate from which the villi extend and gradually divide. On the maternal side are the smallest villi, near the attachment to the mother's decidua. A small thin layer of decidua always goes along with the placenta when

it separates. It is in this area that most of the maternal-fetal interchange occurs. The villi are covered by a fine brush border of microvilli which are seen under the electron microscope to fulfill the function of engulfing the various requirements in the interchange.

FULL-TERM PLACENTA

On the maternal side is the decidua, the compacta and the spongiosa, and the myometrium. The coiled arteries come up to the surface to eject blood into the intervillous space, the maternal circulation. The mother's component has the function of anchoring the placenta and furnishing blood to the intervillous space. On the opposite side of the placenta is the cord with the vessels coming down, dividing and dipping down into the various portions. A term placenta has a maternal and a fetal side. It looks like a flat cake and hence the original Latin word *placenta* was given to it. It is normally 15–20 cm in

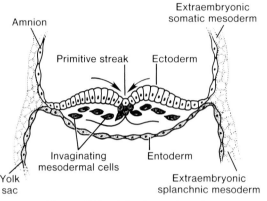

Figure 5.5.   The formative plate.

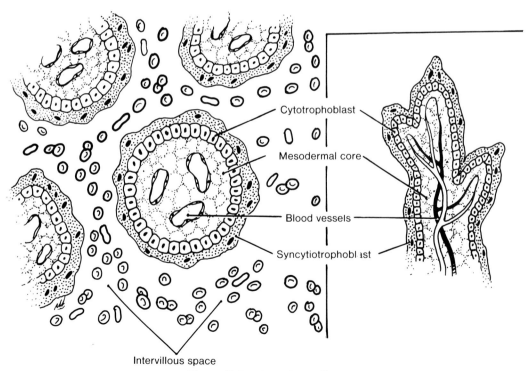

Figure 5.6.   Immature villus.

diameter and 2–3 cm in thickness. The maternal side is divided into a number of compartments, usually 15–20 in number, called *cotyledons*. They are formed by the extensions of the decidual septa into the placenta proper. The fetal blood comes down the umbilical cord in the arteries, which divide and dip down into the various cotyledons, and flows out to the terminal villi. The villi are classified as *primary*, *secondary* and *tertiary*. The tertiary villi are near the attachment to the mother where most of the interchange occurs and where there are microvilli. The placenta is held in place by two different mechanisms, namely the villi that anchor it to the decidua and the decidual septa that occasionally extend through and anchor to the chorionic plate. Beneath the placenta there is a layer of mucopolysaccharide called *Nitabuch's layer*, which limits the downgrowth of the villi, preventing them from continuing any deeper than the decidua spongiosum. Blood is ejected into the intervillous pool or lake at 70–80 mm Hg pressure and works its way toward the chorionic plate, guided along the various villi and the decidual septa. The flow is for the most part directly across to the chorionic plate, where it reaches a pressure of 7–9 mm Hg when the patient is lying down. When the patient is sitting or standing, the pressure is generally 30 mm Hg in the intervillous lake. This is a very low pressure but there is about 500 ml of blood per minute flowing from the maternal side into the intervillous pool or lake so that the volume of blood that goes through makes up for the low pressure. The volume of the intervillous space is normally 175–250 ml during relaxation of the uterus. However, as the uterus contracts, the intervillous space is compressed and there is a reduction in the intervillous space as well as an accompanying decrease in the maternal blood flowing into the intervillous space and fetal blood coming to the villi.

The umbilical cord has two arteries and one vein. The umbilical arteries come off the hypogastric arteries through the umbilicus, carry the less oxygenated blood to the placenta, and dip down into the cotyledons; after the gaseous interchange at the intervillous pool, the oxygen-rich blood goes back via the umbilical vein. Blood flows down the umbilical artery at 48 mm Hg and returns via the umbilical vein at a pressure of 24 mm Hg, which is a very low pressure. However, there is about 400 ml of blood per minute flowing from the fetal side into the placenta.

If the villi were laid end to end, it is estimated they would be 30 miles long! The exposed surface is approximately 16 sq m or 150 sq ft. The increased surface area of the villi combined with the blood volume flowing through the intervillous pool more than compensates for the poor intervillous and umbilical blood flow pressures. The cord is normally 55–60 cm long. The placenta is usually spontaneously expelled from the uterus by one of two methods. When the placenta is expelled with both the maternal and fetal sides visible simultaneously, it is known as the *Duncan method* (Fig. 5.7). If the membranes or fetal side is expelled and emerges first, it is known as the *Schultz method*, after Schultz who described it (Fig. 5.7). The placenta normally weighs 400–600 gm, depending on how much of the membranes and how much of the cord are left attached to the placenta.

For the first 3 weeks and up to 6 weeks, the placenta weighs substantially more than the embryo. After the 16th week, the fetus outstrips the growth and size of the placenta. At term, the placenta usually weighs about one fifth to one sixth of the fetus. The fetal weight is approximately 650 gm at 24 weeks. Thereafter, the fetal weight increases approximately by multiples of 650 gm every 4 weeks until 40 weeks.

ENDOCRINE PHYSIOLOGY OF THE PLACENTA

The placenta produces 1) protein hormones such as human chorionic gonadotropin (hCG), human placental lactogen (hPL), placental thyrotrophin (TSH), pla-

Maternal   **Fetal**

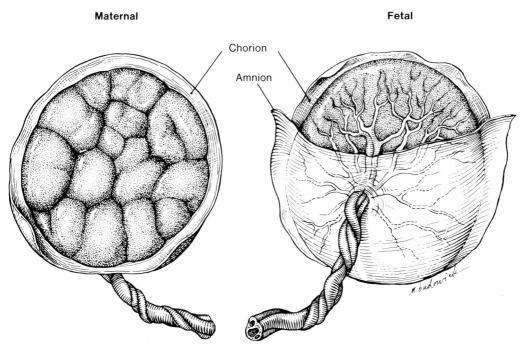

Figure 5.7.   Term placenta. Maternal surface (*left*) and fetal surface (*right*).

cental adrenocorticotrophin (ACTH), placental luteinizing hormone-releasing hormone (LH-RH) and 2) steroid hormones such as estrone (E_1), estradiol (E_2), estriol (E_3), progesterone and some androgens. The amounts of hPL, estrogens and progesterone produced increase with gestational age and reach maximum levels at term, while hCG reaches a peak level at 10–12 weeks pregnancy and declines after 14 weeks to remain at a relatively constant level until delivery. Both the protein and the steroid hormones are produced in the syncytiotrophoblast. However, some studies indicate that the cytotrophoblast is responsible for the synthesis of hCG. It should be noted that the cytotrophoblast undergoes change to become the syncytiotrophoblast. The protein hormones and progesterone are produced by the placenta with no participation by the fetus, whereas E_3 requires both the placenta and the fetus for its synthesis to be completed. Thus hCG and hPL reflect trophoblast mass and viability, while E_3 reflects the viability of

the fetoplacental unit (see chapter on "Endocrinology of Pregnancy and Parturition").

AMNIOTIC FLUID

The volume of amniotic fluid varies with gestational age. In early pregnancy, there is very little amniotic fluid. At term, amniotic fluid generally averages about 1000 ml. *Hydramnios* and *polyhydramnios* refer to an excess of amniotic fluid above 2000 ml.

FUNCTIONS OF THE PLACENTA

1. It provides nutrients such as essential amino acids, fatty acids, glucose and oxygen from the mother to the fetus.
2. It acts as an organ that clears the metabolites and waste products generated by the fetus.
3. It provides immunoprotection of the fetus and transfers antibodies against

infection from the mother to the fetus, thus conferring the latter with passive immunity.

4. It is an endocrine organ with a profound capacity for hormone synthesis. It synthesizes hCG, hPL, estrogens and progesterone.

5. It produces a variety of enzymes such as alkaline phosphatase and oxytocinase.

6. It may fulfill other functions which are yet to be defined.

Suggested Reading

1. Novak, E.R., and Woodruff, J.D. *Novak's Gynecologic and Obstetric Pathology with Clinical and Endocrine Relations*, 8th edition. W.B. Saunders, Philadelphia, 1978.
2. Gruenwald, P. *The Placenta and its Maternal Supply Line*. University Park Press, Baltimore, 1975.

CHAPTER 6

Endocrinology of Pregnancy and Parturition

M. YUSOFF DAWOOD, M.D.

Pregnancy brings about progressive and profound changes in the endocrine milieu of the maternal organism which is related to the maintenance of the pregnancy and its subsequent termination with the onset of labor. The endocrine changes are due to hormone production from three major sources, namely 1) the mother, 2) the fetus and 3) the placenta. The hormone changes found during pregnancy are an interaction between these three sources. In some instances, the placenta and the fetus function as a single endocrine unit which is referred to as the *fetoplacental unit*. From the time of implantation to the time of expulsion, the placenta continuously produces a variety of hormones either by itself or together with the fetus. The hormones produced by the placenta are:

Protein Hormones
1. Human chorionic gonadotropin (hCG)
2. Human chorionic somatomammotropin (hCS)
3. Placental specific proteins or pregnancy associated proteins
4. Human chorionic thyrotropin (placental hCT)
5. Human adrenocorticotropic hormone (placental ACTH)
6. Luteinizing hormone-releasing hormone (placental LH-RH)

Steroid Hormones
1. Estrogens
2. Progesterone
3. Androgens

HORMONAL CHANGES IN EARLY PREGNANCY

It is generally agreed that hCG is detectable in the maternal circulation shortly after implantation on about day 23–25 of the menstrual cycle. Some investigators have demonstrated the presence of hCG or hCG-like material in the circulation prior to implantation but this is still open to question. hCG levels continue to rise rapidly after implantation. hCG stimulates the corpus luteum to become a gestational corpus luteum and maintains it. Consequently, the corpus luteum continues to increase its production of estrone and estradiol, progesterone, 17α-hydroxyprogesterone, all of which continue to increase in the maternal circulation. Thus hCG is the signal from the implanted blastocyst to the corpus to continue to survive.

PROTEIN HORMONES

Human Chorionic Gonadotropin (hCG)

hCG is a glycoprotein hormone containing 8–15% of sugars and sialic acids. It has a molecular weight of about 30,000 and is made up of two subunits, namely, the alpha and beta subunits which are noncovalently linked by a disulfide bond. The alpha subunit of hCG shares similar amino acid sequence to the alpha subunits of follicle stimulating hormone (FSH), luteinizing hormone (LH) and thyroid stimulating hormone (TSH), while the beta subunits of these four hormones are dissimilar

43

and therefore confer hormone immunologic specificity. Thus, antibodies generated against the beta subunit of hCG will be more specific in detecting and measuring hCG than will the antibodies raised against the whole hCG molecule. hCG is produced by the placenta and specifically by the syncytiotrophoblast. hCG is cleared by the kidneys at a rate of 1 ml/minute, which remains constant throughout pregnancy. More than 90% of it is inactivated in the body prior to excretion.

About 500,000–1,000,000 IU of hCG are produced per day during the first trimester of pregnancy. The amount of hCG produced parallels the number of viable trophoblast cells. Hence, the most rapid increase in circulating hCG levels occurs during the first trimester, which is the period of rapid and accelerated multiplication of the trophoblast. After the 100th day of pregnancy (14 weeks) and during late pregnancy, the production rate of hCG declines tenfold to 80,000–120,000 IU per day. In general, hCG levels in the plasma would be cleared and reach low or undetectable levels at 3–4 weeks after expulsion of the placenta. However, with the more sensitive measurement techniques for hCG, it is sometimes detectable as late as 12–14 weeks after delivery. hCG may be detected as early as day 26 of the fertilized cycle or shortly after implantation. The blood and urine levels of hCG run parallel throughout pregnancy. hCG levels reach a peak between the seventh and twelfth weeks of pregnancy, to be followed by an equally sharp decline to levels that remain fairly constant from the 15th week onward.

The concentration of hCG in the urine varies throughout the day and is inversely related with fluid volume, but the level in the blood remains fairly constant. Therefore, as a clinical parameter, the 24-hour urine excretion rate of hCG is preferable to measuring the concentration in random samples. However, for a routine pregnancy test, a morning sample of urine, which is usually more concentrated than that from the rest of the day, may suffice. On the fetal side, hCG has recently been demonstrated in a variety of tissues from the brain to the skin. In the amniotic fluid, hCG is present but the levels are about one tenth of those found in maternal serum. The origin of amniotic fluid hCG is unclear but it has been suggested that there is direct seepage from the trophoblast through the fetal membranes.

There are several physiologic roles of hCG during pregnancy. 1) hCG is *luteotrophic*. It stimulates the corpus luteum of the menstrual cycle to become a gestational corpus luteum which remains highly functional, produces more progesterone and maintains the pregnancy until the synthesizing ability of the trophoblast is fully established. This luteotrophic function is vital up to about 8 or 9 weeks, after which removal of the corpus luteum does not always cause loss of the pregnancy due to a reduction in plasma progesterone. 2) *Differentiation of fetal gonads in early pregnancy*. By the eighth week of pregnancy, the fetal testes are formed and Leydig cells are present. The Leydig cells show maximum differentiation by the 15th week, but the fetal pituitary gland does not secrete biologically active gonadotropins until well beyond the 20th week. During the 8–12th week, hCG levels are maximal and thus hCG is probably necessary for differentiation of the fetal testis at this stage. 3) *Immunoprotective role*. hCG has been credited with being immunoprotective and responsible for preventing rejection of the fetus, which is a heterograft. Most of the studies supporting this role have been based on acceptance of skin heterograft in the presence of hCG but many investigators now believe that this is due to impurities in the hCG used, since highly purified hCG is not able to fulfill this role (see Chapter 8: "Immunology of Pregnancy"). 4) *Stimulation of the fetal adrenal cortex in early pregnancy*. This is based on the same reasoning as differentiation of the fetal testis. Additionally, the fetal adrenal cortex has been shown to have hCG receptors.

CLINICAL APPLICATIONS

Measurements of hCG in plasma or urine have been used for: 1) detection and diagnosis of early pregnancy, 2) as an aid in the prognosis of *threatened* abortion and 3) as an index of trophoblast activity as in ectopic pregnancy and in the diagnosis and follow-up of trophoblastic tumors. hCG can be measured by 1) bioassay, examples of which are the Hogben, the Galli-Manini and the Friedman test, 2) immunoassay as in the slide agglutination test and the hemagglutination inhibition test, 3) the more sensitive radioreceptorassay and 4) the sensitive and specific radioimmunoassay using antibodies generated against the beta subunit of hCG.

Human Placental Lactogen (hPL)

hPL is also known as human chorionic somatomammotropin (hCS). It is produced by the syncytiotrophoblast. The factors regulating hPL synthesis are not known, but hPL secretion is diminished if placental blood flow is compromised. hPL is a single chain polypeptide (cf to hCG) consisting of 190 amino acids with 2 intrachain disulfide bonds. It has a molecular weight of about 19,000–30,000 and shows some immunologic similarities to but is distinct from growth hormone. The half-life of hPL is 20–30 minutes, which indicates that hPL is more rapidly eliminated from the circulation than is hCG. The daily secretion rate at term is 0.5–3.0 gm/day. The mode of metabolism of hPL is poorly understood.

Most of the hPL found during pregnancy is present in the circulation or in the placenta. Very negligible amounts of hPL are found in the amniotic fluid, fetal circulation and maternal urine. hPL levels in the maternal circulation increase to reach maximum levels at 34 weeks of pregnancy and remain thereafter until term. The amniotic fluid has a higher hPL concentration than does the fetal circulation, thus suggesting that hPL reaches the amniotic fluid from the placenta or maternal decidua rather than via the fetus. Amniotic fluid hPL levels are lower than the maternal circulation levels. Spellacy and his colleagues have developed the concept of a "fetal-danger" zone, which is entered if serum hPL falls below 4 μg/ml after the 30th week of pregnancy (Fig. 6.1). They

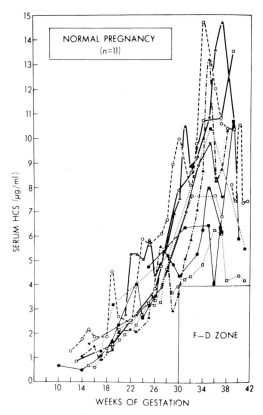

Figure 6.1. Serial maternal serum hPL in 11 women with normal pregnancies. There is an increase in maternal serum hPL with gestational age in normal pregnancy. After the 30th week of pregnancy, when fetal well-being is compromised and there is a likelihood of imminent fetal demise, serum hPL levels enter and remain in the fetal-danger (F-D) zone. (After Spellacy, W.N., Teoh, E.S., and Buhi, W.C. *Obstetrics and Gynecology, 35*:685, 1970.)

found that there was a higher incidence of perinatal morbidity and mortality if the maternal serum hPL enters and remains in this zone.

CLINICAL APPLICATIONS

Measuring maternal serum hPL can be useful in the following conditions: 1) *Threatened abortion*: A subnormal or declining serum hPL indicates an unfavorable prognosis in threatened abortion but is less accurate than serum hCG. 2) *Trophoblastic disease*: Serum hPL is low in choriocarcinoma but is elevated in patients with hydatidiform mole as long as the molar pregnancy is intact. 3) *Multiple pregnancy*: Serum hPL is increased. 4) *Hypertensive disorder of pregnancy*: Serum hPL is either normal or low. When the hPL levels are low, there is an increased risk to the fetus. There is a stillbirth rate of 24% if hPL levels are in the fetal-danger zone in pregnancies complicated by hypertension. There is also a higher incidence of up to 75% of neonatal asphyxia or infants small for dates if serum hPL is significantly below the normal mean for that period of pregnancy. 5) *Fetal distress or asphyxia*: The incidence of fetal distress and/or neonatal asphyxia increases progressively when serum hPL levels remain persistently in the fetal-danger zone. 6) *Fetal growth retardation and death*: Serum hPL is low if the cause of fetal death is related to placental dysfunction. Serum hPL is low in fetal growth retardation. 7) *Diabetes mellitus and rhesus isoimmunization*: There is disagreement on the levels of hPL in both conditions but it is generally agreed that if there is superimposed hypertension in these disorders, then serum hPL can be helpful and would be low.

FUNCTIONS OF hPL

hPL has several biological properties which include: 1) *Lactogenic*—prepares the breast for successful lactation by increasing growth of mammary alveoli and by mediating milk production in an estrogen/progesterone primed breast. 2) *Luteotrophic*—not proven in human beings. 3) *Somatotrophic*—a) hPL has a maternal *glucose-sparing effect* which is seen in late pregnancy because the fetus is able to utilize glucose only for its energy needs. b) hPL increases maternal plasma free fatty acids by mobilizing free fatty acids, i.e., it has *lipolytic* effect. c) hPL increases resistance to endogenous and exogenous insulin and may be protective in insulin-induced hypoglycemia. d) hPL when given in high doses increases nitrogen retention but in low doses it does not. e) hPL has a diabetogenic effect.

STEROID HORMONES

Estrogens

More than 20 different estrogens have been demonstrated in the urine of pregnant women. The three main estrogens are estrone (E_1), estradiol (E_2) and estriol (E_3). In the nonpregnant state, estriol constitutes a smaller proportion of the total estrogens with an $E_3:E_1:E_2$ ratio of $3:2:1$ but becomes the major estrogen with an $E_3:E_1:E_2$ ratio of $30:2:1$.

ESTRONE AND ESTRADIOL

During the first trimester of pregnancy, the major source of E_1 is the corpus luteum of pregnancy but, thereafter, the fetoplacental unit is the primary source. While more than 90% of E_3 is formed by the fetoplacental unit from the fetal dehydroepiandrosterone sulfate (DHEAS), only 40–50% of the E_1 and 50–60% of E_2 are synthesized in the fetoplacental unit from fetal DHEAS (Fig. 6.2). Thus, because the maternal DHEAS provides a significant contribution toward E_1 and E_2 production in late pregnancy, measurements of these two estrogens are not as informative as E_3 determinations in the assessment of fetal well-being in late pregnancy. About 15–20 mg of E_1 and E_2 are produced daily in late pregnancy. The fetus is protected from the undue biologic effects of these two estrogens by metabolizing E_2 to E_3 and 15 α-hydroxyestradiol in the fetal liver.

Plasma unconjugated E_2 is more informative than E_1 in high-risk pregnancies but is less valuable than E_3 in their management. Serial plasma E_2 concentrations which are consistently in the subnormal range or declining into the subnormal range indicate fetal growth retardation or intrauterine fetal demise, but normal E_2 values have also been found under these clinical circumstances (Fig. 6.3).

ESTRIOL

For E_3 to be formed, the fetus and the placenta have to function as a single fetoplacental unit. This is necessary because the placenta possesses certain enzymes

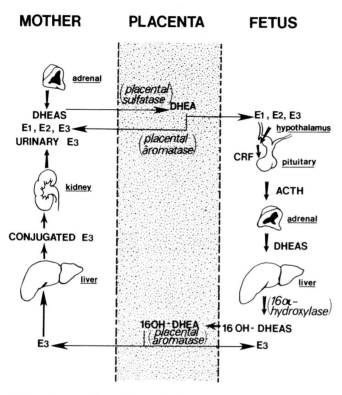

Figure 6.2. Simplified scheme of the pathway for biosynthesis of estrone (E$_1$), estradiol (E$_2$), and estriol (E$_3$) in the fetoplacental unit. The enzyme involved in the biosynthesis is written in brackets. ACTH = adrenal corticotropic hormone, CRF = corticotropin releasing factor, DHEA = dehydroepiandrosterone, DHEAS = dehydroepiandrosterone sulfate, 16α-OH DHEA = 16α-hydroxy dehydroepiandrosterone, 16α-OH DHEAS = 16-hydroxy dehydroepiandrosterone sulfate.

(sulfatase and 3β-ol-dehydrogenase) which the fetus does not and the latter has 16α-hydroxylase which the former does not have. This arrangement protects the fetus from undesirable masculinizing or feminizing effects. The pathway for the synthesis of E$_3$ is shown in Figure 6.2. DHEAS is produced from the adrenal cortex in response to ACTH released from the anterior pituitary gland, after stimulation by corticotropin releasing factor (CRF) from the hypothalamus. DHEAS is converted to 16α-OH DHEAS in the fetal liver. The 16α-OH DHEAS is desulfated by sulfatase in the placenta to 16α-OH DHEA. 16α-OH DHEA is aromatized under the influence of aromatizing enzymes to 16α-OH testosterone and then to E$_3$. E$_3$ is passed into both maternal and fetal circulations. In the fetal circulation, 15α-hydroxylation of estrogens, including E$_3$, occurs in the liver as a protection against the feminizing effects of estrogens. Thus, E$_3$ is converted into 15α-hydroxyestriol or estetrol (E$_4$). In the maternal circulation, E$_3$ is conjugated to E$_3$-sulfate and E$_3$-glucuronide, which are collectively referred to as *conjugated estriols*. Conjugated E$_3$, which is more water-soluble than is unconjugated E$_3$, is therefore more easily excreted by the kidneys and constitutes a major component of urinary E$_3$. Only about 10% of circulating E$_3$ is in the unconjugated form, while 90% is in the conjugated form. Both unconjugated and total E_3 in maternal circulation increase progressively during pregnancy, with the rate of increase being maximal in the third trimester. Plasma E_3 is measured by radioimmunoassay. Plasma unconjugated E_3 increases slowly from 0.23 ng/ml at 14 weeks to 2.6 ng/ml at 20 weeks, 6.3 ng/ml at 30 weeks, and 14.2 ng/ml at 37 weeks (Fig. 6.4). Most of the E_3 in amniotic fluid is in the conjugated form. Therefore, the concentrations of unconjugated E_3 of amniotic fluid are low, with 1.1 ng/ml in mid-trimester and 10–19 ng/ml at 34–42 weeks. Measurements of E_3 in plasma or urine are valuable for screening and evaluation of high-risk pregnancies (Tables 6.1 and 6.2).

If properly used, plasma E_3 determinations can be helpful in the management of high-risk pregnancies. It is preferable to measure plasma unconjugated E_3 rather than total E_3. The trend in the serial E_3

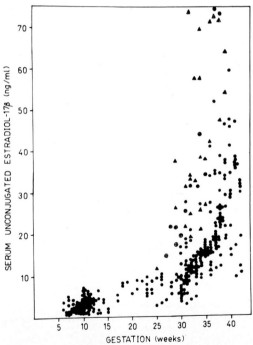

Figure 6.3. Maternal serum unconjugated estradiol (E_2) throughout normal pregnancy. There is a rapid increase in E_2 from 30 weeks until term. (After Dawood, M.Y., and Ratnam, S.S. *Obstetrics and Gynecology, 44,* 1974.)

levels is more important than a single value. Measurements of plasma unconjugated E_3 have been helpful in the diagnosis of 1) fetal death in utero, 2) anencephaly, 3) fetal adrenal hypoplasia, 4) placental sulfatase deficiency, and 5) fetal well-being in the third trimester. In the second and third trimesters, plasma unconjugated E_3 levels consistently less than 1 ng/ml and 2.5 ng/ml, respectively, are found 4–6 hours after fetal demise in utero. The major usefulness of plasma unconjugated E_3 determinations is in the assessment of fetal well-being in the third trimester. Generally, good correlations have been found between plasma E_3 and clinical conditions with hypoxia and malnutritive placental insufficient, as in pregnancy-induced hypotension and idiopathic growth retardation. With diabetes mellitus, caution is necessary in interpreting plasma E_3 since the placenta is larger and in the absence of hypertension the mean plasma E_3 levels may be higher. Low urinary E_3 may be found in the following situations: 1) placental sulfatase deficiency when all other clinical indices of the pregnancy indicate that it is normal, 2) when the patient is taking corticosteroids, 3) when the patient has been taking ampicillin for some time, and 4) when the patient is taking phenolphthalein. Plasma E_3 will be low in the first two conditions but not in the last two. Amniotic fluid E_3 is useful in the monitoring of fetal well-being in patients with isoimmunization who receive intrauterine transfusion. A rising level of amniotic fluid E_3 after intrauterine transfusion indicates a favorable response.

Long-term follow-up of children who had low urinary E_3 during intrauterine life indicates that there is a significantly higher incidence of cerebral damage in this group (51.5%) than in children who had normal urinary E_3 during their intrauterine life.

ESTETROL

It has been suggested that plasma estetrol (E_4) is superior to E_3 in indicating fetal well-being since E_4 is almost exclusively a fetal product compared to E_3. Plasma E_4

concentratons are lower than that of E_3. The concentration of plasma E_4 at term is 1.2 ng/ml. Preliminary studies of plasma E_4 have produced conflicting conclusions about its value in monitoring fetal well-being.

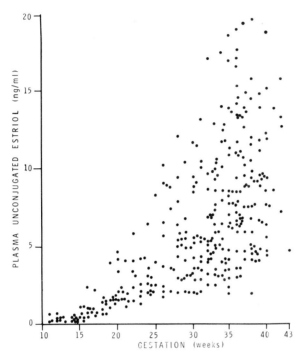

Figure 6.4. Maternal serum unconjugated estriol (E_3) as determined by radioimmunoassay throughout pregnancy.

Table 6.1. Comparison of the Advantages and Disadvantages of Determining Urinary Estriol Versus Plasma Estriol

Plasma E_3	Urinary E_3
Advantages 　1. Rapid to perform, results obtained within a few hours and therefore reflects fetoplacental status of a few hours previously 　2. Does not require patient compliance; only a small amount of blood required 　3. Not affected by phenolphthalein or mandelamine if plasma unconjugated E_3 is measured 　4. Small day-to-day coefficient of variability (16%) and, therefore, appreciable "drops" may reflect pathology rather than physiologic variation 　5. Plasma unconjugated E_3 levels are not affected by urine output or renal function Disadvantages 　1. Requires expensive hardware in initial laboratory set-up 　2. Expertise in radioimmunoassay necessary 　3. Involves blood collection	Advantages 　1. Simple to perform; does not require expensive equipment 　2. Noninvasive 　3. Reflects a 24-hour period of fetal welfare Disadvantages 　1. 24-hour urine collection is not easy. In the most well supervised groups of patients, 22% have incomplete urine collection 　2. Affected by drugs such as mandelamine, phenolphthalein, ampicillin and corticosteroids 　3. Fastest result available reflects fetoplacental status at best 36 to 12 hours previously 　4. Wider day-to-day coefficient of variation than plasma E_3 　5. Affected if urine volume is less than 600 ml 　6. E_3 excretion affected if renal function is severely compromised

Table 6.2.   Shortcomings of Estriol Determination

1. Low levels may mislead the clinician into unnecessary fear and intervention.
2. Fall in E_3 levels may be late sign and may occur after irreversible damage has occurred.
3. Normal E_3 does not necessarily indicate normal fetal health, e.g., rhesus isoimmunization.
4. Accuracy of E_3 in predicting fetal distress is about 70–80%.
5. Unconjugated E_3 may fall abruptly and sharply without apparent associated pathology, only to be followed by a rise within a matter of hours.
6. Normal and abnormal values often overlap.

FUNCTIONS OF ESTROGEN DURING PREGNANCY

1. Estrogens stimulate uterine muscle hyperplasia and hypertrophy, thus accounting for the greatly increased size and thickness of the uterus as pregnancy advances.
2. Estrogen increases the excitability of myometrial cells by altering the membrane potential.
3. Estrogen increases the adenosine triphosphate (ATP) and actomyosin content of the myometrial cells in preparation for the work required at parturition.
4. Estrogens cause an increase in the water content of the cervix, thus giving rise to the softening of the cervix as pregnancy advances.
5. Estrogen stimulates ductal development of the mammary glands in preparation for lactation.
6. Estrogens increase the pelvic and peripheral blood flow.

PLACENTAL DHEAS CLEARANCE

The clearance of DHEAS by the placenta has been suggested as a test of placental hormone biosynthesis. The test involves giving a loading dose of DHEAS (50 mg) intravenously to the pregnant woman and drawing blood samples at regular intervals for E_2 and E_3 determinations. Controversy still exists as to which estrogen is more reliable for determination in this test, which is used in a few centers as a research tool. The advantages of this test include: 1) it is a dynamic evaluation of the actual reserve capacity of placental estrogen biosynthesis, 2) it is a more specific placental function test since the fetus is bypassed, and 3) it may become abnormal several days before a significant drop in plasma E_3. Preliminary studies indicate that the DHEAS loading test is useful in pregnancies in which placental function is compromised, placental sulfatase deficiency is present, and in pregnancy-induced hypertension. In placental sulfatase deficiency, there is no significant increase in plasma estrogen after a loading dose of DHEAS because the placenta is deficient in the enzyme sulfatase.

The metabolic clearance of DHEAS increases throughout pregnancy in normal women. In women who develop pregnancy-induced hypertension, the metabolic clearance of DHEAS before the onset of hypertension is somewhat greater than that of normal pregnant women who will not develop pregnancy-induced hypertension. With the onset of pregnancy-induced hypertension the metabolic clearance of DHEAS is reduced.

Progesterone

Progesterone is known as the gestational hormone. It is initially produced by the corpus luteum during the luteal phase of the menstrual cycle. If pregnancy occurs, hCG is secreted and stimulates the corpus luteum into a gestational corpus luteum which continues to secrete progesterone. Thus, serum progesterone continues to rise. Up to about the eighth or ninth week of pregnancy, the corpus luteum is the primary source of circulating maternal progesterone, but after the ninth week the trophoblast becomes the principal source until delivery. In the placenta, progesterone is synthesized in the syncytiotrophoblast. The mechanism regulating placental production of progesterone is unknown but it appears that oxygen tension of placental blood flow and perhaps the fetus may modulate it. Progesterone is synthesized in the placenta from cholesterol, which is the main precursor via the intermediate pregnenolone (Fig. 6.5). The

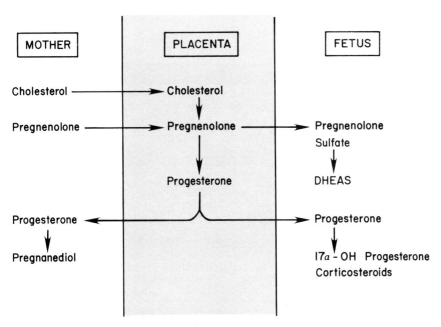

Figure 6.5   Simplified scheme of the pathway for the biosynthesis of progesterone in the placenta.

amount of progesterone secreted during pregnancy increases from 92 mg/day during the first trimester to 263 mg/day during the second trimester and 322 mg/day during the third trimester. In late pregnancy, about 75 mg of progesterone produced per day is transferred to the fetus and the rest goes into the maternal circulation. In the fetus, progesterone is metabolized 1) by the fetal adrenals to deoxycorticosterone sulfate and other corticosteroids, 2) by the liver to pregnanediol glucuronides and 3) by the gonads to 17α-hydroxyprogesterone. The fetus is unable to produce progesterone from pregnenolone because it lacks the enzyme 3β-ol dehydrogenase, which is present in the placenta. The fetus and the placenta act jointly to conserve progesterone: while the placenta can convert 20α-dihydroprogesterone to progesterone, the fetus can convert mainly progesterone to 20α-dihydroprogesterone.

The fetus is unique in having the enzyme 15α-hydroxylase which converts progesterone to 15α-hydroxyprogesterone. Thus 15α-hydroxyprogesterone is found almost exclusively during pregnancy. 15-Hydroxylated steroids are more easily ex-

creted by the fetal kidneys than is the parent steroid. Most of the progesterone during pregnancy is metabolized to pregnanediol and then excreted. Excretion of progesterone and its metabolites during pregnancy is mainly via the kidneys into the urine, via the gut into the feces, via the lungs into the breath and via the skin into the sweat.

Serum progesterone in the maternal circulation increases throughout pregnancy to reach peak levels at term (Fig. 6.6). In the amniotic fluid, the concentration of progesterone is highest in early pregnancy and decreases with gestational age. Umbilical venous blood has a higher concentration of progesterone, about 4 times higher than that in umbilical arterial blood, indicating that the fetus uses progesterone that it receives from the placenta. Progesterone is rapidly cleared from the maternal circulation after removal of the placenta. The physiologic roles of progesterone during pregnancy include : 1) increasing the maternal basal body temperature, 2) increasing the body fat stores, 3) decreasing the smooth muscle tone as in the gut where there is slower intestinal transit time, in the ureters where there is dilatation and in the sphincters which are more relaxed, 4) decreasing the excitability of myometrial cells by altering the membrane potential, 5) depressing the thalamic and medullary centers and giving rise to tiredness and lethargy, 6) stimulating the respiratory center and therefore causing a mild tachypnea and an increase in oxygen consumption, 7) together with estrogen, having a synergistic effect on the development of the breast in preparation for lactation (progesterone stimulating mainly alveolar glandular development) and 8) acting locally to prevent rejection of donor skin grafts. Thus the increased quantities of progesterone present in the placenta could be a factor in preventing rejection of the fetus.

PROGESTERONE AND ABNORMAL PREGNANCIES

As a diagnostic and a predictive index, plasma progesterone has not proven to be reliable in abnormal pregnancies. 1) *Threatened abortion:* Plasma progesterone

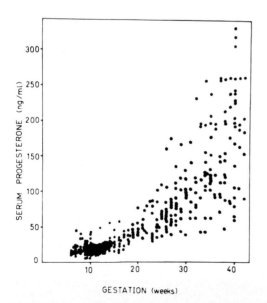

Figure 6.6. Maternal serum progesterone throughout normal pregnancy. Serum rogesterone levels increase with gestation. (After Dawood, M.Y. *American Journal of Obstetrics and Gynecology, 125:*832, 1976.)

may be low or normal. A low plasma progesterone is often the result of the threatened abortion that is becoming inevitable, rather than the cause of the abortion. 2) *Trophoblastic disease:* Plasma progesterone is elevated in patients with hydatidiform mole, due to increased progesterone production by both the trophoblast and the hyperstimulated ovaries. 3) *Multiple pregnancies:* Plasma progesterone is increased but not diagnostic in multiple pregnancies. 4) *Placental insufficiency:* Plasma progesterone is not helpful as an index of placental insufficiency in high-risk pregnancies since the placenta continues to produce and secrete progesterone even after removal of the fetus as long as the placenta is still attached to the uterus.

Other Steroid Hormones

During pregnancy there is an increase in the level of cortisol in the maternal circulation. However, the level of free cortisol, i.e., unbound cortisol, is similar to the levels found during the nonpregnant state. An increase in maternal plasma cortisol occurs as a result of an increase in the circulating level of corticosteroid-binding globulin, which is due to an increase in circulating estrogen. Likewise, plasma testosterone is increased in early pregnancy and remains at about the same level thereafter until delivery. The level of unbound testosterone is unchanged during normal pregnancy. Thus, the increase in plasma testosterone (total) is due to an increase in the circulating level of testosterone-binding globulin (TeBG) which is secondary to the increase in circulating estrogen levels. Hence, caution should be exercised when interpreting levels of plasma cortisol or plasma testosterone in pregnancies complicated by endocrinopathies.

THYROID ACTIVITY

Basal metabolic rate (BMR) rises during pregnancy because of the increased oxygen uptake which is needed by the fetus. Therefore, BMR is unreliable for assessing thyroid function during pregnancy. Thyroid binding globulin (TBG) is greatly increased during pregnancy, due to the increased levels of estrogens. More thyroxin becomes bound to TBG and the pituitary responds by a compensatory increase of thyroid-stimulating hormone (TSH). This stimulates the thyroid gland, which enlarges twofold to threefold. In view of these changes, thyroid function tests during pregnancy should be interpreted with caution. During pregnancy the following changes occur: 1) serum TSH is increased; 2) BMR increases slowly until the eighth month, when it reaches the maximum increase of 15-20% over the nonpregnant state; 3) protein bound iodine (PBI) is increased due to the increased TBG; 4) resin uptake of triiodothyronine (T_3 uptake) is in the hypothyroid range, due to the rise in TBG resulting in a marked increase in the number of unsaturated binding sites; 5) serum T_3 is increased; 6) it is claimed that the free thyroxin index, which is a measure of the relationship between serum T_4 and T_3 uptake, is normal; and 7) serum free thyroxin concentration is normal.

Recent findings indicate that the fetal pituitary-thyroid axis functions as early as 11 weeks of pregnancy. At 100 days of gestation, fetal serum TSH values are in the range of term infants. Placental transfer of both T_3 and T_4 is limited.

It has been suggested that the placenta secretes a protein hormone which is similar to pituitary thyrotropin (TSH). This hormone, which is known as human chorionic thyrotropin (hCT), is thought to be partially responsible for stimulating the thyroid during normal pregnancy and in pregnancies with hydatidiform mole where hyperthyroidism may occasionally result. However, other workers have maintained that hCT is a form of hCG which has the biological property of being able to stimulate the thyroid gland.

Renin-Angiotensin-Aldosterone System

During pregnancy, renin levels in the plasma are essentially within the same range as those found in the nonpregnant state. However, there is a much higher concentration of renin in the amniotic fluid than in the maternal plasma. The significance of this is unclear. In the primigravid woman there is a progressively greater resistance to the pressor effect of infused angiotensin, beginning early in pregnancy. This suggests that in the normal pregnant woman a threshold sensitivity to angiotensin is set at a higher level and continues to be reset at a still higher level as pregnancy progresses. However, in women destined to develop pregnancy-induced hypertension, there is a loss of the normal pregnancy resistance to angiotensin and, therefore, increased vascular sensitivity to infusions of angiotensin occurs some time before the onset of hypertension. Thus, some investigators have suggested using the response to angiotensin infusion in early pregnancy for predicting the subsequent development of pregnancy-induced hypertension.

ENDOCRINOLOGY OF PARTURITION

Many of the hormonal changes in late pregnancy contribute to the preparatory processes that result in parturition. Endocrine changes in the pregnant woman are known to be associated with or to lead to the onset and maintenance of labor. However, the precise sequence of endocrine changes and the actual endocrine trigger that starts labor have not been unequivocally established. It is conceivable that the endocrine mechanism regulating the onset of parturition in women consists of multiple systems that back each other up in the event that one system fails or breaks down. Nevertheless, it is clear that both the maternal and the fetal endocrine systems are involved in the preparation for, onset of and maintenance of labor.

Progesterone Withdrawal Theory

It has been proposed for a long time that progesterone withdrawal was a major factor in initiating human labor. However, most studies on human beings have been unable to demonstrate a convincing or dramatic fall in progesterone levels in the peripheral maternal blood before or during labor. Nevertheless, a fall in progesterone at a local level in the myometrium or in the retroplacental site may play an important role indirectly in either controlling the length of gestation or in triggering a chain of events which ultimately result in labor. Indeed, a fall in progesterone level in the fetal membranes or decidua may be crucial to the generation of precursors for prostaglandin production, which appears to play a significant role in human labor (see below—Prostaglandin Theory).

Fetal Cortisol

In sheep, it has been found that an intact hypothalamohypophyseal-adrenal system is mandatory in the maintenance of normal gestational length and parturition. Hypophysectomy or adrenalectomy would result in prolonged gestation, while administration of corticosteroids would result in premature parturition. Such findings in sheep have been used to explain the observations made in human beings that prolonged gestation is encountered with an anencephalic fetus in which the fetal pituitary may be faulty or totally absent, resulting in understimulation of the adrenal glands and, therefore, in adrenal hypoplasia. It is now known that human pregnancies with anencephalic fetuses complicated by hydramnios, a common association, are not prolonged. Further, the degree of hypothalamus-pituitary absence is variable. Against this theory, however, is the fact that neither cortisol nor ACTH injection into the fetus has been shown to cause premature parturition. Measurements of cortisol levels in maternal plasma showed no significant change with the onset of labor, while amniotic fluid cortisol (which represents fetal cortisol) is increased in instances of spontaneous labor but not when labor is absent. The finding of elevated cortisol levels in cord blood with spontaneous labor has been recently challenged and, at best, indicates that the fetus releases cortisol at the end of spontaneous labor and not necessarily prior to the onset of labor.

Oxytocin Theory

It is clear that administration of oxytocin at term will initiate or augment uterine contractions, but it is not clear if endogenous oxytocin will trigger or initiate the onset of human parturition. The difficulty in proving whether oxytocin is the obligatory factor in the onset of human parturition is compounded by the difficulty in measuring oxytocin levels in human beings, due in part to the low levels of oxytocin present in the circulation. At present, both direct and indirect evidence seem to indicate that oxytocin does play a role in human parturition. Indirect evidence for the role of oxytocin in human labor includes: 1) the claim that hypophysectomy and diabetes insipidus result in prolonged gestation. However, in one review, patients with diabetes insipidus were found to have normal gestation length and labor. Nevertheless, a surge in plasma oxytocin similar to that in normal pregnancy has been reported in diabetes insipidus recently. 2) The occasional association of milk ejection, which is due to release of oxytocin, with labor. Nipple manipulation has been claimed to induce uterine contractions and to have been used with some success for the induction of labor. 3) The use of alcohol to treat premature labor. It is thought to act by inhibiting the release of oxytocin from the neurohypophysis.

Direct evidence for the role of oxytocin in human parturition includes: 1) The significant increase in circulating maternal oxytocin levels throughout pregnancy, with peak levels at 39 weeks. While the uterus is relatively refractory to the effect of oxytocin in early pregnancy, it becomes increasingly sensitive to small doses of oxytocin at or near term. 2) The sharp increase in the maternal plasma oxytocin level from the first to the second stage of labor, followed by a sharp drop during the third stage of labor. There is a significant increase in the level of maternal plasma oxytocin during the second stage of labor consistent with the greatest uterine activity observed throughout labor (Fig. 6.7). 3)

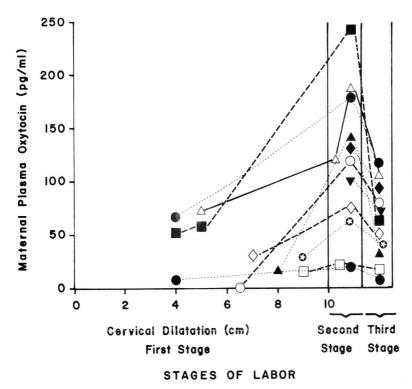

Figure 6.7. Serial maternal plasma oxytocin during the first, second and third stages of labor in 11 women with normal labor and spontanous vaginal delivery. Note the significant rapid increase in oxytocin levels during the second stage followed by a rapid decline during the third stage of labor. (After Dawood, M.Y., et al. *Obstetrics and Gynecology, 51:*138, 1978).

In spontaneous labor, the remarkable increase in the concentration of oxytocin in umbilical arterial blood, giving rise to a significant increase in the umbilical arterial-venous difference in oxytocin concentration. This indicates that the fetus releases significant amounts of oxytocin during spontaneous labor. 4) The release of oxytocin in spurts during pregnancy and labor. The frequency and amplitude of the spurts increase during labor.

The indication is that oxytocin is released during labor and that both the maternal and fetal pituitaries contribute to the increased oxytocin levels found during parturition. It is unclear what stimulates the release of fetal oxytocin. The amount of oxytocin transferred from the fetal to the maternal side during spontaneous labor amounts to about 3.0 MU/min; this is consistent with the amount of oxytocin which, when given as an intravenous infusion at or near term, results in uterine contractions and has been used for induction of labor. Therefore, the fetus acts as an oxytocin injection system to the mother's uterus during spontaneous labor.

Prostaglandin Theory

Since the observation that prostaglandin $F_2\alpha$ (PGF$_2\alpha$) and prostaglandin E_2 (PGE$_2$) were capable of causing contraction of both the pregnant and the nonpregnant uterus, it has been suggested that prostaglandins play an important role in the endocrine regulation of labor. However, it is not clear whether prostaglandins initiate labor or are merely responsible for its maintenance. There is an increase in the concentration of PGF$_2\alpha$ and PGE$_2$ in the amniotic fluid as labor progresses. In the maternal blood, both $PGF_2\alpha$ and its metabolite have been shown to increase at or around the time of labor. These observations indicate that endogenous prostaglandins probably play a crucial role in human parturition. Prostaglandins are synthesized from a polyunsaturated essential free fatty acid, namely arachidonic acid, under the influence of a group of enzymes collectively called *prostaglandin synthetase*. The rate-limiting step in the biosynthesis of prostaglandins is the availability of the precursor, arachidonic acid. Hence, the generation and thus the availability of arachidonic acid is the principal regulator of prostaglandin biosynthesis. Arachidonic acid is generally stored as phospholipids and released from its stored form under the influence of the enzyme phospholipase A_2. Both the decidua and the fetal membranes are rich in this enzyme and have a greatly increased capacity for prostaglandin production at term. Phospholipase A_2 is a lysosomal enzyme, and destruction of the lysosomes will result in release of this enzyme. Since this enzyme liberates arachidonic acid from phospholipids and, therefore, increases the availability of the essential precursor for prostaglandin synthesis, phospholipase A_2 is the earlier and perhaps initial controlling factor in the rate of prostaglandin synthesis. It has been observed that progesterone binds to the cellular fraction corresponding to lysosomes and maintains the stability of the latter. Thus, a fall in progesterone locally within the decidua and/or the fetal membranes will result in a breakdown of the lysosomes, thereby setting off a chain of events which leads to the biosynthesis of prostaglandins. During spontaneous labor, an eightfold increase in the level of arachidonic acid has been found in the amniotic fluid compared with the level in term pregnancies which were not in labor. Hence it is clear that prostaglandin is generated and released during labor and it is important to the maintenance of labor. It is unclear whether stretch which occurs during contractions and which is a stimulus for prostaglandin production could be partially responsible for the prostaglandins found during labor. While the generation and release of prostaglandins appear to be important for producing uterine contractions in human parturition, the initial triggering factors in the cascade of enzymatic and endocrine changes that lead to prostaglandin production have not been clearly defined.

Estrogen and Labor

Based on the work in animals, it was concluded that estrogen increases the excitability of the myometrium to oxytocics. During human pregnancy, there is an increase in circulating estrogens, in particular estradiol and estriol. The rate of increase is maximal during the third trimester. In the human, it has been observed that the gravid uterus becomes increasingly sensitive to oxytocin as pregnancy progresses and this sensitivity is maximal at or near term. The increase in sensitivity to oxytocin has been attributed to the increase in circulating estrogens, in particular estradiol. In the rabbit, estrogens have been shown to increase the number and activity of oxytocin receptors in the myometrium, while progesterone produces the opposite effect. Therefore, it is possible that the rapid increase in circulating estrogen in maternal circulation brings about an increase in the activity and number of oxytocin receptors in the myometrial cells, thus resulting in an increased sensitivity to oxytocin. Another mode of action of the rising concentration of estradiol is through increased prostaglandin production. Estrogens have been shown to stimulate prostaglandin production. Hence, the rise in circulating estrogen at the approach of term not only increases the sensitivity of the myometrium to oxytocin but also increases the production of prostaglandin which itself is stimulatory to the uterus.

Changes at Cellular Levels in Parturition

While the endocrine changes may explain some of the factors regulating the onset of uterine contractions in human parturition, the final pathway of action is at the myometrial cellular level. The uterine contraction brought about by prostaglandins and oxytocin is a calcium-dependent process. Prostaglandins have been shown to inhibit the ATP-dependent calcium binding to the sacroplasmic reticulum in the myometrial cells, thus rendering a higher intracellular level of free calcium. The rise in intracellular free calcium results in activation of the contractile proteins in the muscle fibers. In addition to its influence on intracellular calcium, oxytocin also exerts its uterine contractility effect by an alteration in the intracellular and extracellular sodium ion movement.

The Fetus and Parturition

Ultimately, most of the endocrine changes related to human parturition may be traced to the central nervous system of the fetus as the primary central regulatory mechanism. The fetal hypothalamus secretes corticotropin releasing factor (CRF) which stimulates the release of ACTH from the anterior pituitary gland. ACTH in turn stimulates the adrenal to secrete DHEAS, which is the precursor for estrogen production. Estrogen stimulates prostaglandin production and increases the activity and number of oxytocin receptors in the uterus, thereby increasing the sensitivity of the uterus to oxytocin. Oxytocin is produced in the hypothalamus and stored in the fetal neurohypophysis. The release of fetal oxytocin is increased during human labor. Although the fetal hypothalamus appears to be the common primary center that governs the release of all the hormones that could influence labor, the factor that controls the activity of the fetal hypothalamus at or near term has not been elucidated.

It is evident that many of the pieces of the complex jigsaw in the cascade of endocrine changes that regulate the onset of labor are, at present, available. However, a definitive pattern has not been worked out.

Suggested Reading

1. Fuchs, F., and Klopper, A. (eds.) *Endocrinology of Pregnancy*, ed. 2. Harper & Row, Hagerstown, MD, 1977.
2. Dawood, M.Y. Hormone assay of plasma and amniotic fluid. In *Laboratory Diagnosis of Fetal Disease*, edited by Barton, A.J. John Wright and Sons, Ltd., London, 1980.

CHAPTER 7

Physiology of Pregnancy

LUCIEN ARDITI, M.D.
RONALD M. CAPLAN, M.D.
MAURICE L. DRUZIN, M.B., B.Chir.
NORTON M. LUGER, M.D.

CARDIOVASCULAR CHANGES DURING PREGNANCY

Profound changes occur in the cardiovascular system of the pregnant woman (Table 7.1) that influence preexisting cardiac and renal disease states and hypertension. As well, these changes are implicated in the pathogenesis and course of the hypertensive disorders of pregnancy (see Chapter 20: "Hypertensive Disorders of Pregnancy").

In the first 8 months of pregnancy, body water increases[1, 7] in proportion to the increase in body solids and represents 50–55% of body weight.

The body water turnover rate, which is the percentage of body water exchanged with the environment each day, remains normal during pregnancy. Eight percent of body water is exchanged each day, including the exchange between mother and fetus and the exchange between the mother and the amniotic fluid, which is 600 cc/hour at term.

At delivery, a maternal water loss occurs. The fetus, with its body water, becomes an independent entity. The amniotic fluid is lost, and there is blood loss as well.

In the 24 hours following delivery, the water turnover rate tends to be slow and

then increases to twice the antepartum level and is accompanied by diuresis. Between the second and sixth day postpartum, a normal turnover rate is reestablished. In the patient with a hypertensive disorder commencing beyond the 24th week of pregnancy (preeclampsia), the body water turnover rate is slower than in the normal pregnant patient.

The cardiac output normally increases 30–40% during pregnancy.[5] It is elevated to or near peak levels by 24–28 weeks of gestation. There is a plateau in cardiac output as term approaches. In a supine position the gravid uterus partially occludes the inferior vena cava. When the patient turns on her side, the resting cardiac output is higher than in the supine position, but it is still lower at term than at its peak level. In labor, the cardiac output increases by 20% during contractions. Following delivery, there is a large transient peak in cardiac output due to the decrease in uterine size and the uterine venous plexus and the restoration of normal flow through the inferior vena cava.[13, 14]

The stroke volume increases early in pregnancy, secondary to increased myocardial contractility. The initial increase in cardiac output during pregnancy is due to an increase in stroke volume. Later during pregnancy it is due to an increase in heart

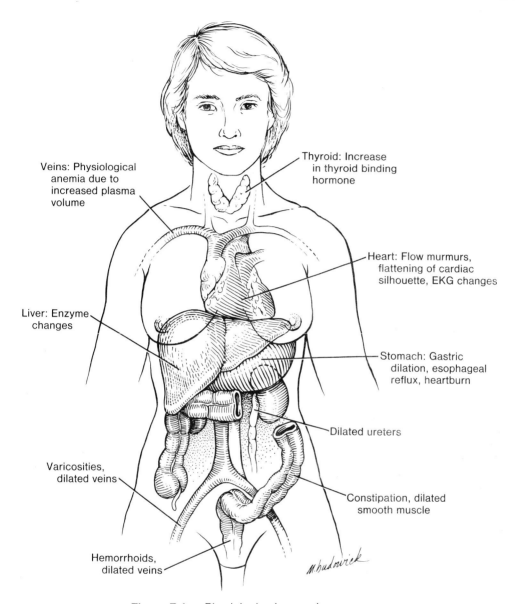

Veins: Physiological
anemia due to
increased plasma
volume

Thyroid: Increase
in thyroid binding
hormone

Heart: Flow murmurs,
flattening of cardiac
silhouette, EKG changes

Liver: Enzyme
changes

Stomach: Gastric
dilation, esophageal
reflux, heartburn

Dilated ureters

Varicosities,
dilated veins

Constipation, dilated
smooth muscle

Hemorrhoids,
dilated veins

Figure 7.1.   Physiologic changes in pregnancy.

rate as the stroke volume declines. Hypervolemia begins early in pregnancy and the increase in maternal blood volume continues until the 30th week and then stabilizes. The increment averages 40% over the pregestational level. Plasma volume increases earlier in pregnancy and proportionately more than the red cell mass, hence the dilutional physiologic anemia of pregnancy. The plasma volume returns to normal within 6–8 weeks postpartum. Both estrogen and progesterone promote sodium and water retention during pregnancy.

Estrogen stimulates the hepatic production of a renin substance, which then adds through the renin-angiotensin-aldosterone cycle to increase production of aldosterone, which in turn promotes increased renal sodium retention. Progesterone also

Table 7.1.   Circulatory and Ventilatory Changes in Pregnancy

Parameter	Type of Change	Pregnancy Value
Cardiac output	Increase	+ 40%
Blood velocity	Increase	
Circulation time	Decrease	12 seconds
Plasma volume	Increase	+ 50 to 60%
Blood volume	Increase	+ 50 to 60%
"Effective" blood volume	Decrease	
Heart rate	Increase	+ 10 beats/minute
Arterial pulse pressure	Increase (slight)	
Diastolic blood pressure	Decrease (slight)	
Systemic peripheral resistance	Decrease	
Pulmonary artery pressure	Increase (slight)	
Right ventricular end diastolic pressure	Increase	
Venous pressure lower extremities	Increase	
Oxygen consumption	Increase	+ 10–20%
Expiratory reserve capacity	Decrease	− 8–40%
Residual volume	Decrease	− 7–22%
Functional residual capacity	Decrease	− 18%
Resting ventilation	Increase	

relaxes venous tone, and estrogens are known to have a vasodilating effect on the maternal vasculature. Placental lactogen stimulates aldosterone as well.

The increased capacitance of the vasculature combined with increased sodium and water retention leads to an increased plasma volume. However, normal pregnancy results in a reduced *effective* blood volume, despite the high levels of aldosterone, desoxycorticosterone, and estrogen and their sodium-retaining effects. Therefore, the use of diuretics is contraindicated in pregnancy.[9] Erythropoiesis lags in its rate of acceleration early in pregnancy, hence the drop in hematocrit. Starting about the 16th week, the reticulocyte count increases, reaching 6% by 25–30 weeks at which level it plateaus until delivery. After the 30th week, the red cell mass continues to rise, while plasma volume has stabilized, hence the rise in hematocrit. The increase of the red cell mass is 300–400 cc for a single pregnancy and is due to increased production of erythrocytes in the bone marrow. Placental lactogen, erythropoietin, and renin stimulate marrow activity, while estrogen has an inhibiting effect.

Iron supplementation during pregnancy may reduce or prevent hemodilution. Twin pregnancies impose a greater burden on the heart rate, in part because the increased blood volume associated with twin pregnancies exceeds that of single pregnancies. A single pregnancy is associated with a 1000 cc increase in plasma volume, and a twin pregnancy is associated with a 1500 cc increase.

Despite this "physiological anemia," most women do not notice any significant distress associated with the lower hemoglobin. Significantly below the physiologic level there is an increase in prematurity and stillbirth, and even moderate anemia may lead to an increased incidence of fetal growth retardation.

Due to the increased blood volume and cardiac output, systolic ejection flow murmurs are commonly heard in pregnancy and must be distinguished from pathologic murmurs.

Positional changes occur in the electrocardiogram of the pregnant woman, due to the elevation of the diaphragm and an exaggerated transverse position and rotation of the heart around its anteroposterior axis. The electrical axis of the heart is deviated to the left by 15 degrees (Fig. 7.1).

The peripheral vascular resistance is lowered in pregnancy. This seems to occur as a result of an increased number of pelvic arterioles with increased caliber, an increased arteriolar flow, and an arteriovenous shunt effect in the placental circulation.

The supine hypotensive syndrome is noted late in gestation when the weight of the gravid uterus may compress the inferior vena cava as the patient is lying down. This will cause a fall in venous return and a subsequent drop in cardiac output. The reduction of venous return may then be compensated by a rise in peripheral vascular resistance. In some patients, on the other hand, the fall in venous return is followed by a sympathetic response with bradycardia and a further fall in blood pressure. This sequence of events ends in a syncopal attack unless these untoward physiologic changes are altered by simply having the patient turn on her side—thus relieving the pressure on the inferior vena cava. Particularly during the third trimester, the patient should be encouraged to sleep on her side and warned about the possibility of difficulties associated with her lying supine.

The blood loss for normal vaginal delivery is probably about 500 cc and is doubled in the case of cesarean section. In view of the increased blood volume of pregnancy, this is well tolerated.

RESPIRATORY CHANGES DURING PREGNANCY

There are no significant alterations in the lung volume parameters until the second half of pregnancy. Airway resistance and respiratory muscle function are not changed (Table 7.1). Prostaglandin $F_2\alpha$ causes constriction of bronchial smooth muscle and increased airway resistance, but prostaglandins E_1 and E_2 as well as increased cyclic nucleotides have a bronchodilator effect.[15] The diffusing capacity of the lungs is unaffected, and the intrapulmonary distribution of gas is not disturbed.

In the first trimester, minute and alveolar ventilations begin to increase. This hyperventilation is stimulated by progesterone which increases the respiratory center sensitivity to carbon dioxide. The resultant respiratory alkalosis is compensated for by renal excretion of bicarbonate.[10]

The actual oxygen consumption increases in pregnancy by 10 to 20%, reflecting the increased oxygen requirement. The cardiac output, however, shows a greater increase in pregnancy, resulting in a fall in the arteriovenous oxygen difference.

In the second half of pregnancy the expiratory reserve capacity of the lungs is reduced and the residual volume is decreased to a lesser extent, so that the functional residual capacity is decreased by 18%. However, the vital capacity is unchanged; therefore, the total lung capacity is only slightly decreased at most. The forced expiratory volume is normal.

Due to the elevation of the diaphragm during pregnancy and the increase in heart volume, changes are seen in the chest roentgenogram. There is an increase in the transverse diameter of the heart and a straightening of the left upper cardiac border. The pulmonary artery segment is prominent in some cases because of increased pulmonary blood flow. Because of increased vascularity, there are increased markings at the lung bases.

RENAL CHANGES DURING PREGNANCY

The renal plasma flow increases by 50 to 85%[2, 3] in early and mid pregnancy and possibly decreases by 13 to 22% between the second and third trimesters.

The glomerular filtration rate increases by 50% throughout most of pregnancy. This results in a decrease of serum uric acid by at least 25% in early pregnancy and a fall in plasma creatinine to two thirds of normal. The glomerular filtration rate falls toward normal in the last 2 weeks of pregnancy. Thus the tubular reabsorption of uric acid decreases in early pregnancy, followed by a progressive increase. Significant hyperuricemia in late pregnancy seems to correlate with the presence and severity of preeclampsia.[2]

The filtration fraction is reduced in early

pregnancy. It rises to at least the nonpregnant level in the third trimester.

Because of the increased glomerular filtration rate, some women develop glycosuria in pregnancy, as the tubular function is overwhelmed. It is also possible that there is an actual change in the reabsorptive capacity of the proximal tubule. In spite of this phenomenon, glycosuria should be an indication for assessment of blood glucose values following a carbohydrate load. This simple procedure will differentiate the patient with gestational diabetes from the one with glycosuria due to maximal reabsorptive capacity of the tubule being exceeded.

Increased amounts of amino acids are passed by the kidney in pregnancy. Significant clinical proteinuria, however, is not usually in evidence unless the pregnant woman has a hypertensive disorder of pregnancy or renal disease.

Because of hormonal effects on smooth muscle leading to its relaxation, a certain degree of hydroureter develops in pregnancy (Fig. 7.1). This can be a significant factor in renal disease in pregnancy.

COAGULATION CHANGES DURING PREGNANCY

Blood coagulation in the human body is a dynamic process: coagulation and lysis at various sites are continually taking place and are in a state of equilibrium.

Thrombin activity increases during normal pregnancy and is significantly raised at the time of placental separation.[6]

Table 7.2. Coagulation Factors Elevated in Pregnancy

Factor I	(Fibrinogen)	Counteracted by increased plasminogen
Factor II	(Prothrombin)	
Factor VII	(Proconvertin)	
Factor VIII	(Antihemophilic globulin)	
Factor IX	(Plasma thromboplastin component)	
Factor X	(Stuart—Prower)	
Factor XII	(Hageman)	

Puerperium
  Platelets

Those factors that are elevated in pregnancy are listed in Table 7.2. The greatest rise occurs in factors VII and X, which are necessary for the conversion of prothrombin to thrombin.

Antithrombin III, the main inhibitor of thrombin, increases during the puerperium. Plasminogen and antiplasmin concentration increases, but plasminogen activator is lost. The net result is an increased coagulant and decreased fibrinolytic capacity.[6]

HEPATIC CHANGES DURING PREGNANCY

The maternal hepatic blood flow is normal during pregnancy, but the relative perfusion of the liver is decreased due to the enhanced cardiac output.[11]

No specific histologic changes occur in the liver. However, some tests of liver function are altered in pregnancy.

Due to the placental component, there is an increase in alkaline phosphatase[12] and leucine aminopeptidase activity. 5-nucleotidase, however, is normal and thus is useful in distinguishing hepatobiliary disease in pregnancy.[4]

Total serum proteins decrease, due to the decrease in serum albumin and in spite of a slight rise in α- and β-globulins. Serum cholinesterase activity is decreased. An abnormal retention of bromsulfophthalein is noted in the last month of pregnancy.

Because of the increased circulating estrogen, certain signs generally associated with liver disease (specifically spider nevi and palmar erythema) are normally seen in pregnancy.

GASTROINTESTINAL CHANGES DURING PREGNANCY

Gastric dilatation occurs in pregnancy. The esophagus is slightly retrodisplaced, and esophageal reflux occurs. Heartburn is often a resultant symptom, necessitating the use of antacid preparations for relief.

Because of general smooth muscle relaxation, the large intestine is somewhat dilated, resulting in constipation. This can generally be overcome by altering the diet to include more fiber or by the use of natural vegetable laxatives.

Smooth muscle relaxation on a hormonal basis and increasing intraabdominal pressure account for the marked incidence of hemorrhoids in pregnancy (Fig. 7.1).

References

1. Carey, H.M. *Modern Trends in Human Reproductive Physiology "1"*. Butterworths, Washington, D.C., 1963.
2. Davison, J.M., and Dunlop, W. Renal hemodynamics and tubular function in normal human pregnancy. *Kidney Int. 18*:152, 1980.
3. Dunlop, W. Renal physiology in pregnancy. *Postgrad. Med. J. 55*:329, 1979.
4. Freidman, R.B., Anderson, R.E., et al. Effects of disease on clinical laboratory tests. *Clin. Chem. 26*:416D, 1980.
5. Guzman, C.A., and Caplan, R.M. Cardiorespiratory response to exercise during pregnancy. *Am. J. Obstet. Gynecol. 108*:600, 1970.
6. Howie, P.W. Blood clotting and fibrinolysis in pregnancy. *Postgrad. Med. J. 55*:362, 1979.
7. Little, B. Water and electrolyte balance during pregnancy. *Anaesthesiology 26*:400, 1965.
8. Milne, J.A. The respiratory response to pregnancy. *Postgrad. Med. J. 55*:318, 1979.
9. Nolten, W.E., and Ehrlich, E.N. Sodium and mineralocorticoids in normal pregnancy. *Kidney Int. 18*:221, 1980.
10. Prowse, C.M., and Gaensler, E.A. Respiratory and acid-base changes during pregnancy. *Anaesthesiology 26*:381, 1965.
11. Scholtes, G. Liver function and liver diseases during pregnancy. *J. Perinat. Med. 7*:55, 1979.
12. Seymour, C.A., and Chadwick, V.S. Liver and gastrointestinal function in pregnancy. *Postgrad. Med. J. 55*:343, 1979.
13. Ueland, K. Heart disease and pregnancy. In *Advances in Obstetrics and Gynecology*, edited by Caplan, R.M., and Sweeney, W.J. Williams & Wilkins, Baltimore, 1978, pp. 174–176.
14. Ueland, K. Pregnancy and cardiovascular disease. *Med. Clin. North Am. 61*:17, 1977.
15. Weinberger, S.E., Weiss, S.T., et al. Pregnancy and the lungs. *Am. Rev. Respir. Dis. 121*:559, 1980.

CHAPTER 8

Immunology of Pregnancy

RONALD M. CAPLAN, M.D.

It has long been considered that one way to look at the developing fetus is as a homograft. The fetus obtains half of its genetic material from its father, yet lives unmolested in the maternal uterine environment for some 266 days. The reason for its survival, unscathed by maternal immunologic attack except under special circumstances such as Rh incompatibility (see Chapter 24: "Rh Isoimmunization"), is an interesting study in itself. However, there are more interesting broader questions that are raised, such as the implications for survival of other homografts in the human body and the comparison of "invading" trophoblast to malignant tumors.[7] The understanding of the rapid "aging" process that occurs in the placenta could lead to a more complete knowledge of aging itself and to a better understanding of various degenerative and "immunologic" disease states.

THEORIES OF FETAL SURVIVAL

The classic theories that attempted to explain the survival of the fetus in the uterus were advanced by Billingham. He thought that the fetus was immunologically immature, a concept that is gradually being modified and at least partially disproved. Instead of believing that the fetus is immunologically immature, the opposite has been postulated: the immunologic competence of the fetus destroys migrant maternal lymphocytes. On the other hand, there is some evidence that fetal cell surfaces have a smaller concentration of histocompatibility antigens than do those of an adult. It has also been postulated that these histocompatibility antigens in the fetus differ qualitatively from their adult counterparts.[16]

A finding that may have some significance is the reportedly depressed level of P component[2] in newborn plasma. Amyloid, of which P component is the protein fraction, is found in hyperimmune states. Therefore, it could be postulated that a low level of this substance in the fetus is related to its survival.

Billingham conceived of the uterus as a privileged site. This idea has been gradually updated, so that Freedman and Gold[6] speak of the "unique milieu" of the uterus. Certainly, the fact that the fetus is not a vascularized allograft and is sequestered in the uterus is of help to it. Even if defects do occur, allowing "mixing" of the fetal and maternal circulations, the resultant exposure of the mother to fetal antigen in necessarily small amounts could on occasion result in the development of immunologic tolerance to fetal antigen by the mother, rather than an immune rejection response. The opportunity for such mixing of fetal and maternal circulations is evident from the structure of the placenta close to term. Fetal blood circulates through each placental villus, and the villi in turn are bathed in a dynamic "pool" of maternal blood. Normal exchange occurs through the villus. In this relationship near term, the membrane separating the fetal and maternal circulations is only two cells thick. In fact, it has been clearly shown that disruptions frequently occur. Utilizing the Kleihauer technique, stained fetal cells can be demonstrated in the maternal circulation after delivery: the so-called fetomaternal transfusion that is implicated in the development of Rh isoimmunization.

Billingham proposed a physiologic barrier between mother and fetus. The demonstration of trophoblastic sialomucin and the relatively weak reactivity of the trophoblast itself corroborate this idea. Low molecular weight antibodies (most notably IgG as seen in Rh isoimmunization) can cross the placental barrier and attack fetal erythrocytes but larger weight antibodies cannot, accounting for example for the relative innocuousness of ABO incompatibility between mother and fetus, where the operative antibodies are IgM.

In the maternal decidua, antihuman immunoglobulin binding has been demonstrated. This reaction, which is maximal in the first trimester, could protect the fetus from the onslaught of maternal serum immunoglobulin.

Billingham stated that the pregnant woman herself had a "weakened" immunologic reactivity. This theory does have merit,[7] although animal studies have shown that the pregnant female will reject skin grafts from the fetus.[6] Moreover, the pregnant woman in the third trimester does not have significant alterations in circulating T and B lymphocytes.[4, 15] Thus the concept of impaired cellular immunity is not completely supported. There are studies that suggest, however, that the pregnant woman is less inclined to reject paternal skin grafts in the gestational period.[12] IgG and IgA concentrations in human pregnancy serum decrease significantly in the second and third trimesters, and some decrease in IgM has been documented as well.[1]

Recently, the concept of maternal serum blocking antibodies has been advanced.[3] A maternal serum factor produced by the fertilized ovum and known as *early pregnancy factor* (EPF)[17] appears hours after fertilization and prior to implantation. This factor suppresses or blocks the maternal immune response in pregnancy by suppressing lymphocyte activity. The EPF titer falls prior to delivery. Such observations lead to the realization that a multiplicity of factors are probably operative in the protection of the fetus from immunologic rejection.

IMMUNOLOGIC FACTORS IN OTHER EVENTS

It can be postulated that fetal protection may be temporary and that immunologic factors may be implicated in spontaneous abortion, stillbirth, placental aging and abruption, and even in labor itself. There is little evidence at present in support of immunologic factors in the initiation of labor, but it has been suggested that the facilitation reaction and rejection reaction balance each other until term.[2, 3]

MATERNAL LYMPHATIC SYSTEM

The physiologic changes that occur in the thymolymphatic system during pregnancy are significant. Atrophy of the maternal thymus glands occurs.[19] The lymph nodes lose their germinal centers,[13] and there is a depressed level of circulating lymphocytes[13] which is proportional to the titer of human chorionic gonadotrophin (hCG). This observation suggests that the hCG may have a role in inhibiting lymphopoiesis, resulting in a decreased level of immunologically competent cells.[2, 8]

INTERPLAY OF FACTORS

A key to understanding immunologic mechanisms in pregnancy may be the crucial alterations in the *amounts* and *reactivity* of various factors. Thus, minute breaks in the fetomaternal circulation allow the passage of small amounts of fetal antigen, possibly resulting in maternal tolerance rather than rejection. Decreased numbers of immunologically competent maternal cells coupled with the presence of the placental barrier lead to diminished ability on the part of the mother to reject the fetus, because of an insufficient attack. Humoral maternal antibody that is demonstrably cytotoxic in vitro can be absorbed by the fetus, seemingly with no effect.

PROTECTION OF THE FETUS
(Table 8.1)

The protection of the fetus from rejection may be considered in stages, beginning even prior to fertilization, always remembering that, as in all physiologic mechanisms, this is not a series of "steps" but is a gradually evolving process with overlapping of the various mechanisms in the time sequence.

It has long been known to medical observers that inbreeding is injurious to the viability of the human species. This infers that immunity that develops in the mother might be advantageous.[5, 10, 16] In any case, previous childbearing can result in histoincompatibility between mother and fetus.

The fetus does not remain immunologically incompetent for a long period. By 9 weeks of gestation, cellular immune responsiveness has been demonstrated in fetal liver cells.[3] Although maternal and fetal circulations are in close proximity, especially near term, connection between the two systems is rare in the crucial early gestational period.

On the maternal side, under the influence of estrogen, progesterone,[9] and hu-

Table 8.1. Immunologic Protection of the Fetus

I.	Ovum and Placenta	1. Zona pellucida
		2. Trophoblast: low immunogenicity
		3. Fetal circulation
		4. Sialomucin
		5. Maternal circulation
		6. Fetus: not a vascularized allograft
II.	Fetus	1. Altered histocompatibility antigens
		2. Immunologic competence (9 weeks)
III.	Mother	1. Serum blocking antibodies
		2. Early pregnancy factor
		3. Antihuman immunoglobulin binding (decidua)
		4. hCG (see Table 8.2)
		5. Depressed lymphopoiesis
		6. Altered thymolymphatic system
		7. Depressed reticuloendothelial system
		8. Decreased antigen uptake
		9. Histoincompatibility: advantageous aspect

Table 8.2. Possible Role of hCG in Suppression of Maternal Immunity

hCG: depression of lymphopoiesis → fewer immunologically competent cells

hCG + estrogen + progesterone + corticosteroids: altered thymolymphatic system

hCG + estrogen + progesterone: depression of maternal reticuloendothelial system → reduced antibody formation

hCG + cortisol: decreased antigen uptake by macrophages

man chorionic gonadotrophin,[2, 8, 19] as well as corticosteroids[2] from the adrenal gland, the morphologic changes previously described in the thymolymphatic system occur. Human chorionic gonadotrophin, possibly in conjunction with estrogen and progesterone, may have a role in depressing the maternal reticuloendothelial system, leading to a reduction in antibody formation, although the contribution of purified hCG has recently been questioned. Human chorionic gonadotrophin also works in conjunction with cortisol to block the uptake of antigen by macrophages (Table 8.2). The early fertilized ovum is antigenic but is protected by its coating, the zona pellucida. Weak histocompatibility antigens are thought to be present in the blastocyst trophoblast.[5, 11, 14, 20] Later, as placental development occurs, the fetus and placenta itself are protected by the low immunogenicity of the trophoblast, although trophoblast does contain a full complement of histocompatibility antigens[6] as well as the fibrinoid[5] or sialomucin layer at the implantation site. The sialomucin,[18] which is a negatively charged mucopolysaccharide surrounding the cell surface, probably is one of the more important mechanisms that protects the fetus from rejection. The cell surface antigens of the placenta are masked by this material.

The developing fetus is protected because it is not a vascularized allograft. Fetal histocompatibility antigens may differ from those of an adult. Moreover, migrant maternal lymphocytes can be destroyed.

Once breaks in the integrity of the fetal and maternal circulations do occur, with resultant mixing, the repeated small doses of fetal antigen to the mother may result in the development of immunologic tolerance by the mother for her fetus. Maternal serum blocking antibodies are formed. When these connections between the maternal and fetal circulations do occur, maternal immunocytes can enter the fetus against the hydrostatic gradient, but if they are in insufficient numbers the fetus may be unaffected.

LABOR

There is no substantial evidence at present that the onset of labor is an immunologically defined event or that it is related in any way to the immunologic phenomenon of graft rejection. There is, however, a striking similarity of the placental "aging" process to the pathologic changes observed in transplanted organs undergoing rejection.

It is of interest that the maternal leukocytes in the circulation of the primigravida only become reactive to placental antigens in the fourth month of gestation.[20] On the other hand, it is in the first trimester that vascular changes and lymphocytic infiltration of the decidua are most marked. These changes, in a lesser fashion, occur again at the time of delivery in conjunction with antihuman immunoglobulin binding. The gravida in the third trimester does have an increased percentage of IgG-bearing B lymphocytes and an increased number of these cells, as compared with the nonpregnant woman.[4] This may infer a somewhat enhanced humoral immunity in the third trimester.

SPONTANEOUS ABORTION
(Table 8.3)

Approximately 12% of all human pregnancies terminate spontaneously in the first trimester. It has been noted that vascular changes and lymphocytic infiltration characteristic of a hypersensitivity reaction are most marked in the decidua in the first trimester, when spontaneous abortion is most apt to occur.

Table 8.3. Steps at which Pregnancy may be Terminated by Immunological Onslaught

1. Histoincompatibility (previous matings), eg, Rh isoimmunization
2. Loss of uterine "protected site," eg, ectopic gestation
3. Transplantation immunity (vs. placenta)
4. Maternal immunocytes → fetal circulation (break in integrity of circulatory systems)
5. Absent enhancing antibody → abortion
6. Diminished enhancing antibody → toxemia

On the other hand, the lack of reactivity to placental antigens by the leukocytes of the primigravida at this early stage might lead one to suspect that miscarriage is more common in multiparous parents, and such is not the case.

The multitude of immunologic factors that may be operative in protecting the ovum and embryo from rejection have already been discussed. In essence, probably one third of all spontaneous abortions occur in conjunction with a "defective ovum." It could be argued that a defective ovum might well have a defective zona pellucida or defects in other protective mechanisms previously described. On the other hand, it could be argued that some of these defective ova result from immunologic attack, although there is at present no clear evidence to support this.

"SUBCLINICAL ABORTION"

Specific, sensitive techniques recently evolved to detect small amounts of human chorionic gonadotrophin in maternal serum have been used to study women at the time of, or shortly after, a "first missed" menstrual period. These techniques involve either radioreceptor assay of hCG or β-subunit assay for hCG.

In many cases, it has been possible to detect levels of hCG in patients who do not display any clinical evidence of pregnancy. Often, this positive pregnancy testing is followed by the clinical appearance of what seems to be a somewhat heavy, delayed "menstrual flow." This "flow" probably represents, in fact, a subclinical spontaneous abortion. The incidence of this phenomenon in the population is unknown, but it probably occurs at a much higher rate than previously suspected. It is possible, although not proven, that a certain percentage of such subclinical abortion is due to immunologic attack, as many of the defensive mechanisms previously described have not been developed at this early stage of gestation.

References

1. Amino, N., Tanizazoa, O., et al. Changes of serum immunoglobulins IgG, IgA, IgM, and IgE during pregnancy. *Obstet. Gynecol. 52*:415, 1978.
2. Burstein, R.H., and Bumenthal, H.T. Immune reactions of normal pregnancy. *Am. J. Obstet. Gynecol. 104*:671, 1969.
3. Centaro, A., and Carretti, N. *Immunology in Obstetrics and Gynecology.* Excerpta Medica/American Elsevier, New York, 1974.
4. Cornfield, D.B., Jencks, J., et al. T and B lymphocytes in pregnant women. *Obstet. Gynecol. 53*: 203, 1979.
5. Edwards, R.G. Immunology of conception and pregnancy. *Br. Med. Bull. 26*:72, 1970.
6. Freedman, S.O., and Gold, P. Immunology as it relates to reproductive biology. *Clin. Obstet. Gynecol. 20*:665, 1977.
7. Gleicher, N., Deppe, G., and Cohen, C. Common aspects of immunologic tolerance in pregnancy and malignancy. *Obstet. Gynecol. 54*:335, 1979.
8. Gruenwald, P. *The Placenta.* University Park Press, Baltimore, 1975.
9. Hulka, J.F., and Mohr, K. Interference of corti-sone-induced homograft survival by progestins. *Am. J. Obstet. Gynecol. 97*:407, 1967.
10. James, D.A. Effects of antigenic dissimilarity between mother and fetus on placental size in mice. *Nature 205*:613, 1965.
11. Kirby D.R.S. The immunological consequences of extrauterine development of allogenic mouse blastocysts. *Transplantation 6*:1005, 1968.
12. Mitchell, G.W., Jr., Bardawil, W.A., and Marchant, D.J. The conceptus as a homograft. *Harper Hosp. Bull. 24*:119, 1966.
13. Nelson, J.H., and Hall, J.E. Studies on the thymolymphatic system in humans. *Am. J. Obstet. Gynecol. 93*: 1133, 1965.
14. Palm, J., Heyner, S., and Brinster, R.L. Differential immunofluorescence of fertilized mouse eggs with H-2 and non H-2 antibody. *J. Exp. Med. 133*: 1282, 1971.
15. Scott, J.R. T- and B- cell distribution in pregnancy. *J.A.M.A. 239*:2769, 1978.
16. Simmons, R.L., Ivaskova, E., et al. Symposium on pregnancy and transplantation. *Transplant. Proc. 1*:47, 1969.
17. Smart, Y.C., Roberts, T.K., et al. Early pregnancy factor: Its role in mammalian reproduction—research review. *Fertil. Steril. 35*:397, 1981.
18. Urbach, G.I. Fetal-maternal placental immunologic relationship. *Fertil. Stril. 21*:356, 1970.
19. Younger, J.B., St. Pierre, R.L., and Zmijewski, C.M. Effect of human chorionic gonadotropin on antibody production. *Am. J. Obstet. Gynecol. 105*: 9, 1969.
20. Youtananukorn, V., Matangkasombut, P., and Osathanondh V. Onset of human maternal cell-mediated immune reaction to placental antigens during the first pregnancy. *Clin. Exp. Immunol. 16(14)*:593, 1974.

CHAPTER 9

Physiology and Endocrinology of Lactation

ANNA-RIITTA FUCHS, D.Sc.

Lactation is an essential part of reproduction in most mammals. Failure to lactate means failure to reproduce. Fortunately, the human infant can survive on milk from animal species. Indeed, technological advances during the past half century have made formulas based on cow's milk or other milk substitutes so safe that artificial feeding has become an accepted way of raising babies in large parts of the world.

When artificial feeding is practiced under less favorable conditions, as presently is the case in many third world countries, the disadvantages are often quite marked. Attention has therefore been refocused on the benefits of breast-feeding, and many epidemiological and clinical studies have recently demonstrated the superiority of breast-feeding vs. artificial feeding as nutrition for human infants. Spurred by these findings, increasing numbers of women in the Western World now want to breast-feed their babies. Contributing to this change in attitudes is the decline in birth rate. Approaching zero population growth we want to provide every individual with optimal conditions for growth and development.

Human milk satisfies the specific nutritional requirements of human infants better than does cow's milk or formula, and it provides protection against bacterial as well as viral infections by supplying antiviral factors and antibodies that are absent in formulas. Psychologically and emotionally, breast-feeding also promotes close bonding between mother and infant and provides the infant with security and well-being.

First-time parents represent an increasing proportion of all expectant parents. Since the prospective grandmothers of today are as ignorant of breast-feeding practices as are the first-time mothers, it is the responsibility of the obstetrician or the midwife to guide the expectant mother and her family in preparation for breast-feeding. Since successful lactation is very dependent on attitudes and customs, it is important to inform the prospective parents not only of the benefits of breast-feeding but also of the difficulties to be expected and to provide psychological support to overcome these difficulties.

Although a period of 6 months is an optimal duration for breast-feeding, any period of lactation is beneficial to the infant and mother. Employment of the mother does not have to preclude breast-feeding altogether. Working women, who constitute a growing number of the pregnant population, should be encouraged and informed about initiation and maintenance of lactation in relation to their employment plans.

Prematurity does not preclude breast-feeding. On the contrary, the mother should be advised to express milk manually for the baby until it is capable of nursing at the breast.

BREAST-FEEDING VS. BOTTLE-FEEDING

Breast milk is much more economical than the various formulas. The extra calories needed for the production of milk, about 500 kcal/day, can be obtained from a couple of peanut-butter sandwiches and a glass of milk per day. This consideration is of special concern for women of lower socioeconomic classes and for women in the third world, where food is scarce. The powdered milk products distributed by many organizations to infants in developing countries would be more useful if given to lactating mothers instead of being used for infant formulas.

Breast milk is always available and needs no sterilization. Human milk is free of pathogenic organisms, whereas formulas easily become contaminated. Moreover, the heating process used for sterilization of cow's milk or in the preparation of formulas causes denaturation of many enzymes and proteins, such as growth and resistance factors as well as immunoglobulins. All these factors contribute to the protective effect of human milk against bacterial and viral infections and to the significantly reduced incidence of gastrointestinal and respiratory tract infections in breast-fed infants compared with the incidence in bottle-fed infants.

The composition of human milk provides a better balance of the energy-yielding constituents, lipids, proteins, and carbohydrates than do formulas in which a much larger proportion is derived from proteins. Moreover, these constituents are present in human milk in a more easily digested form than in cow's milk or in most formulas. About 95–99% of the fat present in human milk is absorbed in the gut, and a high proportion of the fat in human milk is composed of unsaturated, essential fatty acids. In human milk, about 25% of the nitrogen content is present as nonprotein nitrogen providing an immediate source of many essential amino acids. A large proportion (75%) of the proteins in human milk consist of the easily digested whey proteins, lactalbumin, and lactoglobulin, in contrast to cow's milk in which casein is the principal protein.

The bioavailability of many other constituents of human milk is also superior to that of cow's milk or formulas. Thus, iron is present in quite low concentration in human milk, but breast-fed infants accumulate iron at the same rate as do infants on iron-fortified formulas, in spite of an approximately 20-fold difference in concentration. As a result, a smaller volume of human milk with a smaller caloric content satisfies the needs of an infant better than do formulas. This may be the reason breast-fed infants are usually not overweight nor underweight, and subsequent growth curves indicate that fewer breast-fed infants become overweight children and adults. Contributing to this may be that human milk is not uniform in composition; the last milk expressed usually has a higher fat content than does the early milk, leading to the sense of satiety at the end of the nursing period.

The salt and electrolyte content is considerably higher in bovine milk and in formulas than in breast milk. This can pose a burden on the immature kidney function of newborn infants who are unable to concentrate urine to the same extent as adults. Paradoxically, although the calcium concentration in formulas is much higher than in breast milk, hypocalcemic tetanic episodes are seen exclusively in bottle-fed infants. This is due to the high phosphorus concentration in bovine milk, which results in lowering of serum calcium levels. In addition, the high casein and butterfat concentration in many formulas leads to the formation of insoluble curds which bind Ca^{++} and inhibit its absorption in the gut.

The high ash content together with the high buffering capacity of casein in cow's milk and formulas results in a more alkaline intestinal pH in bottle-fed than in breast-fed infants. The lower pH favors the growth of beneficial lactobacilli and inhibits the growth of harmful pathogens such as *Escherichia coli*, whereas the higher intestinal pH in formula-fed babies has the opposite effect. The lactose present in human milk, but absent in most formulas, also promotes the growth of lactobacilli. In addition, human milk contains a high concentration of the so-called bifidus factor which also promotes the growth of *Lactobacillus bifidus*. The *Lactobacillus* flora provides the infant with many resistance factors against intestinal infections caused by several pathogens. Another factor present in human milk, lactoferrin, inhibits the growth of *E. coli* by restricting the availability of free iron and, at the same time, promoting the uptake of iron by the gut.

Human milk provides the infant with soluble maternal antibodies that are secreted into the milk. Human milk also contains cellular elements such as macrophages and lymphocytes which contain antibodies. These confer passive immunity to the newborn infant during the period of 4–6 months until its own immune system becomes competent. Colostrum, the milk-like substance secreted by the alveoli during the first few days of lactation, is especially rich in immunoglobulins and cellular elements; mature milk also contains significant amounts of these substances. Milk is especially rich in IgA which resists destruction by the digestive enzymes. Besides providing protection against infections of the gut, these antibodies also gain access to the systemic circulation. In the newborn period, large proteins can pass through the epithelium of the gut and antigen-bound antibodies actually promote uptake of proteins. High concentrations of IgA have been found in the nasal epithelium of breast-fed infants; this probably contributes to the much lower incidence of respiratory tract infections in breast-fed than in bottle-fed infants. These antibodies are probably inhaled during nursing and absorbed through the nose. It is also believed that during nursing infections affecting the infant may be transmitted to the mother, who then forms antibodies against them. The antibodies are in turn transferred to the baby via the mother's milk and help to protect the infant against the infection.

DRUGS IN MILK

Drugs ingested by the mother may reach the baby via the milk, just as drugs ingested by the pregnant mother can pass through the placenta and affect the developing fetus. The passage of various drugs into milk depends on their molecular weight, their lipid solubility, the degree of protein binding, as well as their pH. The higher the lipid solubility, the greater will be the concentration in human milk. Nonionized drugs enter the alveolar cells more easily than do ionized drugs, hence weakly basic drugs that are mostly nonionized at the plasma pH of 7.4 enter milk more easily than do weakly acidic drugs, and their concentration may occasionally exceed that in maternal serum.

The effect of various drugs on the nursing infant is variable, depending on concentration and toxicity. It is difficult to apply general rules; in each case the benefits of the drug to the mother and its possible harmful effects on the baby must be considered. The concentration of many drugs in human milk has not yet been determined, but generally less than 1% of the ingested dose appears in milk. Exceptions are chloramphenicol, sulfanilamides, and thiouracil which are present in higher concentration than in plasma.

Anticoagulants warfarin and dicumarol appear safe, as do most antihistaminics.

Of antihypertensive drugs, propranolol and guanethidine are minimally excreted in milk and appear safe, whereas reserpine has been reported to cause nasal congestion, lethargy and diarrhea in suckling infants.

A large number of acidic antimicrobials are only minimally excreted in breast milk and appear safe, such as penicillin, ampicillin and aminoglycosides. On the other hand, chloramphenicol (Chloromycetin) and metronidazole (Flagyl) appear in milk in high concentration and are definitely contraindicated. Tetracycline causes permanent discoloration of the teeth and may cause enamel hypoplasia. Many sulfonamides are excreted in milk at levels equal to those in plasma and should therefore be used cautiously.

Most drugs that affect the central nervous system are lipid-soluble and are therefore excreted in milk, although their relative concentration may vary depending on the pH and protein binding. Meprobamate is two to four times more concentrated in milk than in plasma and should not be used by lactating women. Diazepam is also found in relatively high concentrations in the milk, and clear effects on the baby have been described when mothers were taking 20–30 mg/day in at least 1 week.

Alcohol passes freely into milk, but alcoholic beverages taken in moderation appear to have little effect on the infant, whereas prolonged ingestion of large amounts is hazardous.

Marihuana and heroin are excreted in breast milk and withdrawal symptoms have been described in breast-fed infants of addicted mothers upon weaning. Barbiturates such as phenobarbitol are also excreted in milk in small amounts and may lead to the induction of hydroxylating enzymes in the liver of the infant upon prolonged use.

Nicotine is detected in milk of smoking mothers and causes decreased milk production in mothers smoking 20–30 cigarettes a day.

Antimigraine drugs, especially ergot alkaloids, are excreted into the milk and toxic symptoms have been described in nursing babies. Aspirin and other acidic analgesics are only minimally excreted into milk.

Most laxatives do not enter milk in appreciable amounts and appear safe.

Protein hormones such as insulin are destroyed in the gastrointestinal tract of the infant and are therefore safe. Thyroxin is excreted in milk only in insignificant amounts, but iodine passes freely into milk. Iodine and iodocompounds are known to induce thyroid dysfunction in breat-fed babies. Thiouracil also passes into milk in relatively high concentrations

and is contraindicated in lactating women.

Steroid hormones are lipid-soluble and enter the milk in measurable quantities. There is as yet no consensus on the safety of oral contraceptive drugs when taken by lactating mothers. While animal studies have shown that the use of synthetic estrogens and progestins carries a serious risk for the offspring of lactating mothers, few adverse effects have been found in women using steroidal contraceptives during lactation. Development of gynecomastia has been noted in some infants, and growth of the infants may be decreased by some contraceptive steroids. Due to the possible long-term effects, estrogens should not be used during lactation. On the other hand, low-dose progestins are very effective contraceptives in lactating women, and in the absence of any reported side effects their use may not be contraindicated.

Environmental chemicals such as pesticides, etc. do occur in breast milk in women exposed to these agents. A national survey conducted in 1975 by the Environmental Protection Agency demonstrated detectable levels of several chlorinated hydrocarbon insecticides in human milk. The average concentrations varied from none to 3500 parts per billion (fat basis). Another survey in 1980 showed that the average concentration of polychlorinated biphenyls in breast milk was 1.7 ppm, with a range of 0–10.6 ppm. Although the level of these contaminants is low, the possible toxicological impact of multiple contaminants is not known. A Michigan State Department of Health Services panel reviewed these findings and unanimously recommended that women from the general population *not* be discouraged to breast-feed on this account. It ought to be kept in mind that the levels of these contaminants in cow's milk are similar or often higher than those found in human milk.

THE MAMMARY GLAND AND ITS SECRETORY FUNCTION

Lactation depends on five processes that are all hormonally controlled and that must be synchronized for the establishment of adequate milk flow. These are:

1. Mammary development or mammogenesis
2. Initiation of milk secretion or lactogenesis
3. Maintenance of milk secretion or galactopoiesis
4. Milk removal or galactokinesis
5. Involution of the gland

All aspects of lactation depend on the action of multiple hormones, and probably no other organ in the body has more complex requirements for its endocrine control than does the mammary gland. Ovarian hormones, anterior and posterior pituitary hormones, adrenal steroids as well as insulin and thyroid hormones are needed for the growth and function of the mammary gland.

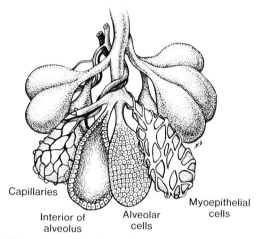

Capillaries

Interior of alveolus

Alveolar cells

Myoepithelial cells

Figure 9.1. Basic unit of the parenchyma of the mammary gland. Diagram of a cluster of alveoli. (From A.T. Cowie, in *Reproduction in Mammals, No. 3,* edited by R. Short. Cambridge at the University Press, 1972, p. 111.)

ANATOMY AND MORPHOLOGY OF THE MAMMARY GLAND

The adult breast consists of glandular tissue or parenchyma and of stroma consisting of connective tissue and fat. The two stromal elements give the mature, nonpregnant breast its shape and size; in the resting state the glandular tissue occupies only a small fraction of the volume of the breast.

Figure 9.1 shows a diagram of the basal unit of the mammary gland. The parenchyma consists of small saclike structures called *alveoli*. The alveoli occur in clusters; each opens to a small duct, which joins with others to form larger ducts and finally they form the 12–20 galactophores that lead through the nipple. The alveoli of a fully developed breast are lined by a single layer of alveolar cells, the milk secreting cells. Surrounding each alveolus is a network of myoepithelial cells. They are contractile in nature and are concerned with the expulsion of milk from the lumina of the alveoli and the small ducts. Surrounding the basket-like layer of myoepithelial cells is a dense network of capillaries.

Being of cutaneous origin, the mammary gland shares its blood supply and nerve supply with the contiguous skin. It receives the major part of its blood supply from the mammary artery, the internal thoracic and the lateral thoracic arteries, but other thoracic and intercostal arteries also contribute to its blood supply. Innervation is provided by somatic sensory and autonomous motor nerves. The innervation of the nipple and the areola is abundant, whereas it is very sparse in the corpus mammae. The nerve fibers accompany the mammary blood vessels and only rarely do nerves impinge on the glandular cells. The myoepithelial cells are without innervation. The sensory innervation of the areola plays an important part in lactation as it mediates the activation of the neurohumoral reflexes responsible for the removal of milk from the gland and for the release of prolactin that is essential for the maintenance of lactation. The intraglandular innervation of the vasculature may influence the mammary blood flow and thus indirectly the milk secretion.

Microscopically, the appearance of the alveolar cells in fully developed glands have all the characteristics of a secretory cell (Fig. 9.2). The cells are columnar and tall when the alveolar lumen is empty and become flattened when the lumen is full. They abut on myoepithelial cells and on

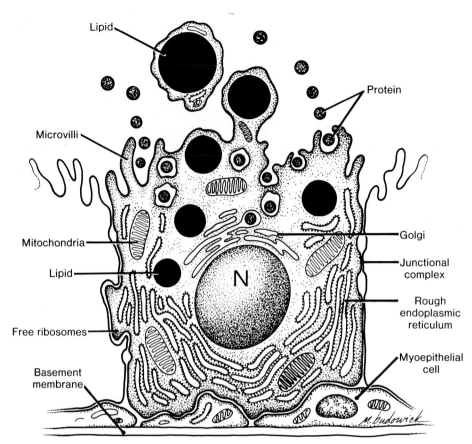

Figure 9.2. Ultrastructure of the secretory cell. (From A.R. Findlay, *Research in Reproduction.* International Planned Parenthood Federation, 6 (6), Nov. 1974.)

the basement membrane which is folded, providing a large surface for the uptake of precursors for the secretion of milk. The nucleus is large, rounded and centrally located. The clear cytoplasm contains abundant rough endoplasmic reticulum, a conspicuous paranuclear Golgi apparatus, large mitochondria with prominent christae, and secretory granules and fat droplets in various stages of development. On the luminal surface of the cells, numerous microvilli are seen. Each cell is firmly joined to its neighbors by tight junctional complexes. Very few cells in mitosis are seen in the lactating gland. In contrast, resting alveolar cells from nonpregnant adult women are flat, the nucleus is located near the base of the cell, the cytoplasm is granulated and contains a very sparse endoplasmic reticulum, few mito-

chondria and minimal Golgi apparatus. Very few fat droplets are seen. In the mammogenic phase of early pregnancy, many of these stem cells are seen dividing, and the alveolar cells occur in two layers.

MAMMOGENESIS

The development occurs in four stages:

1. During fetal life
2. At the onset of puberty
3. In early gestation
4. In early lactation

At birth, a rudimentary mammary gland is present, consisting of a nipple and a primitive duct system which are laid down during fetal life. The gland derives from the ectoderm, which forms two thickenings that appear as a ridge on both sides of the midline. Nodules are formed from this so-called mammary ridge; they sink into the dermis to become mammary buds. They start to elongate into a cordlike structure which in later stages becomes hollow and branches distally into one or two ducts, whose walls are formed of two layers of cuboidal cells.

From birth to the onset of puberty, no glandular development occurs except isometric growth. At puberty there is a rapid proliferation and branching out of the duct system, with the formation of terminal buds from which the alveoli and lobules will later develop. After the onset of regular menstrual cycles a certain amount of lobulo-alveolar development takes place in women, whereas in many animals with short luteal phase only the ductal system develops at this stage. There is also a rapid deposition of fat and connective tissue into the stroma which gives the breast its adult shape and size. The volume of the breast fluctuates somewhat in nonparous, menstruating women during the menstrual cycle, but these changes are mainly due to cyclic retention and loss of water by the connective tissue and not to true growth. In some women, interalveolar secretory material appears in the premenstrual period.

Pregnancy is associated with a remarkable growth of both ductal and the lobulo-alveolar systems. Intense cellular proliferation occurs during the first half of gestation; this can be observed within 3 or 4 weeks of conception. In the earliest phases, ductal sprouting predominates; from the third month on, lobulo-alveolar formation becomes the dominant feature. Around midgestation, the alveolar epithelial proliferation gradually declines; during the second half of gestation, mitosis of alveolar cells is rarely seen. Instead, there is differentiation of the alveolar stem cells, which begin to assume secretory characteristics. The continued increase in breast size during the second half of gestation is due to progressive alveolar distention and dilatation of the mammary vascularization. At the same time, the stromal ele-ments progressively decrease, and only thin septa separate the well-developed lobes of glandular tissue at the end of gestation. The alveoli begin to fill with colostrum, which is composed largely of desquamated glandular and phagocytic cells, but during pregnancy there is no lactose formation, nor is fat or protein released from the cells into the alveolar lumina.

The fourth phase of mammogenesis takes place in the early postpartum period and consists of rapid cellular hypertrophy and differentiation of the presecretory cells into secretory cells. This is associated with a marked increase in the rough endoplasmic reticulum and RNA synthesis and is followed by the synthesis of milk proteins and milk sugar, which are released into the lumen of the alveoli and smaller ducts. This process is fully established 2–5 days after parturition.

HORMONAL REQUIREMENTS FOR MAMMOGENESIS, LACTOGENESIS, GALACTOPOIESIS AND GALACTOKINESIS

Our knowledge about these aspects of lactation derives mainly from laboratory animals and large domestic animals. Recently, tissue culture experiments with mammary transplants have extended this work to primates and human beings. Although certain species differences may exist in these requirements, especially in regard to the maintenance of lactation, the findings made in laboratory animals seem to be applicable to the human breast development and function in general.

ENDOCRINE CONTROL OF MAMMOGENESIS

Ovarian hormones are clearly involved in mammary development, since no breast development takes place in ovariectomized animals or agonadal patients. However, in the absence of anterior pituitary hormones, the ovarian hormones are without effect. It has been established that growth hormone, together with estrogens and glucocorticoids, is required for duct development. The development of the lobulo-alveolar system requires the action of progesterone and prolactin in addition to the triad of hormones causing duct development. In women, lactation is possible in the congenital absence of growth hormone and it thus has been suggested that growth hormone is not involved in human mammogenesis. However, human placental lactogen to which these patients are subjected during pregnancy has both prolactin and growth hormone-like activity, and the study is therefore not conclusive.

ENDOCRINE CONTROL OF LACTOGENESIS

Lactogenesis, or the initiation of milk flow, requires a fully developed mammary gland and the influence of prolactin, growth hormone, glucocorticoids, insulin and thyroid hormones. As already mentioned, placental lactogen can substitute for pituitary prolactin and growth hormone during gestation. The metabolic hormones play a permissive role in this process: in themselves they cause no secretion, but in conjunction with prolactin and cortisol they cause a copious milk flow, provided that the ovarian or placental sex steroids are withdrawn. The lactogenic effects of prolactin and cortisol are held in abeyance during pregnancy by the presence of high levels of progesterone and estrogen. The mechanism of action of progesterone has been established in rodents. It controls the onset of milk secretion by inhibiting the formation of α-lactalbumin, one of the main milk proteins that forms a part of the enzyme galactosyl transferase, which synthesizes the milk sugar, lactose. The withdrawal of progesterone is thus a crucial step in lactogenesis. However, once the differentiation of the presecretory alveolar cells into secretory cells has been completed, progesterone no longer inhibits the synthesis of lactalbumin and lactose. The mechanism of action of estrogen on lactogenesis is not clear; it interferes somehow with the expression of the lactogenic potential of prolactin in the alveolar cells, perhaps by inhibiting prolactin binding to mammary gland cells.

ENDOCRINE CONTROL OF GALACTOPOIESIS

The requirements for the maintenance of established lactation are somewhat less stringent than for the initiation of lactation.

In lactating women, prolactin appears to be the single most important galactopoietic hormone, since selective inhibition of prolactin secretion by bromocryptine can inhibit lactation. Ovarian hormones are not needed for maintenance of lactation. High concentrations of ovarian hormones inhibit the initiation of lactation, but they have little effect once lactation has been fully established. Glucocorticoids and the metabolic hormones are still necessary but they need not be present in higher than normal nonpregnant levels.

MILK REMOVAL AND THE ACTION OF OXYTOCIN

The removal of milk from the gland requires the action of the neurohypophysial hormone oxytocin. In the absence of oxytocin, only a small fraction of the milk stored in the gland is available for the suckling infant, namely the portion of the milk that is present in the distended sinuses of the galactophores. Oxytocin causes the myoepithelial cells surrounding each alveolus to contract, forcing the milk out into the duct system. The myoepithelial cells are very sensitive to the action of oxytocin but are quite insensitive to acetylcholine, adrenergic agents and other biogenic amines.

The release of oxytocin is effected by a neurohumoral reflex, called the *milk ejection reflex*. The afferent part of this reflex consists of neural impulses elicited by the baby's suckling. The sensory nerve endings involved in the initiation of the reflex are located under the areola. The impulses are transmitted along the spinal cord to the hypothalamus and to the neurons of the paraventricular and supraoptic nuclei and down their axons to the nerve endings in the posterior pituitary lobe. This results in the release of oxytocin which is carried by the bloodstream to the mammary gland, causing the alveoli to contract.

The emptying of the gland is of vital importance for the maintenance of lactation. Milk secretion is inhibited if milk is not regularly removed from the gland. The accumulation of milk causes distention of the alveoli which impedes the blood flow through the capillaries and causes mechanical atrophy of the epithelial cells. The elasticity of the gland permits milk storage for about 24–48 hours before secretion declines.

The suckling stimulus plays a key role in the maintenance of lactation. It is essential not only for the milk ejection reflex and the emptying of the gland but also for the maintenance of prolactin secretion through another neurohumoral reflex. During pregnancy, elevated prolactin levels are maintained by the high circulating estrogen levels, but the postpartum fall in estrogens is followed by a fall in plasma prolactin. During lactation, elevated levels of prolactin are maintained by the suckling stimulus. Each nursing episode is associated with an abrupt rise in plasma prolactin; maximal levels are reached in 10–30 minutes, declining thereafter over 2–3 hours to reach baseline levels before the next nursing episode. The neuroendocrine consequences of suckling are illustrated in Figure 9.3.

Frequent nursing promotes prolactin secretion and hence milk secretion and successful lactation. Frequent nursing is also required to maintain the pituitary responsiveness to the suckling stimulus at an optimal level. Studies in laboratory animals indicate that the pituitary response to a given suckling stimulus diminishes as the intervals between suckling episodes are lengthened. If the application of the suckling stimulus is delayed postpartum, the responsiveness of the pituitary to the stimulus declines. Putting the baby to the breast as early as possible is therefore

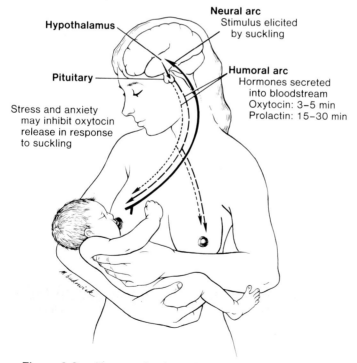

Figure 9.3.   Neuroendocrine reflexes elicited by suckling.

helpful in establishing lactation; clinical studies have borne this out. Lactation was maintained longer and was more successful the sooner after delivery the baby was allowed to nurse.

HORMONAL CHANGES DURING PREGNANCY AND LACTATION

Figure 9.4 summarizes the endocrine changes occurring during pregnancy as reflected in plasma levels. After conception the ovarian steroids produced by the corpus luteum are the first to rise, soon augmented and supplanted by steroids of pla-

cental origin. Plasma prolactin starts to increase between the fifth and eighth weeks of pregnancy and the rise continues progressively toward term, reaching very high levels, often several hundred nanograms per milliliter shortly before parturition. Growth hormone levels do not change during pregnancy; placental lactogen, which has both GH and PRL-like activity, starts to rise around the tenth week of gestation and continues to rise progressively toward term. There is also a moderate rise in both cortisol and plasma insulin levels. The concentration of thyroxine in plasma likewise rises during gesta-

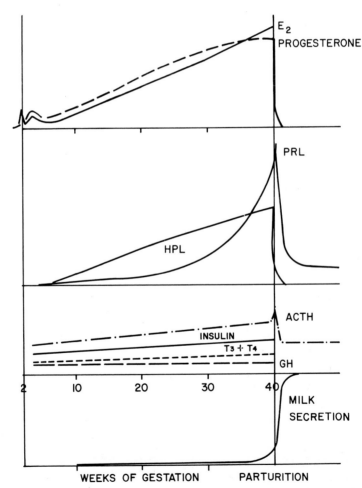

Figure 9.4.   Diagram of hormonal changes during gestation and postpartum in relation to the initiation of lactation.

tion, but the rise is caused by an increase in the protein-bound hormone, free thyroxine, remaining essentially unchanged.

The breast is thus subjected to strong mammogenic influences during pregnancy, reflected in the rapid onset of mammary development. What brings about the cessation in the cellular proliferation at midgestation and brings about the differentiation to presecretory cells is not yet clear. It seems, however, that the lactogenic potential of pituitary prolactin, placental lactogen and the metabolic hormones is held in abeyance by the high estrogen and progesterone levels.

Postpartum, following the delivery of the placenta, plasma progesterone and estrogen levels fall very rapidly, permitting the lactogenic effects of prolactin to be expressed. Prolactin levels are maximal at parturition, and plasma cortisol also rises to maximal levels during and shortly after labor. This is associated with a rapid increase in rough endoplasmic reticulum, RNA synthesis, protein synthesis, and formation of secretory products, the milk proteins, lactose, and fats. In the early postpartum period the differentiation of the presecretory alveolar cells to secretory cells is completed.

During pregnancy the high plasma PRL levels result from the action of estrogens. Estrogens promote the synthesis as well as the release of PRL from the pituitary. With falling estrogen levels, postpartum plasma PRL also declines, although at a less rapid rate than do estrogens. Basal PRL levels are reached in about 2 weeks in nonlactating women. In lactating women, basal PRL levels fall at about the same rate, and the maintenance of prolactin secretion postpartum depends on the suckling stimulus. As has been pointed out earlier, prolactin is the main galactopoietic hormone in man and the baby's suckling is the single most important factor in assuring prolactin secretion and continuation of lactation.

As lactation advances, the increment in prolactin secretion brought about by each nursing episode decreases, eventually bringing lactation to an end. It is not quite clear whether the decrease in pituitary response is due to exhaustion of pituitary PRL or to a refractoriness to the stimulation. In certain cultures, women are known to lactate up to 4 years. Mother's milk is then the main source of nutrition for the infant, which therefore is probably fed at frequent intervals. The decreased pituitary responsiveness mentioned above was observed in European women, and it is possible that it was caused by the lengthening of the intervals between suckling as other baby foods were added. The suckling stimulus may also become less intense as the baby is given supplementary food.

INVOLUTION

Involution of the mammary gland sets in abruptly in nonlactating women, whereas in lactating women it is more gradual as weaning is usually extended over a period of time. Although the withdrawal of prolactin at the cessation of nursing contributes to the involution, this process is mainly controlled by mechanical rather than hormonal factors. Distention of alveoli due to the accumulation of milk causes mechanical atrophy of the epithelial structures. Alveolar distention also impedes the blood flow through the surrounding capillary network and may lead to partial or complete obstruction of the capillaries. Deprived of oxygen and nutrients, the secretory cells disintegrate and desquamate. This induces phagocytic and resorptive processes and leads to necrosis of the lobulo-alveolar structures. Reduction in these glandular elements is followed by formation of connective tissue and deposition of fat. At the end of the postlactational involution, which takes about 3 months to be completed, the breast usually assumes its prepregnant size, although the breast may be somewhat less dense and have less nodular-glandular tissue than in the prepregnant state.

ENDOCRINE CONSEQUENCES OF LACTATION

The resumption of cyclic ovulatory function postpartum is considerably delayed in lactating women in comparison to nonlactating women. In the latter group, the first ovulation occurs on the average 49 days after delivery. In women on full lactation, the first ovulation occurred on the average 112 days after delivery, although with extended lactation the occurrence of first ovulation can be delayed considerably longer. However, in all women the incidence of ovulation increases as breast-feeding continues, and most lactating women ovulate within 1 year of delivery.

In more than half of lactating women the first menstruation is ovulatory. Breast-feeding is therefore not a reliable contraceptive method and after 10–12 weeks of lactation some kind of anticonceptive should be utilized unless another pregnancy is desired.

The lactational amenorrhea is caused by at least two factors: pituitary unresponsiveness and ovarian refractoriness. The response of the pituitary gland to hypothalamic ovulatory stimuli is suppressed during the first weeks, returning gradually to normal in about 6 weeks. This is observed both in lactating and in nonlactating women, although the recovery is somewhat more rapid in nonlactating women.

The ovarian responsiveness to gonadotropin stimulation is suppressed in lactating women. This is due to the elevated plasma prolactin levels. This is supported by the findings illustrated in Figure 9.5 which indicate that in lactating women plasma LH and FSH levels return to the normal nonpregnant range 2 or 3 weeks after delivery. While LH tends to remain at the low-normal range, FSH is in high-normal or even supra-normal range. In spite of high FSH levels, ovarian estrogen production does not increase but remains very low as long as prolactin levels remain elevated over normal nonpregnant values. When breast-feeding is stopped, prolactin declines and ovarian estrogen production is almost immediately resumed, leading to an estrogen surge which is then followed by a LH surge and ovulation as illustrated in Figure 9.5. When lactation is suppressed by a drug, bromocryptine, which selec-tively inhibits prolactin release, ovarian estrogen production responds immediately to the rising FSH levels, resulting in a peak in plasma estrogen. This is followed by LH peak and ovulation which has been detected as early as 14–18 days postpartum, significantly earlier than in nonlactating women who do not receive bromocryptine. In these, plasma prolactin declines more gradually than after bromocryptine treatment.

SUPPRESSION OF LACTATION

Women who do not wish to breast-feed, who have a still-born child, or who suffer from a serious disease are usually given either steroids or, more recently, a drug that specifically prevents prolactin release from the hypothalamus.

The absence of suckling stimuli and not emptying the breast will in itself lead to cessation of lactation within about 1 week without any medication. However, most women will suffer from painful breast engorgement and will experience milk leakage. Although tight binding of the breasts and application of ice packs will relieve the condition after a few days, many patients prefer to obtain relief through medication. The most widely used method depends on the ability of sex steroids to inhibit lactation. As mentioned earlier, estrogens and progesterone are very effective in preventing lactogenesis, but they are without effect once lactation has been established. They are therefore most effective when given just before parturition, in early labor. However, since the use of steroids prepartum may result in long-term adverse effects in the fetus, it is advisable to delay the injection until immediately postpartum.

Estrogens, progestins and androgens in various combinations have been advocated for suppression of lactation over the years. Presently a combination of testosterone enanthate (360 mg) and a long-acting estrogen (16 mg estradiol valerate) (Deladumone) given as a single intramuscular injection immediately after delivery is the most widely used and is effective in preventing lactation in about 80–85% of

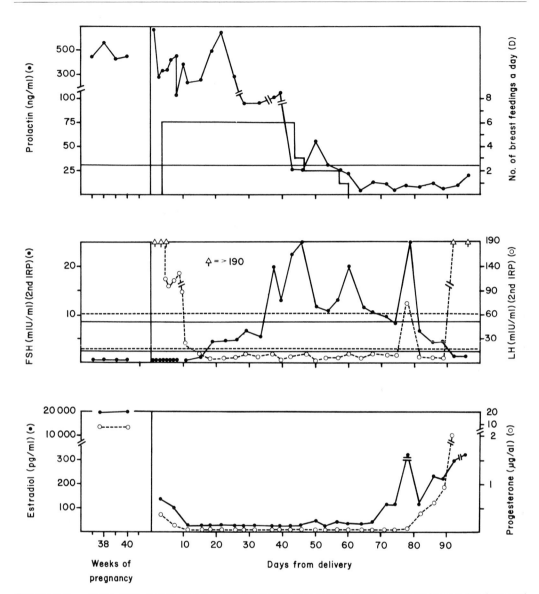

Figure 9.5. Endocrine profile of a lactating woman. The relationship between breast-feeding and the peripheral levels of prolactin, FSH, LH, 17β-estradiol, and progesterone during the puerperium. Horizontal lines indicate the range of normal cycling women. Note that after breast-feeding was discontinued, plasma estrogen levels promptly increased, leading to an ovulatory surge of LH. The woman conceived during this ovulation and became pregnant without experiencing any postpartum menstruation. (From R. Rolland et al., *Clinical Endocrinology*, 4:15–21, 1975.)

women, provided that the breast is not suckled. The testosterone antagonizes the estrogenic effects to a certain degree and reduces the effect of estrogen on uterine involution and endometrial proliferation and on thromboembolic disease. Likewise, any virilizing action of the androgen is neutralized by the presence of the relatively high dose of estradiol. It is usually necessary to give a long-acting preparation; the effect of Deladumone persists for 2–4 weeks.

There are several groups of women in whom the use of estradiol is strongly contraindicated, and therefore another type of drug to suppress lactation is highly desirable. Bromocryptine has been widely used in Europe for this purpose. It is a dopaminergic agonist which inhibits the release of PRL, thus preventing lactation. The drug can be taken orally and it is usually necessary to take it for at least 2 weeks.

Bromocryptine is also effective in other galactorrheic states associated with ovulatory dysfunction. In a high proportion of cases, such treatment results in initiation of ovulation. Side effects of the treatment include nausea and vomiting; these can be minimized by increasing the dose gradually. Bromocryptine has been reported to be 95–100% effective in suppressing postpartum lactation; neither breast pain, breast engorgement nor milk leakage was observed when the drug was given 2.5 mg, b.i.d. for 2 weeks.

CONTRACEPTION DURING LACTATION

As already mentioned, ovulation is often resumed in lactating women while they are still nursing; the first ovulation is often not preceded by menstruation. It is therefore of importance to advise patients to utilize contraception during lactation, beginning about the sixth to eighth week postpartum.

Intrauterine devices may be used and should be inserted at about 8 weeks post-partum. Postpartum expulsion of IUDs is unfortunately relatively frequent, and other methods may have to be utilized. There is still no consensus regarding the safety of contraceptive steroids when given to lactating women. As previously mentioned, the steroids are secreted into the milk and measurable quantities of synthetic progestins have been found in milk. Some adverse effects have been reported; these include accelerated bone maturation and gynecomastia. The quantity and composition of milk is also somewhat affected. A decrease in milk secretion is often associated with the use of conventional oral contraceptives; this is attributed to the estrogenic component of the Pill. The low-dose progestin pills do not appear to influence milk yield and they are effective contraceptive agents in lactating women. The concentration of steroids excreted in milk is too low to have any effect on bone maturation, and they may be used safely even by lactating mothers. Compounds having pure progestational effects are preferable to those having some inherent estrogenic properties.

Suggested Reading

1. Applebaum, R.M. Modern management of successful breast-feeding. *Pediatr. Clin. North Am.* 17:203–225, 1970.
2. Fonion, S.J. *Infant Nutrition.* W.B. Saunders, Philadelphia, 1974.
3. Kon, S.K., and Cowie, A.T. *Milk: The Mammary Gland and Its Secretion.* Academic Press, New York, 1961.
4. Vorherr, H. *The Breast: Morphology, Physiology, Lactation.* Academic Press, New York, 1974.

CHAPTER 10

Anatomy of the Pelvis and Perineum

PAUL S. MILLEY, M.D.

THE BONY PELVIS

General Features

The adult bony pelvis is comprised of four bones joined together by four joints. The two *innominate bones* articulate with each other anteriorly at the *symphysis pubis* and posteriorly they are joined bilaterally to the *sacrum* by the *sacroiliac synchondroses*. The sacrum in turn articulates with the *coccyx*. Each innominate bone is formed by fusion, about the time of puberty, of three separate bones: the *pubis*, the *ilium* and the *ischium*. The *superior ramus* of the pubis passes posteriorly, upward and laterally from the *body*, forms the upper margin of the *obturator foramen* and fuses with the ilium at the *acetabulum*.

Important landmarks of the lateral aspect of the innominate bone should be reviewed (Fig. 10.1). The *anterior-superior iliac spine*, which is readily palpated, gives attachment to the inguinal ligament and marks the anterior boundary of the *iliac crest*. This crest runs backward to the *posterior-superior iliac spine*. The prominent *iliac tubercle* lies on this crest and is an important landmark since it is the highest point on the crest, marks the widest points on the crest and lies on the level of the disc between lumbar vertebrae 4 and 5.

On the medial aspect of the innominate bone the *ischial spine* is of particular significance (Fig. 10.2). This inwardly projecting prominence separates the *greater*

sciatic notch above from the *lesser sciatic notch* below. The *ischiococcygeus* (or coccygeus) muscle is attached to its medial aspect and the *sacrospinous ligament* is attached to its lateral aspect.

The *ischial tuberosity* marks the inferior boundary of the *lesser sciatic notch*. The *sacrotuberous ligament* forms the inferior boundary of the *lesser sciatic foramen*. When the subject is standing the tuberosity is covered by the gluteus maximus muscle, but when the subject is sitting it is separated from the integument only by a bursa.

The *inferior ramus* of the *ischium* fuses anteriorly with the *inferior ramus* of the *pubis* to form the anterior and inferior border of the *obturator foramen*.

Also on the medial surface of the innominate bone the *iliopectineal line* (also known as the arcuate line or linea terminalis) begins anteriorly at the pubic spine and ends posteriorly at the *auricular articular surface* where the innominate bone articulates with the sacrum. This iliopectineal line forms the major part of the *pelvic brim* or *inlet*.

The sacrum forms the posterior wall of the bony pelvis. Generally comprised of 5 fused vertebrae (sometimes 4 or 6), it is a wedge-shaped bone with its base above and apex below. With the patient in the upright position the sacrum lies in an oblique plane that is more nearly horizontal than vertical. The superior surface has

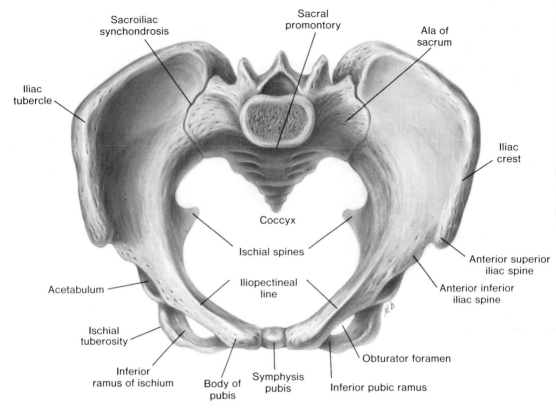

Figure 10.1.   Superior view of an articulated pelvis showing major landmarks.

a specialized area for articulation with the fifth lumbar vertebra. The anterior margin of this articular area is known as the *sacral promontory*. On either side of the promontory are the *alae*, which together with the promontory form the posterior boundary of the pelvic brim or inlet.

The anterior or pelvic surface of the sacrum is concave. On the posterior aspect the inferior opening of the vertically oriented sacral canal is known as the *sacral hiatus*. This opening is of interest to the obstetrician who employs caudal analgesia. Inferiorly the sacrum articulates with the coccyx, which is formed by four rudimentary vertebrae.

The articulated pelvis is divided into *true* and *false* pelvis by the brim or inlet. The false pelvis forms the lower boundary of the abdominal cavity and lies above the pelvic brim. The true pelvis lies below the brim and bounds the pelvic cavity and the perineal space. The obstetrician is mainly concerned with the true pelvis, which consists of the brim, cavity and outlet.

The *inlet* or *brim* of the true pelvis is bounded by the inner surface of the pubis, the iliopectineal line and posteriorly by the anterior borders of the alae and promontory of the sacrum.

The *pelvic cavity* is a curved canal with a deep concave posterior wall which is approximately twice as long as the shallow anterior wall.

The *outlet* of the pelvis is somewhat diamond shaped and is bounded by the *arcuate pubic ligament* and the *pubic arch* anteriorly, the ischial tuberosities and sacrotuberous ligaments laterally, and the tip of the coccyx posteriorly.

Axis of the Birth Canal

This axis is of greatest obstetrical significance since it corresponds to the course taken by the fetal head in its passage through the pelvic cavity and is a guide to

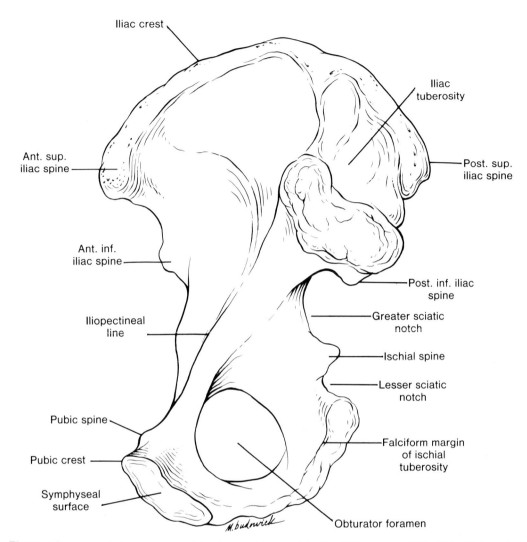

Iliac crest

Iliac tuberosity

Ant. sup. iliac spine

Post. sup. iliac spine

Ant. inf. iliac spine

Post. inf. iliac spine

Greater sciatic notch

Iliopectineal line

Ischial spine

Lesser sciatic notch

Pubic spine

Pubic crest

Falciform margin of ischial tuberosity

Symphyseal surface

Obturator foramen

Figure 10.2. Medial aspect of the innominate bone showing major landmarks. The iliopectineal line forms the main boundary between the false pelvis above and the true pelvis below.

the direction of pull necessary for forceps-assisted delivery (Fig. 10.3). The pelvic brim makes an angle of about 60 degrees with the horizontal, while the plane of the pelvic outlet makes an angle of only about 10 degrees with the horizontal.

The fetal head descends at right angles to the plane of the pelvic brim and continues to descend along this line as far as the level of the ischial spines. At this level the birth canal takes a gentle right-angled forward turn due to the sloping pelvic floor and forwardly directed vagina. The forward turn directs the presenting part of

the fetus into the axis of the pelvic outlet, which corresponds to the center of the vagina.

Internal Measurements of the Pelvis

Three different anteroposterior diameters have been described, all of which have as their posterior point of reference the center of the sacral promontory (Fig. 10.4). Relative to their anterior points of reference, these diameters are from above downward:

The *true conjugate*, which runs from the middle of the sacral promontory to the

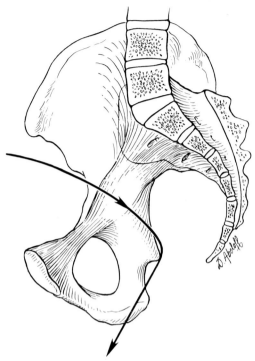

Figure 10.3. The axis of the birth canal is illustrated. The axis turns forward at the level of the ischial spine.

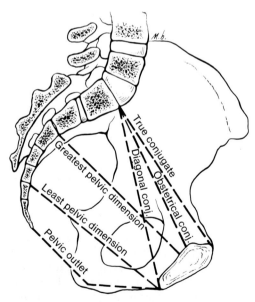

Figure 10.4. Sagittal section through the articulated pelvis showing anteroposterior diameters and major planes.

upper margin of the symphysis pubis. This diameter measures approximately 11.25 cm and is of more anatomic than obstetric significance.

The *obstetrical conjugate*, which has been defined as the shortest distance between the promontory of the sacrum and the symphysis pubis. This represents the shortest diameter through which the fetal head must pass in its passage through the pelvic inlet.

The *diagonal conjugate*, which is the distance between the lower border of the symphysis pubis and the sacral promontory. It can be measured by inserting the index and middle fingers into the vagina and directing them toward the sacral promontory. If the tip of the middle finger fails to touch the promontory or touches it with difficulty, it can be taken that the conjugate is adequate to accommodate a fetal head of average dimensions.[11] If the examining finger touches the promontory, the distance between it and the point on the hand which lies immediately beneath the symphysis pubis may be measured.

Planes of the Pelvis

For convenience the pelvis is described as having four imaginary planes.

The *plane of the inlet* (or superior strait). This plane is bounded anteriorly by the upper margins of the horizontal rami of the pubic bones and symphysis pubis, laterally by the iliopectineal line, and posteriorly by the promontory and alae of the sacrum. Four diameters of the pelvic inlet are described (Fig. 10.5): The *anteroposterior* (which corresponds to the true conjugate described above), the *transverse*, and two *obliques*. The transverse diameter is constructed at right angles to the true conjugate and represents the greatest distance between the iliopectineal line on either side. The oblique diameters extend from one of the sacroiliac joints to the iliopectineal eminence of the opposite side.

The *plane of the greatest pelvic dimensions*. This plane corresponds to the widest part of the cavity of the pelvis and passes through the middle of the symphysis pubis and the junction between the second and

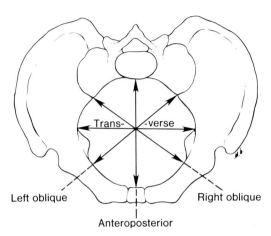

Trans- -verse

Left oblique

Right oblique

Anteroposterior

Figure 10.5. Superior view of the pelvic inlet showing the four major diameters.

third sacral vertebrae.

The *plane of least pelvic dimensions*. In contrast, this plane corresponds to the narrowest part of the pelvic cavity. It passes through the lower border of the symphysis pubis, the ischial spines and the lower border of the sacrum. Failure of the levator ani muscle to relax properly may produce difficulty at this level.

The *plane of the outlet*. This actually consists of two triangles having a common base which is a line drawn between the two ischial tuberosities. These two triangles are not on the same level, due to the slope of the pelvic bones. The tuberosities are lower than either the anterior or the posterior ends of this plane. As soon as the fetal head passes through the pelvic outlet, it becomes extended beneath the subpubic arch. The width of the subpubic angle is, therefore, very important. If the angle is narrow the head is thrust farther back toward the coccyx and extension of the head may be very difficult, leading to outlet distocia and severe perineal laceration.

Internal Pelvic Dimensions

Approximate average dimensions of the pelvis are summarized in Table 10.1.

Descending down the pelvic cavity, the anteroposterior diameters increase and transverse diameters decrease (when allowance is made at the outlet for movement of the coccyx). It should be noted

Table 10.1. Average Internal Dimensions of the Pelvis

	Antero-posterior	Oblique	Transverse
Inlet	11.2 cm	12.5 cm	13.1 cm
Cavity	13.1 cm	13.1 cm	12.5 cm
Outlet	12.5 cm	11.8 cm	11.8 cm

that the greatest diameter of the pelvic inlet is transverse, of the cavity is oblique, and of the outlet is anteroposterior. This explains the mechanism of fetal head rotation during its passage through the pelvic cavity since the largest diameter of the fetal head will always occupy the widest diameter of the pelvis.

Nicholson[9] and Ince and Young[6] feel that there are five main pelvic measurements necessary for evaluating the prognosis of labor. These are:

1. The transverse diameter of the brim
2. The diameter between the ischial spines
3. The plane of the least pelvic dimensions
4. The obstetrical conjugate
5. The subpubic angle

These measurements can be taken accurately only with the use of radiology.

In describing the relationship between the level of the fetal head and the pelvis, the classification introduced by DeLee and Greenhill is frequently used.[4] The level of the tip of the ischial spines is arbitrarily called position O. The position of the fetal head is described in centimeters as being plus or minus as it lies below or above the level of the spines. For example, a fetal head palpated to be 2 cm below the level of the ischial spines would be described as being at "spines plus 2."

Muscular Pelvic Floor

The muscular floor of the pelvis or pelvic diaphragm is a bowl-shaped sheet of muscle with encompassing fascia that is slung around the midline body effluents (the urethra, vagina and anorectal canal) (Fig. 10.6).

This diaphragm is comprised of three separate but continuous muscles that are

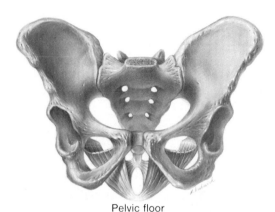

Pelvic floor

Figure 10.6.   The bowl-like or sling shape of the muscular pelvic floor is emphasized in this anteroposterior view.

named from their origins and insertions. They are best considered as one morphological and functional entity. From anterior to posterior these muscles are the *pubococcygeus* arising from the body of the pubis, the *iliococcygeus* which arises from a thickening in the obturator internus fascia known as the white line or tendinous arch, and the *ischiococcygeus* (or coccygeus) arising from the ischial spine. The pubococcygeus and iliococcygeus together are called the *levator ani*. Note that each of these muscles takes origin from a different portion of the innominate bone and that all three muscles insert into either the coccyx or the anococcygeal raphe. From their origins the muscle fibers slope downward, backward and to the midline. The muscular pelvic floor produced in this manner slopes downward and forward.

Phylogenetically these muscles served to wag the tail of the prontograde quadriped. The support of the abdominal and pelvic viscera in these animals is primarily the pubis and anterior abdominal wall. In these lower animals the levator ani arises from the pelvic brim. As man developed the upright posture, the muscles of the pelvic diaphragm assumed a secondary supportive function.[10, 14] In addition, the levator ani acts as an antagonist of the thoracoabdominal diaphragm and the abdominal muscles by contracting when these opposing muscles contract. This pre-

vents inferior herniation of the pelvic viscera when intra-abdominal pressure rises.[5, 13]

The pubococcygeus is a flat muscle whose fibers are in different functional sets. The bulk of its posterior fibers sweep backward and are inserted into the tip of the coccyx and anococcygeal raphe, thus constituting the Y-shaped pubococcygeus muscle proper (Fig. 10.7). Fibers arising more anteriorly swing more medially and more inferiorly around the anorectal junction and join fibers from the opposite side. This results in a U-shaped sling which holds the anorectal junction angled forward. These latter muscle fibers also partially join posterior muscle fibers of the external anal sphincter, and this portion of the muscle is therefore called the *puborectalis*. A similar U-shaped muscular sling known as the *pubovaginalis* passes behind the vagina and into the perineal body. These transverse fibers of the pubovaginalis which insert into the perineal body are known as the "fibers of Luschka." They hypertrophy during pregnancy and can be seen when the perineum is deeply torn at parturition.

The midline opening in the pelvic diaphragm through which the three tubular structures (urethra, vagina and anal canal) pass is known clinically as the *levator hiatus*. That portion of the pelvic diaphragm from just behind the hiatus to the coccygeal insertion is known as the *levator plate*.

Berglas and Rubin[1] using elegant technique studied the functional anatomy of the levator plate in vivo by the direct injection of radiopaque contrast material into the levator plate muscles with simultaneous placement of contrast material in the vagina, cervix and uterus. Radiographs were taken of the patient at rest and while straining. The results showed the horizontal position of the normal levator plate even while the patient was straining. The rectum and vagina rest on this horizontal levator plate (Fig. 10.8). The blood vessels and lymphatics from the hypogastric plexus enter and leave the uterus and vagina along the lateral margins of these organs. Around these vessels, condensa-

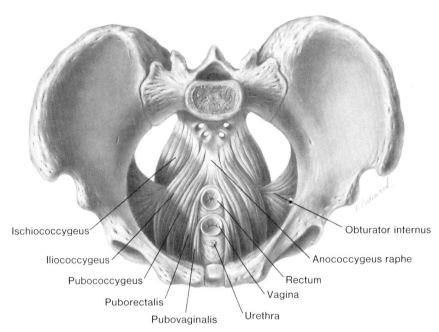

Ischiococcygeus

Iliococcygeus

Pubococcygeus

Puborectalis

Pubovaginalis

Urethra

Vagina

Rectum

Anococcygeus raphe

Obturator internus

Figure 10.7.   Pelvic floor viewed from above showing the muscles forming the main support of the pelvic viscera. Note the U-shaped sling formed by the puborectalis and pubovaginalis muscles.

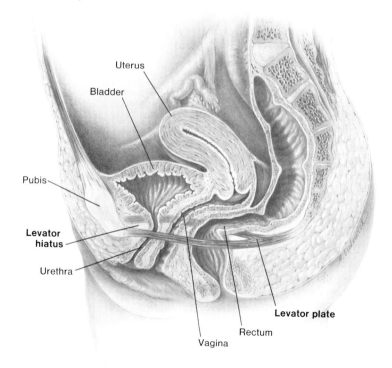

Uterus

Bladder

Pubis

Levator hiatus

Urethra

Vagina

Rectum

Levator plate

Figure 10.8.   Relationships of the rectum, uterus and upper vagina to the levator plate. Note the horizontal position of this plate and the urethra, vagina and rectum passing through the levator hiatus.

tions of connective tissue form the *cardinal* and *uterosacral* ligaments.[3, 8] These ligaments are part of the suspensory apparatus that serves to hold the uterus and upper vagina over the levator plate.

The slope of the muscular pelvic floor plays a role in obstetrical mechanics. The lowest part of the descending fetus is the first to meet this sloping muscular gutter and, therefore, during delivery is mechanically rotated to the front.

When the presenting part reaches a certain point during the second stage of labor, the muscular mass forming the perineal body (or central point of the perineum) bulges downward and becomes markedly attenuated. The pubovaginalis and puborectalis together with the sphincters of the anal canal relax and the levator ani is drawn up over the advancing fetal part. If the levator ani fails to relax at the crucial moment, extensive damage to the pelvic floor may result.

THE PERINEUM

In anatomy the term *perineum* refers to the whole pelvic outlet below the pelvic floor. It is a diamond-shaped space bounded anterolaterally by the inferior rami of the pubis and ischium, laterally by the tuberosity of the ischium, and posterolaterally by the lower border of the sacrotuberous ligament covered by the gluteus maximus muscle. This space is arbitrarily divided by a transverse line immediately in front of the anus into the *urogenital triangle* anteriorly and the *anal triangle* posteriorly.

Spanning across the superior aspect of the urogenital triangle is the *urogenital diaphragm* (Fig. 10.9). This diaphragm is formed by a muscular layer (the deep transverse perineal muscle and the sphincter of the membranous urethra) enclosed between two triangular fascial membranes. The thin superior fascial layer spans the gap between the anterior portions of the levator ani. The inferior fascial layer is considerably stronger and blends posteriorly with the sacrotuberous ligaments.

On the inferior margin of the pubic symphysis, there is a small *arcuate pubic ligament*. Between this ligament and the anterior free margin of the urogenital diaphragm, there is a space through which passes the deep dorsal vein of the clitoris. This vein passes into the pelvis to join a venous plexus at the bladder neck.

Piercing the urogenital diaphragm are the urethra and vagina, blood vessels and nerves passing to the clitoris and bulb of the vestibule, and the posterior labial nerves and vessels passing to the labia. The arteries and nerves are branches of the internal pudendal trunks.

The space between the two fascial layers of the urogenital diaphragm is known as the deep perineal pouch. In contrast, the *superficial perineal pouch* is bounded above by the inferior layer of the urogenital diaphragm and below by Colles' fascia (the deep layer of the superficial fascia of the abdominal wall) (Fig. 10.10).

Contained within the superficial pouch are the superficial transverse perineal muscle (a weak and sometimes absent structure), the crura of the clitoris ensheathed by the ischiocavernosus muscle, the bulb of the vestibule surrounded by the bulbocavernosus muscle, Bartholin's glands and their ducts, the terminations of the vagina and urethra together with blood vessels lymphatics and nerves. The *ischiocavernosus muscle*, innervated by the perineal branch of the pudendal nerve, compresses the crus and by inhibiting venous return assists in clitoral erection. The *bulbocavernosus muscle* blends with the external anal sphincter posteriorly, thus forming a figure-of-eight around the vagina and anal canal. Also innervated by the perineal branch of the pudendal nerve, the muscle arises from the perineal body, passes forward around the orifice of the vagina, surrounds the bulb of the vestibule and is inserted into the body of the clitoris on its dorsal aspect.

The *perineal body* is a fibromuscular and elastic structure found in the midline between the ischial tuberosities. Also known as the central point of the perineum, it is somewhat like the hub of a wheel into which various muscles (the superficial and deep transverse perineal

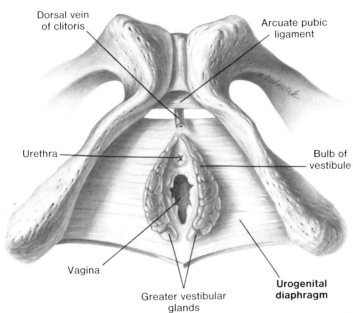

Figure 10.9. The urogenital diaphragm is shown with the overlying bulbs of the vestibule and Bartholin's glands. The dorsal vein of the clitoris enters the pelvis beneath the arcuate pubic ligament.

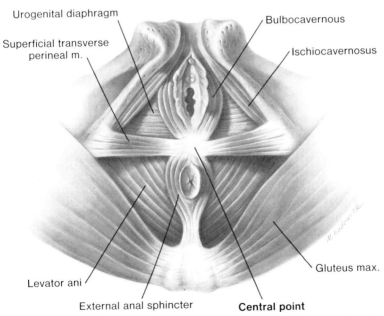

Figure 10.10. The muscles of the perineum as seen from below occupying the superficial perineal pouch.

muscles, the bulbocavernosus muscles, the external anal sphincter and some fibers of the levator ani) are inserted like spokes. When in the standing position, the urogen-ital diaphragm is almost horizontal in sagittal section, and for this reason its fixation to the perineal body contributes to the support of the urethra and vesicourethral junction.[8] The perineal body has some degree of distensibility which if lost through unrepaired perineal laceration may give rise to rectocele and posterior vaginal eversion. The importance of the perineal body to obstetrics is so great that the term *perineum* is applied by clinicians to this localized area of the much larger diamond-shaped anatomic perineum defined above.

The *ischiorectal fossa* is a pyramidal shaped space in the anatomic perineum which lies between the tuberosity of the ischium laterally and the rectum and anal canal medially. The superior apex of this space lies at the origin of the levator ani from the tendinous arch. The lateral wall is formed by the fascia of the obturator internus muscle and in this wall is the pudendal canal containing the internal pudendal vessels and nerves. Anteriorly the fossa is bounded by the posterior edge of the urogenital diaphragm. The posterior boundary is formed by the sacrotuberous ligaments and the gluteus maximus. The ischiorectal fossa contains a supportive pad of fat and is frequently the site of abscess formation secondary to the spread of infection from adjacent organs.

The perineal nerve innervates the whole of the perineum, including the clitoris, labia and perineal body. If a block is done at the main trunk of the nerve near the ischial spine, complete anesthesia in the area of its distribution is produced.[7]

Application of Perineal Anatomy to Episiotomy

The simple operation of episiotomy is frequently performed in order to protect the perineum. The resulting incision is considerably easier to repair than is a traumatic spontaneous irregular laceration. There are two basic types of episiotomy: the midline (or median) and the mediolateral.

The advantages of the midline operation

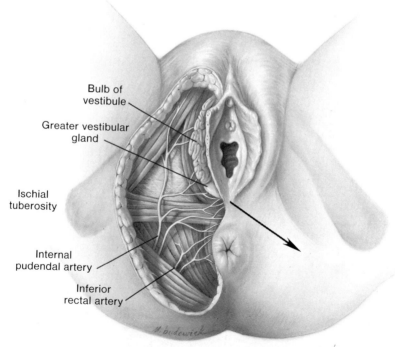

Bulb of vestibule

Greater vestibular gland

Ischial tuberosity

Internal pudendal artery

Inferior rectal artery

Figure 10.11.   Perineal anatomy showing important structures relative to episiotomy. The skin and subcutis have been omitted from one side of the illustration for reference. The *arrow* indicates the direction of incision for a mediolateral episiotomy.

are that it is easier to repair, results in less bleeding and postpartum discomfort, and more readily heals by primary intention. The major disadvantage is that if the wound extends posteriorly the external anal sphincter and rectum may be lacerated.

The mediolateral episiotomy incision is begun at the midpoint of the fourchette and is then directed laterally toward a point midway between the anal orifice and the ischial tuberosity (Fig. 10.11).

References

1. Berglas, B., and Rubin, I.C. Study of the supportive of the uterus by levator myography. *Surg. Gynecol. Obstet.* 97:677, 1953.
2. Caldwell, W.E., and Moloy, H.C. Anatomical variations in the female pelvis and their effect in labor, with a suggested classification. *Am. J. Obstet. Gynecol.* 26:479, 1933.
3. Curtis, A.H., Anson, B. J., Ashley, F.L., and Jones, T. Blood vessels of the female pelvis in relation to gynecological surgery. *Surg. Gynecol. Obstet.* 75:421, 1942.
4. DeLee, J.B., and Greenhill, J.P. Diameters of the pelvis. *Br. Med. J.* 2:737, 1950.
5. Dickinson, R.L. Studies of the levator ani muscle. *Am. J. Obstet.* 22:997, 1889.
6. Ince, H., and Young, M. The bony pelvis and its influence on labor. *J. Obstet. Gynecol. Br. Emp.* 47:130, 1940.
7. Klink, E.W. Perineal nerve block, an anatomic and clinical study in the female. *Obstet. Gynecol.* 1:137, 1953.
8. Nichols, D.H., and Milley, P.S. Clinical anatomy of the vulva, vagina, lower pelvis and perineum. In *Davis' Gynecology and Obstetrics.* Harper & Row, Hagerstown, MD, 1972, vol. 1, chap. 4.
9. Nicholson, C. The interpretation of radiological pelvimetry. *J. Obstet. Gynecol. Br. Emp.* 45:950, 1938.
10. Power, R.M.H. Embryological development of the levator ani muscle. *Am. J. Obstet. Gynecol.* 55:367, 1948.
11. Smout, C.F.V., Jacoby, F., and Lillie, E.W. *Gynecological and Obstetrical Anatomy, Descriptive and Applied.* Williams & Wilkins, Baltimore, 1969.
12. Steer, C.M. Clinical examination of the pelvis. In *Gynecology and Obstetrics,* edited by Sciarra, J.J. Harper & Row, New York, 1979, vol. 2, chap. 2.
13. Sturmdorf, A. *Gynoplastic Technology.* F. A. Davis, Philadelphia, 1919.
14. Thompson, P. On the arrangements of the fasciae of the pelvis and their relationship to the levator ani. *J. Anat. Physiol.* 35:127, 1901.

Section 2
Perinatology

CHAPTER 11

Diagnosis of Pregnancy: Amenorrhea

ROBERT LANDESMAN, M.D.

The diagnosis of pregnancy may be definitive or suggestive, depending on the clinical criteria. The history, physical examination and laboratory results will usually reveal sufficient information for a definite diagnosis. The earlier in pregnancy that the diagnosis is attempted, the fewer modalities may be positive. Although the pregnancy test for the presence of human chorionic gonadotropin (hCG) is the most accurate of all the findings, the physician must provide the final diagnosis by proper synthesis of all the clinical data. The findings may be divided into the following three groups: history, the objective physical examination and laboratory data.

History: Menses
Basal body
temperature
Breast changes
Nausea—distention
Bladder function
change
Fatigue
Quickening: fetal
movement
Objective signs: Hegar's sign
Goodell's sign
Chadwick's sign
Breast examination
Fetal sounds by
doptone
Fetal movements
Ballottement of fetus

Laboratory tests: Roentgenographic
examination
Ultrasound
Human chorionic
gonadotropin—
pregnancy test

HISTORY

Menses

Normal menses may vary in frequency from an interval of 19 to 60 days; the usual interval is 26 to 32 days. If the cyclic pattern[4] is regular, delay in the cycle is always suggestive of pregnancy. Frequent irregularities detract from the menstrual cycles as an aid in diagnosis. Unprotected intercourse on or about the time of ovulation associated with a delayed cycle increases the possibility of pregnancy. Rapid loss or gain of weight, episodes of emotional tension, travel or infection may result in periods of amenorrhea. Following months or years of contraceptive pill ingestion, amenorrhea may persist for months and sometimes as long as a year. This confounds the patient and physician concerning the possibility of pregnancy. With associated protected or unprotected intercourse, on occasion a menstrual cycle may be replaced by minimal staining without cramps or pain. This may be indicative of an early normal pregnancy or a threatened or missed abortion. Weekly observations with pregnancy tests will crystallize the diagnosis. Early continuous staining in pregnancy may be a sign of ectopic pregnancy, and further appropriate tests (culdocentesis, laparoscopy and sonography) may be necessary to rule out this complication.

Basal Body Temperature

In a normal ovulatory cycle, a temperature elevation of 0.4–0.8°F is sustained during the last 14–16 days of the cycle. If this elevation is maintained for more than 18 days, pregnancy is a likely diagnosis. The ingestion or injection of progesterone will produce a similar effect without pregnancy. The temperature is frequently used to confirm ovulation in infertility studies. A useful basal body temperature record requires that the temperature be determined accurately at the same time before rising from bed in the morning. Oscillations may be confounding if precise timing is not adhered to each day.

Breast Changes

The patient frequently may complain of breast pain, tenderness and fullness. Rapid enlargement may be noted 7–10 days after ovulation, particularly in the primipara. Darkening of the areola, enlargement of the nipple and protuberant Montgomery's glands are noted in some instances. The tenderness may subside after the end of the seventh week of pregnancy although the enlargement will be maintained. After the sixth week, colostrum may be expressed; the finding of colostrum in a multipara is of limited significance in making the diagnosis of pregnancy. Enlarged veins about the nipple in fair skinned individuals is not unusual. Swelling of the axilla from ectopic breast tissue is on occasion a most prominent complaint; in an initial pregnancy this is highly indicative of gravidity and usually requires considerable reassurance, for the patient may suspect a lymph gland tumor.

Nausea and Distention

Nausea and distention due to pregnancy may be the only symptom and sign and may lead to unnecessary gastrointestinal investigation, including radiological examinations which may be detrimental to the fetus. Nausea as a single symptom in a woman in the childbearing period should always suggest the possibility of pregnancy. A urine or blood test for hCG of the proper sensitivity will usually rule out a gravidity. Nausea in pregnancy is extremely variable. Usually it is not severe enough to prevent the ingestion of nourishing fluids. Distention of the abdomen and constipation are related to the reduced peristalsis of early pregnancy. The patient may point to an enlarged lower abdomen thinking that this is a growing uterus. However, in the first 8 weeks of pregnancy, the uterus is only a pelvic organ. The bloating of the abdomen is extremely variable and unreliable as an indication of pregnancy. More than half of patients do not notice this change. If persistent vomiting occurs, intravenous feeding may be necessary. The exact mechanism of the nausea is unknown; it appears more frequent in the group that will carry successfully to term. Staining in the absence of nausea may be a symptom of an impending abortion. Although the exact mechanism of the nausea has not been elucidated, the sudden elevation of estrogen and progesterone, particularly the former by the corpus luteum and placenta, reduces peristalsis.

Bladder Function Changes

Bladder function changes may be due to pregnancy. In the early months, relaxation of the bladder and ureteral muscle occurs as well as enlargement of the cystic and urethral vessels. This may result in low-grade infection, urethritis and cystitis, that may be characterized by tenesmus and burning. After its presence has been substantiated by culture and examination of the sediment, urinary infection should be treated by antibiotics with minimal fetal toxicity. Later during the third trimester, direct bladder pressure produces reduced capacity and frequency. During the first 6 weeks of pregnancy, bladder symptoms may be absent in the majority of patients and in general they are not rewarding criteria for determining the presence of pregnancy.

Fatigue

Episodes of fatigue are a frequent symptom of early pregnancy. Office or industrial workers are unable to arise at the usual morning hours and find themselves losing their ability to concentrate during the course of the day. This lassitude usually ceases after the first trimester. Periods of drowsiness and faintness are common during the early pregnancy. They are accentuated by rushing to work and traveling in crowded trains and buses. On occasion, loss of consciousness may occur. The onset of fainting may be rapidly and successfully terminated by lowering the head or by any stimulus such as spirits of ammonia. At times this faintness may be related to transient hypoglycemia, which may be relieved by ingestion of sugar. On occasion, extensive neurological work-ups have been undertaken with such syncope; this approach is abandoned if pregnancy is the cause.

Quickening

Quickening is the perception of fetal movement by the patient. The earliest this may be perceived is 14 weeks and by some as late as 20 weeks. In women with long periods of amenorrhea and in some who have taken the pill, the first sign of pregnancy may be lower abdominal movements. Patient's observations must be confirmed by the obstetrician who will palpate for an abdominally enlarged uterus, attempt to ballote the fetus and listen with ultrasound fetoscope for fetal tones to confirm the pregnancy.

OBJECTIVE SIGNS

The pregnant uterus is virtually unchanged in size until 6 weeks. The perception of increased size is far more accurate if a baseline examination has been performed. The multiparous uterus tends to be slightly hypertrophied and the multiparous uterine cavity and cervix may vary in length from 6 to 8.5 cm. The change in consistency of the uterine muscle is an earlier sign. The first change is a softening of the upper cervix (Hegar's sign); this is associated with softening of the cervix itself (Goodell's sign) and finally the cervix and vaginal mucosa may have a bluish hue (Chadwick's sign). None of these historical signs are consistent or reliable. Parity or fibroids may enlarge and soften the uterus. Increased venous enlargement or capillary dilation may account for a blue color. A frequent cause of vascular engorgement may be cervicitis of bacterial or fungal origin.

Breast enlargement and engorgement are frequently noted. In a nullipara, a darkening of the areola and prominence of Montgomery's glands are visible by 4-6 weeks. In a multipara, these changes are less marked and increased density of the breasts may occur as a normal variant in the secretory phase of the menstrual cycle. Colostrum does not usually occur until the 6th-8th week and is only significant in the nullipara. High prolactin values in prolonged amenorrhea may also be associated with spontaneous breast secretion.

The ultrasound fetoscope, with the maternal bladder emptied, may pick up a fetal heartbeat by 9-11 weeks. This may be delayed if the placenta is on the anterior uterine wall or if the uterus itself is deeply set in the pelvis or is in the retroverted position. If a small-for-date fetus or a multiple gestation (twins or triplets) is present, delay in recognition of fetal heart sounds may be anticipated. The maternal vessel sound or uterine souffle may be easily distinguished by the lower rate 60-90, whereas the fetal heart is at 110-160. The maternal pulse may be taken while listening with the "doptone" to distinguish the two cardiac rates.

Fetal movements may be seen and may be palpated abdominally from 14 to 20 weeks. The onset of such positive observations are highly variable, depending on the character of maternal abdominal and uterine walls, placental site and fetal movement pattern at time of observation.

Ballottement of the fetus may be performed as early as 16 weeks but usually after 20 weeks. With both hands the fetus is displaced from one position to the other across the amniotic sac. The hard larger cephalic pole may be distinguished by its density and spherical shape.

LABORATORY TESTS

Roentgenographic diagnosis of pregnancy is now almost completely avoided with the development of highly improved and precise sonography because of danger to the fetus from radiation exposure. At the present time, radiographs performed on the fetus will detect the fetal skeleton at 14–16 weeks. X-rays for other indications accidentally may demonstrate fetal bony structures during a barium enema or intravenous pyelogram or films of the hips, spine and sacrum.

The earliest pregnancy may be detected by ultrasound at 5–6 weeks (see Chapter 15, "Ultrasonography"). If after 8 weeks no fetal pole is visualized or if no fetal motion is observed with a real time scanner, a missed abortion may be present. If the presence of a fetus is doubtful, the procedure may be repeated in 1 week; if the fetal sac is smaller and if no fetal pole is recognized, pregnancy loss may be anticipated. If no fetal sac is visualized after 6 weeks with a positive pregnancy test, an ectopic pregnancy may be likely. In the diagnosis of ectopic pregnancy, the absence of a fetal sac in the uterus is important. The finding of a sac outside of the uterus in the tube is infrequent and is usually late in the process of implantation. The pelvic examination, quantitative hCG testing, laparoscopy and culdocentesis together are helpful aids in confirming or denying the diagnosis of ectopic pregnancy.

The most important method for the diagnosis of pregnancy is the detection of chorionic gonadotropin, which was first described 53 years ago by Aschheim and Zondek[1] (Table 11.1). In the intervening period, there has been a continuous effort to increase the sensitivity, specificity, speed, and simplicity of the pregnancy test. Over this period, four different techniques for determining hCG have been utilized. These include: 1) bioassays with intact animals, 2) immunological methods with hemagglutination or latex agglutination, 3) radioimmunoassay (RIA) requiring labeled hormone and antiserum, and 4) radioreceptorassay (RRA) requiring labeled hormone with biological activity and specific receptor.

The improvements in the techniques for measuring hCG have been primarily related to the purification of the molecule and isolation and elucidation of the amino acid sequence of the hormone nonspecific α-subunit and hormone specific β-subunit. The bioassay of hCG as a pregnancy test was first described in 1927 by Aschheim and Zondek[1] in mice (Table 11.1), by Friedman in rabbits, by Frank and Berman and by Kupperman in rats. Urine or serum was injected in the various animals; ovarian hypertrophy, hyperemia or hemorrhage was used as the indication of a positive assay. Galli-Mainini developed another rapid assay, injecting urine or serum in the male toad; the presence of hCG caused the discharge of sperm in the urine in 1–5 hours. This bioassay had the advantage of speed and the toads would usually be reused. The supply and maintenance of animal colonies became difficult and costly; infection and disease interfered with the accuracy of the bioassay.

The second phase of the development of pregnancy tests in 1960 was possible after additional purification of the hCG molecule and the achievement of potent anti-hCG serum raised in rabbits. Wide and Gemzell and Brody and Carlstrom developed independently the binding of hCG to red cells and latex particles providing the basis of hemagglutination and latex agglutination. The sensitivity of the agglutination tests was not an improvement over the original bioassays, but the cost and time of performance were reduced. The biological and immunological tests provided a sensitivity of 500–1500 IU/liter (42–125 ng/ml) which meant that pregnancy could be detected 6 weeks after the last menstrual period with a 95% accuracy. However, a large number of early normal pregnancies (prior to the eighth week), ab-

Table 11.1.   Four Generations of Pregnancy Tests

Type of Test	Investigators	Endpoint	Time	Days of Detection After Ovulation	Specimen
Biologic	Aschheim and Zondek 1927	Luteinization (mouse ovary)	5 days	25	Urine
	Friedman 1929	Ovulation (rabbits)	48 hours	25	Urine
	Kupperman 1943	Hyperemia (rat ovary)	2 hours	25	Urine
	Galli-Mainini 1947	Ejection of sperm (frogs)	2 hours	25	Urine
Immunologic	Brody and Carlstrom 1960	Latex particle slide test	2 minutes	25	Urine
	Wide and Gemzell 1960	Hemagglutination inhibition	2 hours	25	Urine
					Serum
Radioimmunoassay	Wide 1969	Competition with immunoreactive ^{125}I-hCG for specific antibodies to hCG	24 hours	12	Serum
	Vaitukaitis 1972	Competition with immunoreactive ^{125}I-hCG for specific antibodies to the β unit of hCG	24 hours	8	Serum
Radioreceptorassay	Saxena 1974	Competition with biologically active ^{125}I-hCG for specific receptor sites	1 hour	8	Urine
					Serum

normal pregnancies, missed abortions, 50% of ectopic pregnancies and trophoblastic tumors with levels of hCG less than 500 mIU/ml were not detected. The patient who was a week late after missing the menses could not affirm or deny the diagnosis of pregnancy with the agglutination or original bioassays. Long episodes of amenorrhea and late ovulation complicated the detection process and often resulted in a false-negative result even after 6 weeks of amenorrhea.

Yalow and Berson introduced radioimmunoassay in 1960 and with further purification of hCG, highly sensitive antibodies were produced resulting in an RIA for hCG with a sensitivity of 6 mIU/ml. The cross-reaction between hCG and luteinizing hormone (LH) was circumvented by development of an antiserum raised against the hormone-specific β-subunit of hCG by Vaitukaitis et al.[6] Originally the RIA required 48–72 hours of incubation. At the present time (in 1980) with highly purified specific antibodies and improved techniques for purification, the incubation time has been reduced to less than an hour. Although the RIA to the β-subunit may be sensitive to 6 mIU/ml, the qualitative pregnancy test has been set at 40 mIU/ml with assay above declared positive and below negative. This provides a positive pregnancy test in a normal quantity during the fourth week following the last menstrual cycle. This reduces some cross-reaction with incomplete hormones and prevents interference with immunoreactive subunits or fragments of these hormones.

In 1974 Saxena[5] introduced the radioreceptorassay (RRA) for hCG, the latest advance in pregnancy testing. The receptor, obtained from the plasma membranes of bovine corpora lutea provided a biospecific binding protein for the biologically active intact hCG molecule. The receptor does not recognize subunits or fragments of hCG. Total incubation with the receptor can be reduced to 15 minutes. Separation is rapid and may be performed by simple centrifugation. The assay is completed in 1 hour and has the same sensitivity as the RIA of 6 mIU/ml. The RRA has the sensitivity of the RIA and the biological specificity of the animal *in vivo* tests.

The RRA does not discriminate between hCG and LH. However, the receptor has an affinity threefold higher for hCG than that for LH. There is no increase in basal LH in pregnancy and the RRA is performed in the presence of serum from the luteal phase of nonpregnant patients. The qualitative RRA test for pregnancy is set at a level of 200 mIU/ml to avoid the LH surge at ovulation and the high LH of menopause. High LH may at times confuse the RRA; the RIA for hCG using the antiserum to the β-subunit will clarify the problem.

The development of the third and fourth techniques for the detection of hCG (the RIA and RRA) has permitted the diagnosis of pregnancy as early as 1 week after documented conception and has greatly improved the management of the first trimester of pregnancy. The quantitative RIA and RRA have provided valuable information in accurately dating the age of pregnancy, helping in early diagnosis of ectopic pregnancy, threatened and missed abortion, multiple gestation and molar disease.

As antisera were produced that were more sensitive and specific for hCG, the pregnancy tests improved in their accuracy and provided a diagnosis at an earlier time (Table 11.2). The slide tests were the least sensitive but could be completed in several minutes. With this technique, hCG was sufficiently elevated to be recognized in a normal pregnancy at 6 weeks from the last menstrual period. Similar agglutination test performed in tubes with a longer incubation period of 1–2 hours provided an earlier positive diagnosis at 5 weeks gravidity. The neocept tube test detected hCG at the low value of 200 mIU/cc which was reached before the first missed menses at about 10 days following conception. The slide or tube test using latex agglutination or hemagglutination required no special equipment and could be accomplished in any office, clinic or small laboratory. The radioimmunoassay and recep-

Table 11.2. Commercially Available Pregnancy Tests

	Sensitivity mIU/ml
Urine-tube tests	
Neocept (Roche)	200
Accusphere (Organon)	750
Pregnostic (Organon)	750
Pregnosis Placentex (Roche)	1000
UCG-Lyphotest (Wampole)	1250
EPT (Warner-Chilcott)	1250
Acutest (Williams)	1250
Urine-slide tests	
Dri-Dot (Organon)	1500
Pregnosis (Roche)	1500
Pregnosticon (Organon)	1500
UCG (Wampole)	2000
Gravindex (Ortho)	3500
Serum-Beta subunit	
Betatec (Wampole)	40
Beta-CG (Monitor Science)	40
Preg-CG (Cambridge Nuclear)	40
Beta-CG (Serano)	40
Serum hCG (RRA)	
Biocept-G (Wampole)	200

torassays required the special use of isotopes, ultracentrifuges and γ-counters. Their sensitivity of 40–200 mIU/cc of serum permitted the diagnosis of pregnancy in the fourth week of pregnancy, before the missed menstrual cycle in the normal gravidity. The RRA and RIA also detected abnormal pregnancies, missed and threatened abortions and some ectopic pregnancies which were formerly overlooked by the less sensitive techniques. The RRA (Biocept G) sensitivity was set at 200 since the receptor also detects LH. At lower levels the receptor will combine with the LH at its peak at ovulation and the sustained LH elevation of the menopause. The RIA for the β-subunit of hCG is set at 40 mIU/ml. Lower values are not practical since hCG in small amounts may be produced by normal cells. These molecules, even though they have no biological activity, will combine with the hCG or β-hCG antibodies. The receptor of the RRA has the special advantage of not combining with the segments of the hCG molecule which may be present in serum of the nonpregnant patient.

Although pregnancy tests in the past 2 decades have become rapid and specific, a positive result demonstrates the presence of human chorionic gonadotropin (hCG) and not the diagnosis of pregnancy. In addition the opportunities for laboratory error are many; they include misread labeling, inadequate incubation, substandard reagents, interfering substances in urine or serum and careless pipeting. The history and objective findings require clinical evaluation together with the laboratory data. With our newest laboratory aid, sonography (gray scale after 6 weeks and real time after 8 weeks), we may provide accurate information concerning the size and location of a pregnancy.

References

1. Aschheim, S., and Zondek, B. Hypophysenvorderlapen hormon und ovarialkormon in Harn von Schwangeren. *Klin. Wochenschr.* 6:1322, 1927.
2. Danforth, D.N. *Obstetrics and Gynecology.* Harper & Row, Hagerstown, MD, 1977.
3. Hobbins, J.C., and Winsberg, F. *Ultrasonography in Obstetrics and Gynecology.* Williams & Wilkins, Baltimore, 1977.
4. Niswander, K.R. *Obstetrics, Essentials of Clinical Practice.* Little, Brown Co., Boston, 1976.
5. Saxena, B.B., and Landesman, R. Diagnosis and management of pregnancy by the radioreceptorassay of human chorionic gonadotropin. *Am. J. Obstet. Gynecol.* 131:97, 1978.
6. Vaitukaitis, J.L., Braunstein, G.D., and Ross, G.T. A radioimmunoassay which measures human chorionic gonadotropin in the presence of luteinizing hormone. *Am. J. Obstet. Gynecol. 113:*751, 1972.

CHAPTER 12

Antenatal Care

RONALD M. CAPLAN, M.D.

Antenatal care is an essential component of preventive medicine. Its institution has resulted in a continuing dramatic fall in fetal and maternal morbidity and mortality.

Pregnancy is a normal physiologic state. The goal of antenatal care is to prevent deviations from the normal and to detect and reverse them when they arise.

The patient should first be seen in early pregnancy, when she suspects that she is pregnant, generally 2 weeks after the first missed period. At that time, assuming a 28-day menstrual cycle, the pregnancy is 4 weeks from conception, or a 6-week pregnancy by convention (counting from the first day of the last menstrual period). The pregnancy is then clinically detectable. (See Chapter 14, "Lie, Position, and Presentation.")

A complete history is taken, and a physical examination including weight and blood pressure is done to rule out any disease states. In the history, attention is given to previous pregnancies and their outcome. Symptoms of pregnancy are elicited. The patient is asked about smoking and about ingestion of alcohol and other drugs that are potentially harmful to the fetus.

A pelvic examination is performed (see Chapter 14). The presence of an intrauterine pregnancy corresponding in size to its age of gestation is confirmed. An evaluation is made of the pelvic architecture.

Blood and urine tests are taken (Table 12.1). Some advocate the inclusion of a 1-hour glucose tolerance test as part of the routine to rule out gestational diabetes. A pregnancy test is taken if the diagnosis of pregnancy is doubtful; if necessary, a quantitative radioreceptorassay or radioimmunoassay for hCG may be done, and ultrasonography may be carried out.

Special tests are taken as required (Table 12.2). For example, black patients should be tested for sickle cell trait, and Jewish patients should be tested for Tay-Sachs disease. The patient who is 35 years of age or older should be advised to undergo amniocentesis to rule out the possibility of Down syndrome.

Table 12.1.   Routine Antepartum Screening

First visit
  VDRL
  Complete blood count
  Blood typing
  Antibody screen (Rh, CDE system, rare group antibodies)
  Rubella titre
  Toxoplasmosis titre
  Microscopic urinalysis
  Urine test for glucose, albumin
  Urine culture and sensitivity
  Papanicolaou smear
  1-hour glucose tolerance test
  Gonorrhea culture

Each subsequent visit
  Urine for glucose, albumin

Sixteen weeks
  α-Fetoprotein

Thirty-two weeks
  Complete blood count
  Blood typing
  Antibody screen (Rh, CDE system, rare group antibodies)

Table 12.2.   Special Antepartum Screening

Tay Sachs (both parents)
Sickle cell
Amniocentesis
   16 weeks for Down syndrome, other genetic defects
   As needed for Rh isoimmunization
   Term for foam test, LS ratio–fetal age
Ultrasonography
3 or 5 hour glucose tolerance test
Tine test

The patient is reassured that she is normally pregnant and told her estimated date of confinement. She is advised about proper rest and is instructed to eat a well-balanced high protein diet, taking into account the increased caloric requirements of pregnancy. With proper diet, the only supplementation needed in normal pregnancy is iron and folic acid, both of which can be supplied in prenatal vitamin tablets given once daily. Nonhazardous exercise is important in pregnancy. Both prospective parents are advised to enroll in childbirth classes, which are widely available.

Subsequent antenatal visits occur at intervals of 4 weeks until approximately the 28th week, then at 3-week intervals until the 32nd week, then at 2-week intervals until the 36th week, and then weekly until labor ensues. At each visit the patient is asked if any new symptoms are present, especially swelling of the feet or hands, changes in vision, or headache; all of which may be related to the development of hypertensive disorders of pregnancy. She is asked the date when fetal movement was first noted. A physical examination is carried out with particular attention to the growing fetus. The height of the uterine fundus in the maternal abdomen is measured. The fetal heart is auscultated. The presentation of the fetus is ascertained. The maternal blood pressure and weight are noted. The urine is checked for glucose and albumin.

At the 16th week of pregnancy, maternal blood is taken for α-fetoprotein, to rule out open defects of the fetal cerebrospinal system.

At 32 weeks, a complete blood count, blood typing and antibody screening are repeated.

At the 36th week of pregnancy or beyond, sterile vaginal examinations may be undertaken, if necessary to more carefully evaluate the pelvic architecture, fetal presentation and engagement, and effacement and dilatation of the cervix.

CHAPTER 13

Evaluation of Fetal Growth

MAURICE L. DRUZIN, M.B., B.Chir.

DEFINITION OF AND IDENTIFICATION OF THE HIGH RISK PREGNANCY

The high risk pregnancy can be defined as that pregnancy in which maternal and/or fetal factors give rise to an increased risk of maternal and/or fetal morbidity or mortality.

Prior to the decade of the sixties, most high risk pregnancy was looked at almost exclusively in terms of maternal risk. The philosophy of the fetus being part of the equation only evolved with newer technologies by means of which the fetus could be observed as a complex and dynamic biological unit. The fetus is now recognized as an independent entity whose fate is closely linked to the health and well-being of its carrier, the mother.

Perinatology, also known as "maternal-fetal medicine," is the term used to describe that subspeciality involved in care of the maternal-fetal unit at risk. The development of this subspeciality in obstetrics has been made possible by remarkable technological advances, by means of which the fetus and its milieu in utero can be observed without disturbance. For example, ultrasonography has been used in many forms to detect the fetal heart, to observe fetal movements and other biophysical variables and to delineate anatomical landmarks. (See Chapter 15, "Ultrasonography.")

Recognition of the high risk pregnancy is dependent on complete knowledge of conditions which may give rise to increased risk factors in both the mother and fetus, singly or in combination.

Any medical condition which affects the mother may give rise to fetal compromise (Fig. 13.1). The classical example is that of diabetes mellitus which has profound effects on both the maternal and fetal organism. Other maternal illnesses such as cardiac disease, hypertension, renal disease, hemoglobinopathies, and collagen vascular disease may have effects on both maternal and fetal outcome.

There are conditions which affect the fetus alone without any recognizable ill effects on the mother. The classical example is that of Rh sensitization. The mother, sensitized to fetal red cells, produces antibodies which cross the placenta and lead to destruction of fetal red blood cells, with subsequent anemia and possible death of the fetus. Chromosomal abnormalities, ingestion of teratogens and subclinical viral infections are other circumstances in which the fetus may be seriously compromised, with little or no ill effects on the mother.

There are other conditions in which the maternal organism will be affected but the fetus will remain free of ill effects. Examples are malignancies such as breast cancer, lymphomas and other tumors in which the fetus is not compromised by the maternal disease. However, in the course of treatment of these serious illnesses, iatrogenic fetal damage may result. In these situations, obviously maternal well-being is of paramount importance. Maternal trauma, excluding major abdominal injury, is another example.

The high risk pregnancy should be identified as early as possible in gestation, so that appropriate measures may be under-

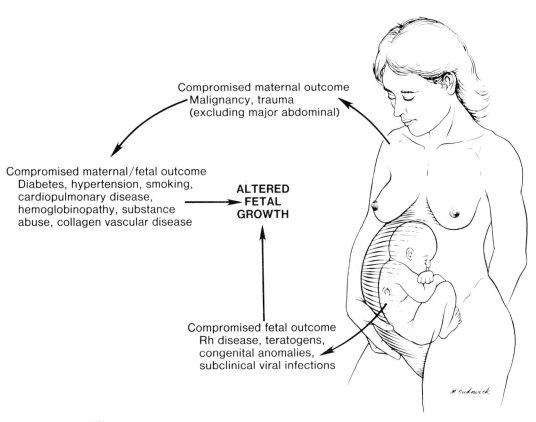

Compromised maternal outcome
Malignancy, trauma
(excluding major abdominal)

Compromised maternal/fetal outcome
Diabetes, hypertension, smoking,
cardiopulmonary disease,
hemoglobinopathy, substance
abuse, collagen vascular disease

ALTERED FETAL GROWTH

Compromised fetal outcome
Rh disease, teratogens,
congenital anomalies,
subclinical viral infections

Figure 13.1. Maternal factors that may lead to fetal compromise.

taken to minimize risks. Eliciting historical data concerning medical conditions as well as prior obstetrical history is the first step in recognition of this entity.

Careful physical examination with close follow-up and appropriate investigations will allow for the detection of the majority of at-risk pregnancies. However, some pregnancies that are so-called low risk will develop high risk factors during the gestational period or perhaps only at parturition. The importance of careful follow-up of all pregnancies cannot be overemphasized. The term *prenatal care* or *antenatal care* is used to denote the appropriate follow up of the pregnant patient prior to the onset of labor. The object of antenatal care is to have the optimal outcome in terms of infant and mother. Detailed knowledge of the physiological changes that occur in pregnancy is essential (see Chapter 7), as these changes might seem abnormal to the inexperienced observer. For example,

there is a so-called physiological anemia in the second trimester, secondary to a relatively increased plasma volume.

Thyroid function tests may mistakenly be reported as abnormal due to the increase of thyroid binding globulin that normally occurs in pregnancy. Lower limb edema is a common entity in normal pregnancy, due to obstruction of venous return by the enlarging uterus and its contents.

Physiological "flow murmurs" occur commonly in the pregnant female and there are other cardiac and electrocardiographic changes that might seem pathological.

There is dilation of smooth muscle due to the effect of high levels of progesterone. This may lead to hydroureter which disappears following delivery. Lower limb varicosities, hemorrhoids and vulvar varicosities are common.

There are conditions which are exclusively related to events of pregnancy and do not occur in nonpregnant females. The classical example is the condition known as preeclampsia/eclampsia, in which hypertension, proteinuria and edema occur, usually in the last trimester of a normal, intrauterine pregnancy. This may occur earlier in gestation in cases of hydatidiform molar disease.

To aid in the recognition of that gestation which if undiagnosed may lead to an increase in maternal and/or fetal morbidity or mortality, various problem-oriented obstetrical records and high risk scoring systems have been devised. The record should fulfill the following requirements: 1) identify problems, 2) provide guidance in the management of these problems, 3) be available for analysis in order to update management, 4) provide for education for health care personnel and 5) fulfill legal audit requirements and research purposes. These various techniques have as their goal the recording of demographic and epidemiologic data, which can be relatively easily obtained by history and physical examination. These data are then assigned various numerical values, with more important risk factors having higher values. The various risk scores are then totalled, and the final score is used to place the patient in a category of relative risk. While numerous schemes have been proposed, the end result of all has been a recognition of the pregnancy destined to be a problem either antepartum, intrapartum or postpartum.

Hobel et al.[3] categorized their patients as group I–IV based on prenatal and intrapartum factors and showed that perinatal morbidity and mortality increase from group I to group IV.

Group I was designated low-low risk, the former term referring to prenatal factors and the latter to intrapartum factors; Group II was high-low risk; group III was low-high risk; and group IV was high-high risk. While this scheme allows the practitioner to focus on the patient with risk factors and will identify most complications, cases which violate all the rules and become high risk due to a condition occurring at an unusual and unpredictable time occur relatively frequently.

In Table 13.1 are listed factors which are universally accepted as being implicated in compromised reproductive performance. It should be emphasized that the list of factors is not complete and that some factors may be historical and may also pertain to the present pregnancy.

A common and serious error is often made in consideration of risk as it applies to socioeconomic status. While certain conditions such as preeclampsia/eclampsia are more common in the underprivileged, poorly nourished population with limited access to medical care, this entity does occur in the wealthy, well-nourished population with excellent medical follow-up, albeit to a lesser degree. Living on the "right side of the tracks" is no protection against the complications of pregnancy,

Table 13.1. Factors Implicated in Compromised Childbearing

Historical	Present Pregnancy
1. Maternal age—extremes	1. Prematurity
2. Socioeconomic status—low	2. Pregnancy-induced hypertension
3. Prior stillbirth or neonatal death	3. Fetal malpresentation
4. Birth interval—decreased interval	4. Multiple gestation
5. Parity—high	5. Lack of prenatal care
6. Smoking	6. Vaginal bleeding
7. Substance abuse	7. Urinary tract infections
8. Diabetes mellitus	8. Exposure to teratogens
9. Organic heart disease	9. Prolonged labor
10. Any chronic medical condition leading to maternal hypoxemia	10. Incompetent cervix
11. Maternal hypertension	
12. Obesity	
13. Rh sensitization	
14. Hemoglobinopathies	

and less than optimal outcomes can result due to failure to recognize these problems at an early and perhaps preventable stage.

The goal of prenatal care should be recognition and prevention of potentially hazardous situations and the competent management of unpreventable situations.

FETOPLACENTAL UNIT

Mammalian development in utero is dependent on a continuing supply of nutrients from the placenta, in contrast to the lower vertebrates in which a store of yolk is available with each egg.

The placenta is an organ composed of a union of maternal and fetal tissues. The basic function is that of exchange of nutrients and waste products between fetal umbilical and maternal uterine circulations.

Chorioallantoic placentation is the principal mechanism of fetal-maternal exchange in the human organism. The basis for this type of placentation is the formation of vascular chorionic villi. These villi are in contact with the maternal endometrial surface. The number of tissue layers involved in the placental membrane gives rise to a classification of chorioallantoic placentas. The hemochorial placenta is composed of three fetal components—trophoblast, connective tissue and fetal endothelium, with the trophoblast exposed directly to maternal blood. This classification did not take into consideration the many factors that have only become possible to observe with recently developed modalities. The ultrastructure of tissues revealed by techniques such as electron microscopy and immunofluorescent staining methods reveals a complex and intricate biological system. However, the classification of placental types based on the number of tissue layers in the placental membrane is useful in understanding the transfer of compounds from the maternal to the fetal circulation and vice versa. In general, the thickness of the membrane layer determines the rate of transfer of compounds across the placenta. This applies to those compounds that cross by simple diffusion but cannot fully explain the transfer of substances by facilitated diffusion and active transport. Transfer of compounds by pinocytosis, placental breaks and bulk flow is obviously by more complex mechanisms.

For compounds moving by simple diffusion and even some compounds transferred by specific carrier systems, there appears to be an inverse relationship between the degree of permeability or rate of transfer and number of placental tissue layers, i.e., rate of transfer increases as number of layers decrease.

Development

The implantation of the blastocyst into a nutritive secretory phase endometrium marks the beginning of the fetoplacental unit which culminates in the birth of a live infant 260 days later.

By day 8, the trophoblast of the blastocyst has differentiated into a placque of syncytium and cytotrophoblast. The syncytium is responsible for local invasion of maternal tissues. The syncytium shows vacuolation with confluence of vacuoles to form laminar spaces which in turn communicate with maternal sinusoids, thus exposing the trophoblast to maternal blood. The trophoblast then proliferates around the chorion, with a resultant villous appearance, while the maternal circulation becomes well established within the intervillous space. When mesenchymal elements invade primary villi, secondary villi are formed and tertiary villi are formed with vascularization of the secondary villi. New villi are added throughout gestation, which increases the surface area of the placenta and thus provides sufficient area for nutrient exchange for the rapidly growing fetus. The permeability of the placenta increases with increasing gestational age, which is related to thinning of the syncytiotrophoblast, attenuation of the basement membrane and decrease in cytotrophoblastic cell numbers.

The structure of the mature placenta consists of cotyledons (see Chapter 5). New cotyledons are not formed after the first few weeks of placental development.

Enlargement of cotyledons occurs through continuous formation of new villi. Each villus is thus the basic unit of nutrient exchange in the placenta.

The umbilical cord is the organ which connects the fetus to its highly specialized nutritive and excretory organ, the placenta. The cord is composed of two umbilical arteries and one umbilical vein. The vein contains blood of pulmonary and portal vein origin and contains the fetal blood with the highest concentration of oxygen and other nutrients. The umbilical vein terminates in the fetal abdomen at its junctin with the ductus venosus. The umbilical arteries are continuations of fetal internal iliac arteries and carry deoxygenated blood to the placenta.

Interruption of any of the structures described above may lead to diminished supplies of nutrients from the placenta to the fetus and thus to compromized fetal outcome.

Function

The most important function of the placenta is that of exchange of substances (Fig. 13.2). Nutrients such as glucose, oxygen and amino acids are transferred by various mechanisms from the maternal to the fetal organism. Excretory products such as carbon dioxide and other metabolic waste products are transferred from the fetus to the mother to be eliminated by the maternal organism.

The transfer rate of a substance across the placenta can be calculated by application of the Fick principle. This states that the quantity transferred across the organ is the product of the arterial and venous concentration differences and the rate of blood flow to the organ. The permeability of the organ to various substances is an additional rate-determining factor in transfer of substances.

The fetal organism has specific adaptations which enable it to function successfully in a seemingly inadequate environment.

For example, the partial pressure of oxygen (pO_2) in the umbilical vein carrying oxygenated blood to the fetus is 29 mm Hg. In the adult, the pO_2 of blood perfusing the body is 95 mm Hg. The fetus has numerous mechanisms which enable it to extract sufficient amounts of oxygen for survival. The higher oxygen affinity of fetal blood is one mechanism by which the

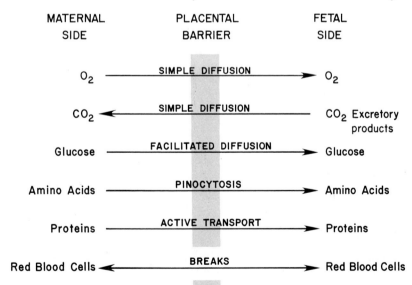

Figure 13.2.   Exchange across the placenta.

fetus accomplishes this. Fetal red blood cells bind more oxygen at a given pO_2 than do maternal red cells. The fetal oxygen dissociation curve (Fig. 13.3) is thus to the left of the maternal curve and allows the fetus to function on its "Mount Everest" in utero.

The exchange of carbon dioxide, sodium, potassium, anions, iron, calcium and magnesium are all in the direction that favors the fetus. Each of these substances has its own specific transfer mechanism. Glucose is the major metabolic fuel of the fetus. Transfer of glucose is by a mechanism of facilitated diffusion which increases the rate of transfer from a high to a low concentration. The transfer rate of glucose is extremely rapid in order to meet the increasing requirements of the developing fetus.

Amino acids are transferred by a mechanism of active transport necessary to accomplish transfer against a concentration gradient. The concentration of most amino acids is greater on the fetal than on the maternal side.

Proteins, substances of large molecular size, are transferred by a process of pinocytosis (Fig. 13.4) in which the membrane engulfs the protein on the maternal side and releases it on the fetal side.

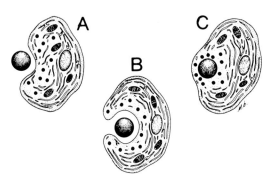

Figure 13.4.   Pinocytosis.

Water crosses the membranes by a process of osmosis, and substances such as red blood cells may cross through "breaks" in the membrane barrier.

The placenta is relatively impermeable to the polypeptide hormones, as a result of which the fetal endocrine system matures early and functions autonomously.

The placental transfer of steroids is dependent on whether these substances are conjugated or unconjugated. Unconjugated estrogens are transferred rapidly, while the conjugation with sulphates and glucosideronates decreases the transfer dramatically. Placental sulphatases cleave the sulphates and again convert these substances to unconjugated forms. Progesterone is transferred rapidly across the human placenta, while cortisone and cortisol have limited transfer potential.

Unconjugated bilirubin is rapidly transferred, while the glucosideronate is not. Glucosideronation in the fetus is suppressed so that the fetus can eliminate potentially harmful levels of unconjugated bilirubin rapidly to the maternal circulation. It is, therefore, only after birth that kernicterus (deposition of bilirubin in the basal ganglia) becomes a potential hazard.

The transfer of all other substances essential for development such as vitamins, lipids and folic acid is accomplished by various mechanisms as previously described. A defect in any of the transport mechanisms may lead to altered metabolic states and growth patterns of the developing fetus.

The term *fetoplacental unit* has been used in discussion of the synthesis of es-

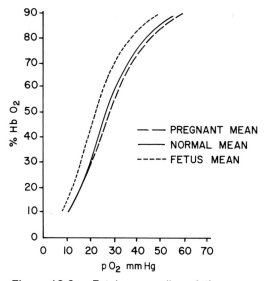

Figure 13.3.   Fetal oxygen dissociation curve.

trogens in human pregnancy. This illustrates the interdependence of the fetus, placenta and maternal circulation (Fig. 13.5). The fetal adrenal produces dehydroepiandrosterone sulphate (DHEAS) which is hydroxylated in the fetal liver to form 16-α OH DHEAS. The 16-α OH DHEAS passes to the placenta where a sulphatase removes the sulphate, allowing the further aromatization of this substance to form estriol. Estriol is then conjugated in the maternal liver and excreted in the urine. Measurements of maternal serum and/or urine levels of estriol are thus used to reflect both fetal and placental function and are interpreted as reliable indices of fetal well-being.

INTRAUTERINE GROWTH RETARDATION (IUGR)

The fetoplacental unit is vulnerable to potential disruption which will substan-

tially alter fetal growth. In general, placental size and birth weight have a linear relationship. At term, the fetal:placental weight ratio is relatively constant at 6:1.

Interruption of nutrient supply to the fetus may occur at many points in the supply line. Decreased placental perfusion occurs with decrease in maternal cardiac output, such as in heart disease, while decreased oxygen-carrying capacity occurs in the hemoglobinopathies and in pulmonary disease. Maternal hypertension and collagen vascular disease cause placental vascular pathology with subsequent compromised placental blood flow. Cigarette smoking and drug abuse cause decreased fetal oxygenation by various mechanisms, while teratogens such as alcohol and viruses exert profound direct effects on developing fetal tissues and lead to developmental abnormalities.

Approximately 7–20% of all neonates are of low birth weight (less than 2500 g).

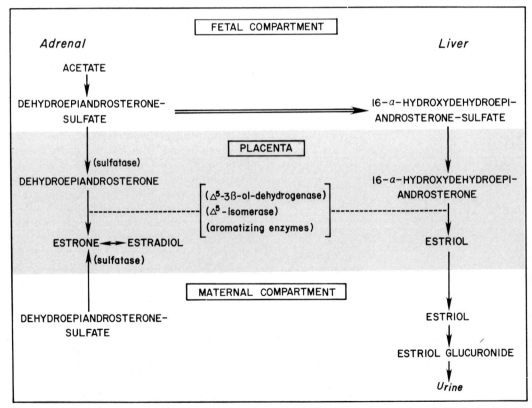

Figure 13.5. Hormone synthesis in the fetoplacental unit, with excretion of estriol in the maternal urine.

However, 30% of these neonates are actually mature, (37 weeks or more gestational age) and can be clearly distinguished from their premature weight peers on clinical, metabolic, morphological, biochemical and developmental grounds.

Gestational age is expressed as time elapsed since the first day of the mother's last normal menstrual period (LNMP>). The variability of the preovulatory phase in any given menstrual cycle makes this landmark unreliable at times but this remains the best single, clinical estimate of gestational age. The normal full-term pregnancy lasts 40 weeks, or 280 days, calculated from the first day of the LNMP. Ovulation age is generally 14 days less than menstrual age and is used to describe actual embryonic age.

Discrepancy between the gestational age and the expected fetal weight at birth has given rise to the concept of the dysmature infant. The classification of infants into SGA (small for gestational age), birth weight <10th percentile, AGA (appropriate for gestational age), birth weight between 10th and 90th percentile, and LGA (large for gestational age), birth weight >90th percentile, has simplified the understanding of altered fetal growth patterns (Fig. 13.6, A and B).

The LGA infant is often the product of a pregnancy of a diabetic mother, in whom high glucose levels lead to fetal hyperinsulinemia and increased fetal weight with profound metabolic effects on the newborn infant.

Although there are multiple factors controlling fetal growth, the dysmature infant, whether SGA or LGA, is at some disadvantage in terms of prognosis for future normal growth and development.

Definition

There are various synonyms used in the discussion of the infant that is of less than expected weight for a particular gestational age e.g., chronically malnourished fetus, light-for-dates or small-for-dates infant, growth retarded fetus, undergrown fetus and SGA fetus.

All of these terms refer to the infant whose weight falls below the 10th percentile for its gestational age[1] or 2 standard

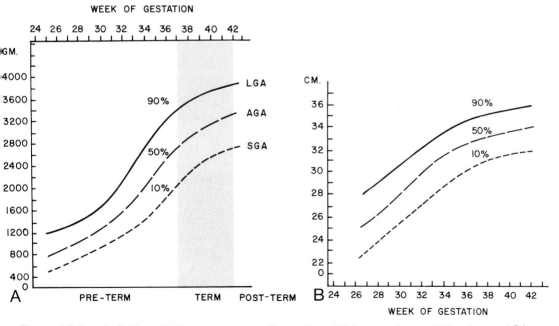

Figure 13.6. *A.* Birth weight at given ages of gestation. LGA, large for gestational age; AGA, appropriate for gestational age; SGA, small for gestational age. *B.* Head circumference of fetus at given ages of gestation.

deviations from the mean of values of birth weight.[4] Rates of perinatal mortality, neonatal hypoglycemia, hypocalcemia, pulmonary hemorrhage and intrapartum asphyxia are all increased in SGA infants. Long-term effects in the form of neurologic handicaps are also increased.

Etiology

Many etiological factors are known to cause IUGR, but there are a substantial number of cases in which no etiological factors are found. The most common and well-known causes of retarded fetal growth are discussed here.

MATERNAL CONDITIONS LEADING TO DECREASED UTEROPLACENTAL BLOOD FLOW

Maternal vascular disease is implicated in approximately 30% of cases of IUGR. Hypertension, collagen vascular disease, cardiac disease and hemoglobinopathies are relatively common causes of decreased placental perfusion. However, any condition leading to decreased oxygen transfer secondary to maternal hypoxemia may result in growth retardation. Treatment of these disorders can result in minimizing the effect on the fetus.

CHROMOSOMAL, GENETIC, INFECTIOUS FACTORS; TERATOGENS

These factors account for approximately 10% of growth retarded fetuses. While chromosomal and genetic factors are not at present amenable to therapy, diagnosis of these cases allows selective termination of the pregnancy, if desired. New techniques may become available for treatment of infections. Exposure to teratogens can be minimized.

NUTRITIONAL FACTORS

The general teaching that malnutrition results in IUGR has not been substantiated in well-controlled studies except in cases of extreme deprivation such as in wartime Holland and Biafra. The studies show that the fetus retains its ability to receive adequate substrate from the maternal organism up to extreme levels of malnutrition.

PLACENTAL FACTORS

Placental and cord defects account for only a small number of cases of IUGR. Infarction, fibrosis, chronic villous inflammation and premature aging are associated with altered fetal growth.

Clinical Considerations

The importance of early recognition of this entity is that the obstetrician can then be alerted to intervene to minimize the effects of any known risk factors. Delivery of the fetus when the intrauterine environment becomes potentially hazardous may be the only option in management.

Antenatal diagnosis of the growth retarded fetus occurs in only 30% of cases.

When identifiable maternal disorders such as hypertension, preeclampsia, substance abuse, smoking, renal disease or hypoxemia are present, up to 75% of cases are identified in the antenatal period.

Diagnosis

The diagnosis of IUGR is difficult and the false-positive rate can be as high as 60%, i.e., only about 40% of newborns expected to be growth retarded turn out to be so. Only about 30% of growth retarded fetuses are diagnosed in the antepartum period.

Any patient with the previously described risk factors should be under surveillance for the possible development of IUGR.

Symmetrical growth retardation, in which the decrease in growth occurs earlier than 28 weeks and affects all organ systems, is seen with chromosomal abnormalities, other congenital anomalies, and maternal cigarette smoking or drug abuse.

Asymmetrical growth retardation, which occurs usually after 28 weeks, is seen with maternal hypertension, hemoglobinopathies and hypoxemia. There is thought to be "head sparing," in which all available nutrients seem to be diverted to that vital organ—the developing brain. This effect is maintained to approximately weeks 34–36, beyond which brain growth is affected.

Clinical factors which lead to the antepartum diagnosis of IUGR include: recognition of risk factors, poor maternal weight gain, lack of fundal growth and previous SGA infants.

Use of sonography has been of great importance, while measurements of serum or urinary estriols and serum levels of human placental lactogen give additional information.

Hobbins and Berkowitz[2] have utilized sonography to calculate the total intrauterine volume (TIUV) by measuring the greatest longitudinal (L) transverse (T) and anteroposterior (AP) diameter and applying the formula for the volume of an ellipse (0.5233 × L × T × AP). The TIUV is then plotted against gestational age and a normogram has been developed. There is a "normal" zone, a "gray" zone and an "abnormal zone" (Fig. 13.7). When TIUV was below the gray zone, the infants were in the 10th percentile for body weight. Those with TIUV above the gray zone were above the 10th percentile for body weight.

Approximately 10% of fetuses with IUGR have anomalies, most commonly trisomy 21, trisomy 18, neural tube defects and Potter's syndrome. IUGR also occurs in fetuses with multiple congenital anomalies. Many of these anomalies can be diagnosed by sonography.

Management of IUGR

Once the diagnosis of IUGR has been made, the following steps should be undertaken:

1. Treatment of any known risk factors such as hypertension, cardiac disease, etc.
2. Substance abusers and cigarette smokers should undergo intensive medical and psychological therapy

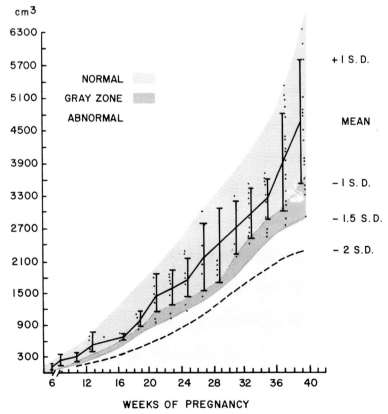

Figure 13.7.   Total intrauterine volume for gestational age. SD: standard deviation.

to reduce their use of these substances.

3. Bed rest in the left lateral recumbent position is thought to increase uterine blood flow.
4. Biweekly determination of serum estriols or 24-hour urinary estriols will give some idea of fetoplacental function.
5. Biweekly antepartum fetal heart rate testing (AFHRT) should be performed. Normal AFHRT is a reliable predictor of fetal health for up to 7 days.
6. If all parameters of fetal well-being are stable, amniocentesis for determination of fetal pulmonary maturity is performed at 36 weeks' gestation.
7. With fetal pulmonary maturity, most authorities would proceed with delivery.
8. Vaginal delivery is undertaken with a favorable cervix and intensive intrapartum fetal monitoring.
9. Cesarean section is performed if safe vaginal delivery cannot be accomplished.
10. Delivery of these neonates should be done in a tertiary care center where intensive neonatal care can be undertaken.

It has recently been shown that intensive management of the IUGR pregnancy and newborn can result in a high percentage of normal, long-term outcomes.

References

1. Battaglia, F.C., and Lubchenco, L.O. A practical classification of newborn infants by weight and gestational age. *J. Pediatr.* 71:159, 1967.
2. Hobbins, J.C., and Berkowitz, R.L. Ultrasonography in the diagnosis of intrauterine growth retardation. *Clin. Obstet. Gynecol.* 20:4, 1977.
3. Hobel, C.J., Hyvarinen, M.A., Okada, D.M., et al. Prenatal and intrapartum high-risk screening: I. Prediction of the high-risk neonate. *Am. J. Obstet. Gynecol.* 117:1, 1973.
4. Usher, R., and McLean, F. Intrauterine growth of liveborn Caucasian infants at sea level: Standards obtained from measurements in 7 dimensions of infants born between 25 and 44 weeks of gestation. *J. Pediatr.* 24:901, 1969.

CHAPTER 14

Lie, Position and Presentation

RONALD M. CAPLAN, M.D.

PELVIC EXAMINATION IN THE FIRST TRIMESTER

The examination of the pelvis when the patient is first seen in early pregnancy serves three purposes: to confirm the presence of an intrauterine pregnancy and its size in relation to the length of gestation; to evaluate the pelvic organs and rule out pathology; and to evaluate the structure of the bony pelvis (see chapter on "Pelvimetry").

The external genitalia are first inspected (see chapter on "Anatomy"). Particular attention is given to palpation of the Bartholin and the Skene glands. The vaginal walls are gently inspected with the aid of a speculum. Any descent of the anterior or posterior vaginal wall is noted. The cervix is visualized. In pregnancy, the cervix is typically cyanosed, giving it a blue or purple appearance. On palpation, the cervix in pregnancy is soft. A Papanicolaou smear should be taken.

With bimanual palpation, the uterus will be felt to be globular and the junction of cervix and uterus, the lower uterine segment, will be soft, giving Hegar's sign—a feeling of partial separation between the uterus and the cervix. Attention should be given to the size, shape, consistency, position and mobility of the uterus. On bimanual palpation of the adnexal regions, one ovary will often be felt to be enlarged and tense, representing the corpus luteum of pregnancy.

EVALUATION OF PELVIC ARCHITECTURE

The fingers of the examiner's hand should be slid posteriorly along the curve of the sacrum from the vaginal introitus to the sacral promontory (Fig. 14.1).

The sacrum will ideally be short and describe a gentle curve. The promontory will not easily be reached in a gynecoid pelvis. The distance from the inferior border of the pubis to the sacral promontory is the diagonal conjugate, and from this manual measurement the anteroposterior length of the pelvic inlet, or true conjugate, can be deduced by subtracting $1\frac{1}{2}$ cm.

The fingers should then be brought around the sacrosciatic notch to the ischial spines. The notch should be wide, and the spines ideally should be blunt and set back. Alternately, the spines may be reached by palpating vaginally from the sacrum along the sacrospinous ligament. An impression should be garnered of the lateral pelvic walls, which should be parallel and not funnelling down toward the vaginal introitus.

The examining fingers should be slid along the inferior pelvic rami, thus evaluating the subpubic angle, which should be greater than 90 degrees.

Lastly, the distance between the ischial tuberosities should be measured. This distance should be greater than 8.5 cm (Fig. 14.2). A rectovaginal examination is an integral part of the pelvic examination, to

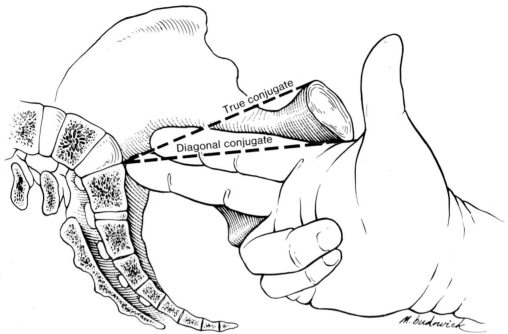

Figure 14.1.   The diagonal conjugate and the true conjugate.

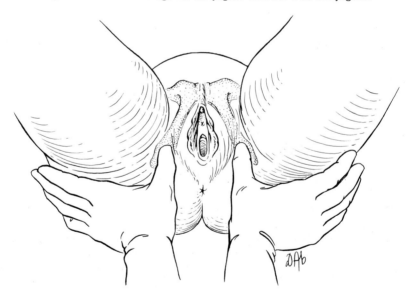

Figure 14.2.   Palpation of the ischial tuberosities.

rule out any masses behind the uterus in the cul-de-sac (pouch of Douglas).

EVALUATION OF FETAL AGE AND SIZE

At the twelfth week of pregnancy (by convention counting from the first day of the last normal menstrual period: that is, approximately 10 weeks from the conception date in a woman with a 28-day cycle) the uterus is large enough to be palpated out of the pelvis. By 14 weeks, the uterine fundus can be palpated two fingerbreadths above the symphysis pubis. It reaches midway between the pubis and umbilicus at

16 weeks, is approximately two finger-breadths below the umbilicus at 18 weeks, and generally reaches the maternal umbilicus at 20 weeks of gestation, midway through the pregnancy. At 24 weeks, by which time the mother should definitely be feeling fetal movement, the fundus is often palpable two fingerbreadths above the umbilicus, at 28 weeks four fingerbreadths, and by 36 weeks it reaches the xiphoid process. In the last weeks of pregnancy, if engagement occurs, some descent of the fundus might be noted.

Various measurements of the size of the uterus have been proposed. Commonly, fundal height is measured from the superior aspect of the pubis to the top of the uterus. This linear measurement has very limited value, as the growing uterus is three-dimensional and the fetus within is only one of several components being measured as a unit.

If there is any question as to the adequacy of fetal growth, other tests must be performed (see chapter on "Evaluation of Fetal Growth").

LIE, PRESENTATION AND POSITION

It is essential to know in what way the fetus will be entering the pelvis in labor. This is defined in terms of lie, presentation and position.

The *lie* refers to the location of the long axis of the fetus in relation to the maternal long axis and is ideally *longitudinal* (Fig. 14.3), so that the long axis of the fetus is parallel to that of the mother. Thus, in a longitudinal lie, either the fetal head or alternately the breech (buttocks) enters the pelvis. *Transverse* and *oblique* lies may also occur. In such abnormal cases, a shoulder, arm, or part of the trunk may enter the pelvis.

The part of the fetus which is entering the pelvis is called the *presenting part*, thus defining the *presentation* which may commonly be *cephalic* (head) or less commonly *breech* (buttocks). Rarely, as previously described, a *shoulder* presentation occurs, in the case of a transverse lie.

The fetal presenting part may enter the maternal pelvis in various *positions* (Figs. 14.3–14.5). These positions are described

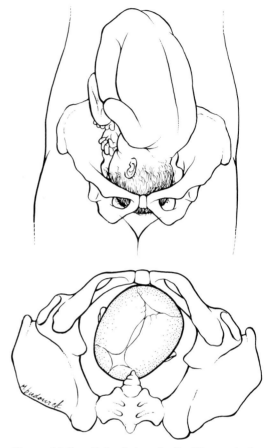

Figure 14.3. Fetus in longitudinal lie, cephalic presentation, left occiput anterior position. With the fetal head well flexed, the posterior (three-sided) fontanelle is easily palpable on vaginal examination, but the anterior (four-sided) fontanelle is not.

by noting the relationship between the leading feature of the presenting part and the pelvis. In the case of the well-flexed fetal head, the *occiput* leads; it is therefore the relationship of the occiput to the maternal pelvis that most commonly is used to denote position. If the head is extended (brow presentation) the brow leads, and the position is defined by the relation of the *frontum* (forehead) to the maternal pelvis. Extreme extension leads to a face presentation, with the *mentum* (chin) leading. This flexion or extension of the fetus is known as its *attitude* (Fig. 14.6).

In a breech presentation, the *sacrum* is

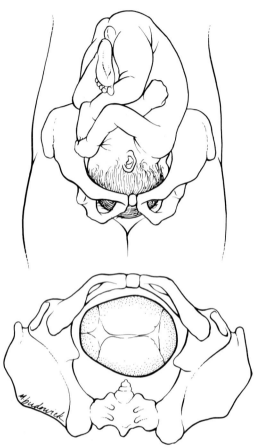

Figure 14.4. Longitudinal lie, cephalic presentation, left occiput transverse position. The fetal sagittal suture is in a transverse position.

used as the reference point to define the position of the fetus in the maternal pelvis. However, in a breech presentation the buttocks lead only in the case of a *frank breech* (Fig. 14.7), where there is complete flexion at the hip joints and complete extension of the knee joints, so that the legs are flexed "straight up" along the body. In the case of a *complete breech*, where hips and knees are both flexed, the buttocks lead but the feet are palpable vaginally. If there is extension at the hips and knees, a foot (or both feet as the case may be) presents: the so-called *footling* (or double footling) *breech*. However, the sacrum is still used in these cases to define position.

In the rarer transverse or oblique lie, as the shoulder often presents, the *scapula* is

used to define position in relation to the maternal pelvis.

LEOPOLD'S MANEUVERS

In order to ascertain the lie, position and presentation of the fetus, abdominal palpation is carried out. Leopold's maneuvers are a systematic way of achieving this. In the first maneuver (Fig. 14.8A), the fetal presenting part is grasped gently between the thumb and fingers. If the presenting part is the head, it will be smooth, hard and globular, as opposed to the buttocks. Moreover, the head is "balloteable" in the amniotic fluid: that is, it can be pushed gently posteriorly and will return. During the second maneuver (Fig. 14.8B), the examiner places one hand abdominally on

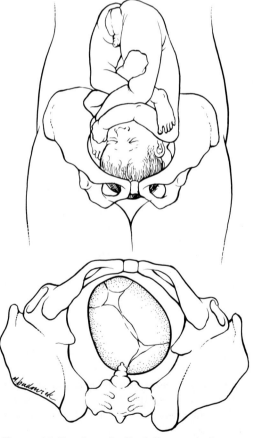

Figure 14.5. Longitudinal lie, cephalic presentation, left occiput posterior position.

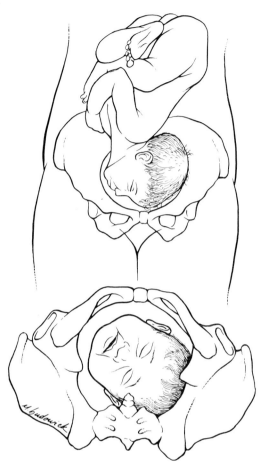

Figure 14.6. Extended attitude, face presentation.

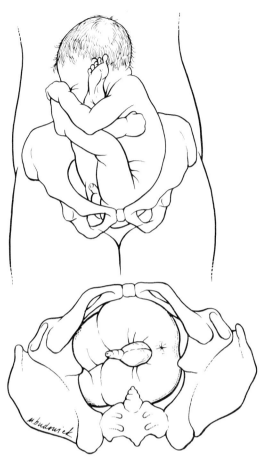

Figure 14.7. Frank breech presentation; left sacrum transverse position.

each side of the uterus from below, thus palpating the fetal spine and limbs and determining their location. In the third maneuver (Fig. 14.8C), both hands are used to examine the fundus of the uterus. During this maneuver the presentation becomes more obvious, because of the difference in palpation of the pole of the fetus here to that palpated in the first maneuver. The fetal buttocks will be found to be softer and less symmetrical. In the fourth maneuver (Fig. 14.8D), the presenting part is palpated from above. If this is the head, the examiner's two hands will diverge as they start around the sphere, then partially converge again if the head is not engaging. Moreover, as palpation downward is done, resistance should first be met by the hand

on the side opposite the fetal spine, if the fetal head is well flexed.

DIAGNOSIS OF MULTIPLE PREGNANCY

The presence of more than one fetus may be suggested by history and be confirmed by physical examination and tests.

There may be a familial tendency to twinning. Multiple pregnancy may be suspected in the previously infertile patient who has taken ovulation-inducing agents. The patient may note an inordinate increase in size and weight, and late in pregnancy she may note shortness of breath. On examination, rapid weight gain may be noted. The fundus may be higher in the

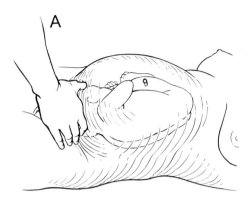

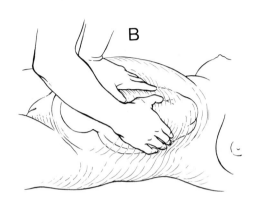

Figure 14.8.   The four Leopold maneuvers.

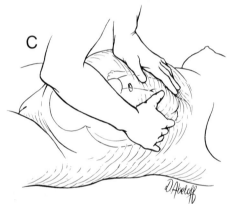

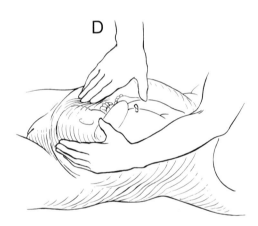

maternal abdomen than the estimated date of confinement would suggest, and the general size of the uterus might on inspection be larger than expected. Leopold's maneuvers should reveal the presence of more than one fetal head, and each palpated fetus should be somewhat small in relation to the total uterine size. If two fetal stethoscopes are used, it may be possible to define separate heartbeats by simultaneously counting and detecting a difference in rate of at least 20 beats per minute.

Ultrasonography can be used to definitively demonstrate the fetuses and to determine presentation and fetal head size.

Bibliography

1. Dennen, E.H. *Forceps Deliveries*. F.A. Davis, Philadelphia, 1955.
2. Oxorn, H., and Foote, W.R. *Human Labor and Birth*, ed. 3. Appleton—Century—Crofts, New York, 1975.
3. Taylor, E. S. *Beck's Obstetrical Practice*, ed. 8. Williams & Wilkins, Baltimore, 1966.

Monitoring the Pregnancy

CHAPTER 15

Ultrasonography

ZOLTAN SAARY, M.D.

The accelerated use of ultrasound in obstetrics has undoubtedly played a major role in improving the quality of prenatal care as well as fetal outcome over the past few years. Since the pioneer work of Donald and Abdulla[2] in the late 1960s, obstetrical applications are ever expanding and no modern prenatal facility can function well without easy access to sonography. Although new technology has made the examinations easy, quick and safe, the interpretation of ultrasound images (sonograms) still requires knowledge and experience.

The higher expectations for better perinatal outcome have necessitated ultrasound scanning of one of every three pregnant women in recent years. The introduction of highly advanced "real-time" equipment has provided the examiner with simple and relatively inexpensive machines for prenatal scanning from the fifth week following the last menstrual period (LMP) throughout the pregnancy.

PHYSICAL BACKGROUND

Sound frequencies above 20,000 cycles per second (cps) are in the ultrasound range. Diagnostic ultrasound equipment generally operates with 1–7 million cps (1–7 MHz). In obstetrics, 3.5 MHz is considered satisfactory.

The high-frequency sound is generated by a disc-shaped piezoelectric crystal based in the center of the transducer. When this crystal is exposed to electrical impulses, it transforms the impulses into acoustical pulses to be transmitted to the patient by the transducer. The high-frequency sound is extremely directional and travels through the body tissues as a narrow beam. Reflection of the sound will occur when it meets an interface between two different tissue densities. The reflections are called "echoes." The strongest echoes are produced by an interface representing the highest tissue density (i.e., bone tissue). The reflected echoes are then converted to electrical signals and displayed as spots of light by the cathode-ray tube of the equipment. The different types of displays are called A, B (cross-sectional) and M-mode, gray-scale and real-time displays. For routine obstetrical work, gray-scale and especially real-time displays are acceptable. M-mode is usually reserved for detection of fetal heart motion in utero. The gray-scale is able to store and display many different levels of brightness simultaneously, adding a "texture" to the scan. Visualization of fine structures becomes possible, together with a better outline of the organs examined. The real-time instruments have the additional advantage of being able to detect motion of certain objects, i.e., fetal motion (FM) and fetal heart motion (FHM). This makes them especially useful in diagnostic obstetrics.

SAFETY OF ULTRASOUND

The two major biological effects caused by ultrasound are *thermal change* and *cavitation* (bubble formation). Ultrasound used for physical therapy can cause significant heat change in tissues but diagnostic equipment works with much less energy. Cavitation will be caused only by intensity levels high above the normal. Based on experimental and human data, it seems that diagnostic ultrasound is harmless to mammalian tissues when used in the conventional way with a justified clinical indication.

ULTRASOUND IN EARLY PREGNANCY

Indications:

1. Uterine bleeding or spotting
2. Pelvic pain
3. Suspected ectopic pregnancy
4. Date/size discrepancy
   Missed or incomplete abortion, multiple gestation, hydatidiform mole, pelvic mass, etc.
5. High risk pregnancy
6. Habitual abortions

The patient's bladder always should be full when ultrasound examination is performed. This will provide the examiner with a "sonic window" to look through. The enlarged bladder will also change the relatively caudal position of the uterus into a more favorable cranial position, allowing better visualization of the adnexal areas as well.

The gestational sac (GS) can be seen in utero between 5 and 12 weeks of pregnancy (Fig. 15.1). The gestational age can

also be estimated by measuring the diameter of the GS. Because of wide variations in size and shape, it is more accurate to measure the crown-rump-length (CRL) of the fetus between 7 and 14 weeks of gestation (Fig. 15.2). After that, the fetal head becomes well defined and the biparietal diameter (BPD) can be taken throughout

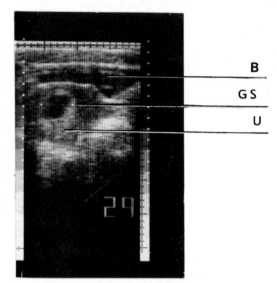

Figure 15.1. 7-weeks gestational sac (*GS*) in utero, with maternal bladder (*B*) showing anterior to uterus (*U*).

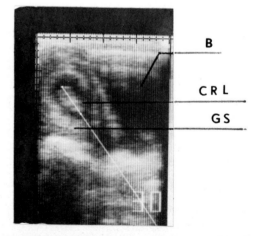

Figure 15.2. 30-mm crown-rump-length (*CRL*) of a 10-weeks fetus within the gestational sac (*GS*).

the pregnancy. At $7\frac{1}{2}$ or 8 weeks, FM becomes visible and from the eighth week on FHM can also be observed with real-time scanning. These fetal functions are considered the most important sonographic signs of fetal viability in utero. At 11 or 12 weeks, early placental formation may be observed and by the 14th week the placental margins can be localized with a clear outline of the chorionic plate (Fig. 15.3).

Differentiation between adnexal enlargements and IUP may be done in the first trimester by identifying the GS with fetal echoes in utero (Fig. 15.4). Slight uterine enlargement with cystic or semicystic adnexal mass might be suggestive of an ectopic gestation. At times, an active fetus can be detected outside the uterus, confirming the diagnosis of an ectopic pregnancy.

Hydatidiform mole can safely be recognized with ultrasound by observing the hydropic villi in utero. The enlarged uterine cavity is completely filled with echoes, resembling an extremely thick, edematous placenta (Fig. 15.5). Enlarged cystic ovaries

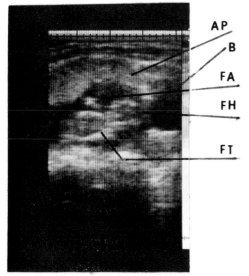

Figure 15.3. IUP at 15 weeks. Anterior placenta (*AP*), fetal arm (*FA*), fetal head (*FH*) and fetal trunk (*FT*) are well outlined.

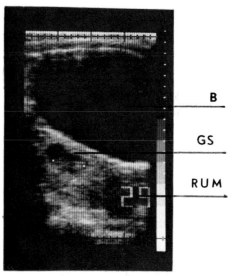

Figure 15.4. IUP at $9\frac{1}{2}$ weeks. Gestational sac (*GS*) with fetal echoes in utero. Retrouterine, semicystic mass (*RUM*) in the cul-de-sac.

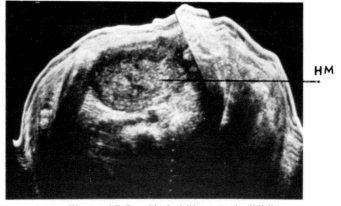

Figure 15.5. Hydatidiform mole (*HM*).

(lutein cysts) may also be observed on either side of the uterus.

Visualization of two or more GSs in utero is no longer considered to be reliable evidence of multiple gestation. Demonstration of more than one fetus is the most precise finding in plural gestation (Fig. 15.6). Follow-up sonograms are always indicated for correct dating and for detection of possible fetal anomalies that are more frequently associated with multiple gestation.

FETAL BIPARIETAL DIAMETER (ULTRASONIC CEPHALOMETRY)

The longest distance between the two parietal bones of the fetal head is called the biparietal diameter (BPD). If taken in the correct plane, the so-called midline echo should be seen as a straight line perpendicular to the BPD in equal distance from both parietal bones. The BPD can be measured directly on the screen with electric calipers, which are built-in to most newly developed models. The midline echo is thought to be caused by an interface between the two hemispheres of the fetal brain (Fig. 15.7).

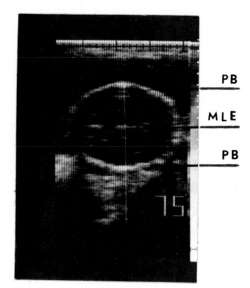

Figure 15.7.   BPD at 30 weeks. Parietal bones (*PB*) with midline echo (*MLE*).

The fetal head is readily recognized from 12 to 14 weeks on. It is estimated that the BPD increases rapidly between 12 and 24 weeks (3 mm/week), slower between 25 and 30 weeks (2 mm/week) and slowest from 31 weeks until term (1.7 mm/week). The growth rate of the fetal head can be followed by serial BPDs (Fig. 15.8). For accurate results the first measurement should be taken between 16 and 24 weeks, then repeated at 2–4 week intervals. Because of biological variations, there is a ±10–14 day range in standard errors during the second and a ±14–21 day range during the third trimester in BPD measurements. The growth rate of twins is about the same until 30–32 weeks and then the combined weight gain of both seems to be the same as that gained by a single fetus.[3] Interestingly enough, the BPD of twins remains just about the same or only slightly below those of single gestations even in the third trimester of pregnancy. This observation is explained by the "sparing" of the fetal brain. (See Chapter 13: "Evaluation of Fetal Growth.")

It has been recognized that intrauterine growth retardation (IUGR) cannot be diagnosed by serial BPDs only. Since IUGR is usually associated with oligohydram-

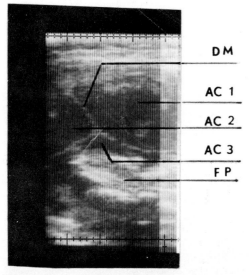

Figure 15.6.   Triplets at 18 weeks. Note the dividing membranes (*DM*) among three amniotic cavities (*AC1, AC2, AC3*), with fetal parts (*FP*) in *AC3*.

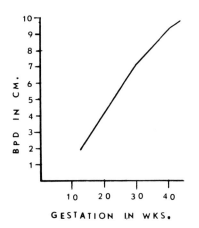

Figure 15.8. BPD growth curve between 12 and 44 weeks of gestation.

nios and microsomia, serial measurement of total intrauterine volume (TIUV) appears to be a more reliable method. Convincing results were found recently by taking head-to-body ratios.[4] It is known that until 34 weeks of pregnancy the circumference of the head is normally larger than the abdominal circumference measured at the level of the umbilical vein. Following that, the abdomen becomes larger. In IUGR this ratio is reversed, resulting in a consistently smaller fetal abdomen after the 34th week of gestation. Therefore, the most reliable way of diagnosing IUGR is to combine the estimated fetal weight with ultrasonic head-to-body ratio measurements. In addition, a number of congenital anomalies may also be detected by ultrasonography.

PLACENTAL LOCALIZATION

Indications:

1. Bleeding during the second or third trimester
2. Amniocentesis (genetic or fetal maturity studies)
3. High risk pregnancy
4. Abruptio placentae

A surprisingly large number of placentas are found in the lower uterine segment during the second trimester, most of them being consistent with different degrees of placenta previa (Fig. 15.9). It is important to note that 80–85% of these low-lying placentas will "migrate" into the upper uterine segment by the end of gestation.[5] This phenomenon is thought to be related to the formation and lengthening of the lower uterine segment, as well as to changes in the fetoplacental ratio during the third trimester. Repeat examinations are therefore necessary to identify true cases of placenta previa.

Localization of the placenta must be done immediately prior to amniocentesis in order to decrease the risk of placental or fetal injury. With sonography, many times a small "window" or a thin placental segment can be found even with anterior implantation. The presence of round echo-free areas within the placenta after 34 weeks may be considered as a sonographic sign of fetal maturity.[6]

Significant *placental thickening* is observed in *diabetes* and *Rh sensitization*. In *abruptio placentae* due to retroplacental blood accumulation, the thickened placenta can be seen bulging into the amniotic cavity. *Polyhydramnios or oligohydramnios* can readily be recognized by ultrasonography. A quick real-time scanning is invaluable in *questionable fetal presentation*.

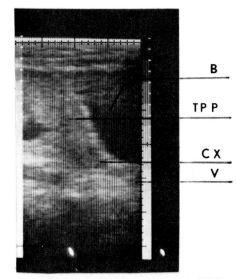

Figure 15.9. Total placenta previa (TPP) at 18 weeks. Cervix (*CX*) and vagina (*V*) also visible.

VISUALIZATION OF FETAL ANATOMY AND DETECTION OF CONGENITAL ANOMALIES

With special equipment, details of the fetal heart (septum, valves and chambers) can be studied from the second trimester on. The fetal spine (Fig. 15.10), spinal canal, kidneys and bladder usually become visible from 16 to 18 weeks together with fetal respiratory movements, the significance of which is yet to be understood.

A number of major congenital anomalies can be uncovered by ultrasound, especially those affecting the shape and/or size of the fetus.

Fetal Head and Spine

For reliable diagnosis of *hydrocephaly* or *microcephaly*, repeat ultrasound is required. *Anencephaly* (Fig. 15.11) or *meningomyelocele* can strongly be suspected by single study. If supported by elevated AFP levels, the sonographic finding should be considered diagnostic, although radiographic confirmation may be necessary. In advanced cases of intrauterine *fetal death*, marked deformity of the fetal head is the leading sign. With real-time scanning the absence of FHM is readily recognized.

Chest, Abdomen and Genitourinary Tract

With high resolution real-time equipment supplemented with M-mode scan,

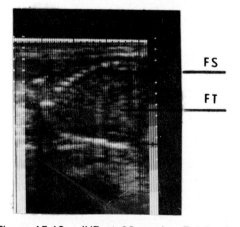

Figure 15.10. IUP at 28 weeks. Fetal spine (*FS*) and fetal trunk (*FT*) are seen.

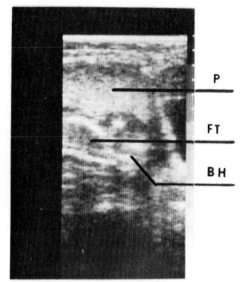

Figure 15.11. Anencephalus at about 19 weeks. Fetal trunk (*FT*) and the base of fetal head (*BH*) are shown. The placenta (*P*) is anterior.

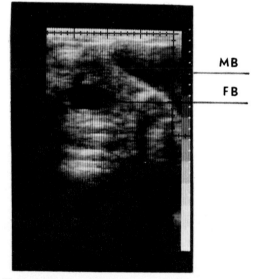

Figure 15.12. Fetal (*FB*) and maternal bladder (*MB*) at 36 weeks in breech presentation.

visualization of the fetal heart can be an important source of information. Occasionally, *cystic structures* may also be seen in the fetal chest. *Fetal ascites* can be detected with ultrasound and is usually associated with obstruction or other anomalies of the GU tract. Increased abdominal circumference with medial displacement of the abdominal organs are suggestive signs in this respect. *Normal kidneys* can easily be seen next to the spine bilaterally. Observation of the *fetal bladder* (Fig. 15.12) speaks for functioning kidneys; however an extremely distended bladder with or without hydronephrosis may suggest *obstruction in the GU tract. Polycystic kidneys* and *solitary cysts* were reportedly diagnosed by ultrasound.[1]

Although much attention has been directed toward determining *fetal sex* in utero, the results are not convincing. Chromosomal analysis of the fetal cells still remains the best method.

References

1. Caffe, S., Rose, J.S., Godmillow, L., Walker, A., Kerenyi, T., Beratis, N., Reyes, P., and Hirshorn, K. Prenatal diagnosis of renal anomalies. *Am. J. Hum. Genet.* 1:241, 1977.
2. Donald, I., and Abdulla, U. Ultrasonics in obstetrics and gynecology. *Br. J. Radiol.* 40:604, 1967.
3. Dow, E., and Walker, J. Growth differences in twin pregnancy. *Br. J. Clin. Pract.* 29:150, 1975.
4. Hobbins, J.C., and Berkowitz, R.L. Ultrasonography in the diagnosis of IUGR. *Clin. Obstet. Gynecol.* 20:957, 1977.
5. King, D.L. Placental migration demonstrated by ultrasonography: A hypothesis of dynamic placentation. *Radiology* 109:167, 1973.
6. Winsberg, F. Echographic changes with placental aging. *J. Clin. Ultrasound* 1:52, 1973.

CHAPTER 16

Prenatal Diagnosis of Genetic Disorders

JOE LEIGH SIMPSON, M.D.
MARION S. VERP, M.D.

GENETIC COUNSELING

The object of genetic counseling is to communicate relevant genetic information to consulting patients. This information should include facts about the specific genetic disorder(s) for which the patient is at risk, estimate of the occurrence or recurrence risks for the disorder, information concerning methods of carrier detection, antenatal diagnosis, and alternative reproductive options.

In order to perform these functions properly, the counselor must first obtain sufficient information to provide an accurate diagnosis. In addition, the numbers and relationship of affected members of a family must be ascertained in order to discern the pattern of inheritance.

After the diagnosis and inheritance pattern have been established, the counselor should convey information about the disorder in understandable language. Anxiety, denial, and repression frequently prevent patients from comprehending the information offered; thus, it may be necessary to repeat the data several times.

Often the counseling session has been requested by a patient who is concerned about future reproductive risks. The counselor must detail these risks, contrasting them with the risks for other genetic disorders and with the risk that any member of the general population has for the dis-

order. Finally, a patient must be told of her reproductive alternatives, e.g., antenatal diagnosis with selective abortion, artificial insemination, and sterilization, and must be allowed to choose the most compatible alternative in a noncoercive atmosphere.

TECHNIQUE AND SAFETY OF AMNIOCENTESIS

In order to diagnose genetic disorders in utero, amniocentesis is usually required to obtain viable amniotic cells that have desquamated into the amniotic liquor. Amniocentesis, the aspiration of amniotic fluid, is best performed at 16 weeks' gestation, because initiating studies then allows sufficient time to culture cells and to exercise options concerning reproductive outcome.

Technique (Fig. 16.1)

Amniocentesis is performed after ultrasonography localizes the placenta, measures the fetal head size, and determines whether an abnormal or multiple gestation is present. A 20- or 21-gauge spinal needle is passed transabdominally into the uterus, from which 35 cc of amniotic fluid is withdrawn. At this stage of gestation, 225 cc are present, with rapid replacement of removed volume. The amniotic fluid can then be directly assayed or, more commonly, its cells can be grown for 3–4

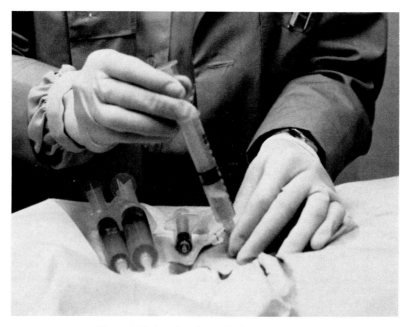

Figure 16.1 Amniocentesis in progress.

weeks, followed by chromosomal analysis or biochemical assay.

Amniocentesis has potential maternal and fetal risks. Maternal risks appear to be very rare. For example, the risk of amnionitis is about 0.1%. Rh-immunization can occur if the mother is Rh negative and the fetus Rh positive. It is thus recommended that anti-Rh (D) immune globulin be administered to Rh-negative women following amniocentesis.

Potential risks to the fetus include bleeding, needle puncture, injuries indirectly induced by aspiration of amniotic fluid and, ultimately, spontaneous abortion or fetal death through several possible mechanisms, such as placental separation. Such injuries have been extremely rare. There is an increased risk of fetal loss secondary to amniocentesis, estimated to be 0.5–1.0% over the background of 2–3% expected for any pregnancy from 16 weeks' gestation until delivery.[25]

CHROMOSOMAL ABNORMALITIES

In North America, about 1 per 160 liveborns has a chromosomal abnormality, with Down syndrome being the most frequent.[12] Among spontaneous abortuses, 50–60% show chromosomal abnormalities;[4] among stillbirths, 5% are abnormal. Cytogenetic (chromosome) studies can be prepared readily from amniotic fluid fibroblasts obtained by amniocentesis. Thus, all chromosomal disorders are potentially detectable in utero.

Cytogenetic Indications for Antenatal Studies

Although technically feasible, it is not appropriate to determine the chromosome complement of every fetus because for many couples the risks of amniocentesis may outweigh the potential diagnostic benefits. However, antenatal studies are certainly appropriate in couples at increased risk for abnormal offspring.

ADVANCED MATERNAL AGE

The most common indication for antenatal cytogenetic studies is increased maternal age. Approximately 90% of all antenatal studies are performed solely for advanced maternal age. The overall incidence of trisomy 21 is approximately 1 per

800 liveborn births in the United States. By contrast, a mother 35 years old at the birth of her child has a likelihood of having a child with trisomy 21 of 1 in 365; at age 39 the risk is 1 in 139; at age 45 the risk is 1 in 32 (Table 16.1).[11] Based on these data, most American authorities believe prenatal diagnosis should be offered to all women who will be 35 years old or greater when their infant is born (expected date of confinement, EDC). However, the choice of a particular age is largely arbitrary because the risk increases steadily from year-to-year even among younger women.

Trisomy 21 is not the only chromosomal abnormality that increases with maternal age. All autosomal trisomies and some X

Table 16.1.   Risk of having a Liveborn Child with Down Syndrome by 1-Year Maternal Age Intervals from Age 20 to 49 Years

Maternal Age	Risk of Down Syndrome
20	1/1923
21	1/1695
22	1/1538
23	1/1408
24	1/1299
25	1/1205
26	1/1124
27	1/1053
28	1/990
29	1/935
30	1/885
31	1/826
32	1/725
33	1/592
34	1/465
35	1/365
36	1/287
37	1/225
38	1/177
39	1/139
40	1/109
41	1/85
42	1/67
43	1/53
44	1/41
45	1/32
46	1/25
47	1/20
48	1/16
49	1/12

Data of Hook and Chambers (11). Because sample size for some intervals is relatively small, 95% confidence limits are sometimes relatively large. Nonetheless, these figures are suitable for genetic counseling.

chromosomal polysomies (47, XXY; 47, XXX) also show an increased mean maternal age. Between ages 35 and 39, limited prospective data indicate that the likelihood a chromosomal abnormality of any type will occur is approximately 1 in 70. Between 40 and 44 the likelihood is 1 in 50. Some of the increased risk is due to sex chromosomal polysomy, which may not be associated with severe phenotypic abnormalities.

The risk figures cited above are based upon *liveborns* with various chromosomal abnormalities. In fact, the prevalence of abnormalities detected by antenatal studies at 16–18 weeks gestation is much higher than expected among liveborn infants.[6] The discrepancy between prevalencies in liveborns and in second-trimester fetuses is generally explained by the fact that some of the chromosomally abnormal fetuses detected at 16 weeks spontaneously abort.

PREVIOUS CHILD WITH AUTOSOMAL TRISOMY

Following the birth of one child with either autosomal trisomy or sex chromosomal abnormality, the likelihood that subsequent progeny will have a chromosomal abnormality has traditionally been considered increased, even if parental chromosome complements are normal. However, the risk is only about 1% and may be increased over levels expected solely on the basis of maternal age only if the mother was 24 years or younger when her child was born.[17] Nonetheless, parental anxiety dictates that antenatal chromosomal studies be offered couples who have had a previous chromosomally abnormal child.

Most geneticists would offer similar counsel if aneuploidy (abnormal chromosome number) were detected in an abortus or stillborn infant; however, the risks following aneuploid abortuses or stillborn infants may or may not be similar to risks following aneuploid liveborn infants. In any case, it would be of immeasurable help in counseling if a blood or tissue sample for chromosome analysis were obtained from every stillborn infant with malformations.

PARENTAL TRANSLOCATIONS OR INVERSIONS

A third, less common, cytogenetic indication for antenatal diagnosis is the presence of a balanced translocation in a parent. The rare detection of an inversion warrants similar attention. The situation is best illustrated by considering translocation Down syndrome. Of individuals with Down syndrome, 2–3% have a translocation, usually between chromosomes 14 and 21. If a child has Down syndrome as a result of such a translocation, e.g., [46, XX, −14, +t (14q; 21q)], the rearrangements will have originated de novo in about 50–75% of cases (i.e., it is not present in either parent). The likelihood of Down syndrome recurring in progeny of parents whose previous offspring had a de novo translocation is probably not greater than for the general population. On the other hand, in about 25–50% of individuals who have Down syndrome as a result of a translocation, one parent has the same translocation chromosomes in a balanced state, e.g., [45, XX −14, −21, +t (14q; 21q)]. The *theoretical* risk that a parent carrying a t(14q; 21q) chromosome will have a child with Down syndrome is 33% (Fig. 16.2). However, *empiric* risks are considerably less. If the father carries the translocation the risk is only 2–3%, whereas if the mother carries the translocation the risk is about 10%.[3] Risks are considered similar for t(21q; 22q), but other robertsonian translocations (translocations involving the acrocentric chromosomes—13, 14, 15, 21, 22) need not necessarily carry similar risks.[3]

Reciprocal translocations (Fig. 16.3), do not involve centromeric fusion and, hence, usually do not involve acrocentric chromosomes. Risk figures are more difficult to obtain because there are many different types of translocations. Empiric data for specific translocations are not available, and generalizations must be made on the basis of pooled data derived from many different translocations. Theoretical risks for abnormal (unbalanced) offspring are greater than empiric risks, which are usually 5–10%.[23]

Ideally, fetal chromosomal abnormalities would be detected without amniocentesis, an invasive procedure. If noninvasive techniques were available, one could screen all pregnant patients, irrespective of prior history or age.

One potential approach is to recover fetal lymphocytes from maternal blood. Fetal lymphocytes are definitely present in the maternal circulation during pregnancy, and analysis of many metaphases from blood samples of pregnant women usually shows some fetal lymphocytes.[22] Assessment of fetal chromosomal status on the basis of cytogenetic studies of maternal blood is, therefore, theoretically possible but currently is impractical and also potentially unreliable because fetal cells can persist from previous pregnancies.

Nonetheless, if a reliable method of isolating and culturing fetal cells were available, a screening approach similar to that utilized for neural tube defects (see below) could be envisioned. A blood sample might be obtained from all pregnant patients. Those women whose blood samples revealed fetal chromosomal abnormalities could be offered amniocentesis for confirmatory chromosomal studies.

MENDELIAN DISORDERS

Mendelian disorders result from mutation at a single genetic locus. The locus may be on an autosome or on a sex chromosome and it may be dominant or recessive in nature. At least 1200 different mendelian disorders are known, and another 1200 disorders could be mendelian. Many mendelian disorders have a frequency of only 1 per 10,000 to 50,000 births. Even the most common examples—cystic fibrosis, sickle cell anemia, Tay-Sachs disease—have frequencies of less than 1 per 1000, although frequencies may be higher in certain ethnic groups. Although individually rare, mutant genes in aggregate cause ab-

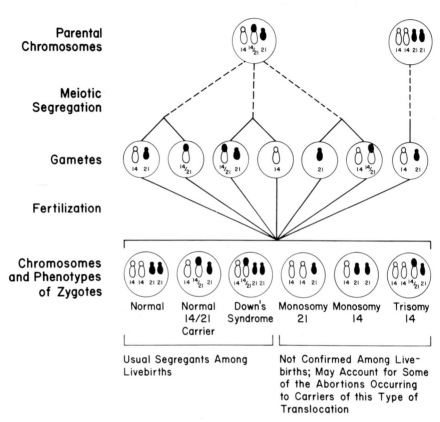

RESULTS OF SEGREGATION IN A HETEROZYGOTE FOR A ROBERTSONIAN TRANSLOCATION BETWEEN CHROMOSOME NUMBERS 14 AND 21 (A FORM OF D/G TRANSLOCATION)

Parental Chromosomes

Meiotic Segregation

Gametes

Fertilization

Chromosomes and Phenotypes of Zygotes

Normal | Normal 14/21 Carrier | Down's Syndrome | Monosomy 21 | Monosomy 14 | Trisomy 14

Usual Segregants Among Livebirths

Not Confirmed Among Live-births; May Account for Some of the Abortions Occurring to Carriers of this Type of Translocation

Figure 16.2 Diagram of possible gametes and progeny of a phenotypically normal individual heterozygous for a translocation between chromosomes 14 and 21. Three of the six possible gametes are incompatible with life. The likelihood that an individual with such a translocation would have a child with Down syndrome is thus theoretically 33%. However, the empirical risk is 10–15% if the mother is a carrier, and it is 2–3% if the father is a carrier. (Reproduced with permission from Gerbie, A., Simpson, J.L. Antenatal detection of genetic disorders. *Postgrad. Med. 59:*129, 1976.)

normalities in approximately 1% of liveborn infants.

Initially, antenatal diagnosis was possible only for certain inborn errors of metabolism, but more recently antenatal diagnosis of hemoglobinopathies, hemophilia, certain renal anomalies, certain skeletal dysplasias, and other disorders has become possible. In addition, fetal sex determination may be helpful to women heterozygous for X-linked recessive traits.

Nonetheless, in most institutions antenatal studies for mendelian disorders are performed less often than chromosomal studies.

Inborn Errors of Metabolism

Antenatal diagnosis is possible for approximately 80 to 100 inborn errors of metabolism. Almost all these traits are autosomal recessive, but a few X-linked recessive and autosomal dominant traits are

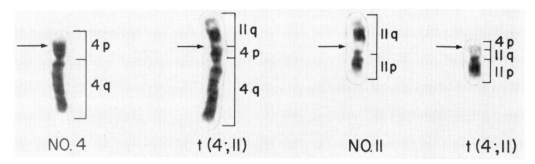

Figure 16.3   Partial karyotypes showing a balanced reciprocal translocation between chromosomes 4 and 11. (Reproduced with permission of the publisher from Simpson, J.L. Genes, chromosomes, and reproductive failure. *Fertil. Steril. 33:*107, 1980.)

known to result from enzyme errors. The diagnosis of errors of metabolism is usually a more difficult prospect than that of cytogenetic diagnosis. Several technical problems deserve mention.

First, a couple will usually be identified to be at risk because a previous child was affected, although screening programs might identify heterozygotes for some traits (Tay-Sachs disease, sickle cell disease). Obviously, the correct diagnosis of previously affected offspring or heterozygous parents must be established in order that appropriate antenatal tests can be offered. Sometimes this is not an easy task. If an affected child is no longer alive, the diagnosis may be impossible to verify.

Second, antenatal detection of metabolic errors requires that the enzyme be expressed in amniotic fluid fibroblasts, a requirement not fulfilled by all metabolic disorders. In general, one analyzes cultured amniotic fluid fibroblasts rather than assaying uncultured cells or amniotic fluid liquor.

Third, for each assayed compound, one must establish normal values for amniotic fluid fibroblasts of comparable gestational age. The enzyme levels may depend on the type of cell cultured (fibroblast-like or epithelial) and possibly on culture conditions.

Fourth, biochemical studies usually require more cells than do cytogenetic studies; thus, 4–6 weeks may be necessary for the former, compared to only 3 or 4 weeks for the latter.

Tay-Sachs disease (GM_2 gangliosidosis type I) is an example of an inborn error of metabolism for which screening programs have been developed and antenatal diagnosis is possible. In this disorder, hexosaminidase A, which is necessary for metabolism of sphingolipid, is virtually absent. The Tay-Sachs gene exists in the general population (1:300) but is much more common among Ashkenazi Jews (1:30). Intensive education programs aimed at this group have resulted in widespread utilization of screening tests for heterozygote detection. If both prospective parents are heterozygous, they have a 25% chance of producing an affected offspring. These at-risk pregnancies can be monitored by assay of the hexosaminidase A level in AF fibroblasts. Affected fetuses are thus recognized and pregnancy termination is offered.

Lists of metabolic disorders detectable in utero have been published.[18]

Chromosomal Breakage Syndromes

Several inherited disorders are characterized by chromosomal breakage. Individuals with these disorders often show increased propensity for neoplasia and, usually, growth retardation and various somatic anomalies. These disorders include Bloom syndrome, ataxia telangiectasia, and Fanconi anemia. A related disorder is xeroderma pigmentosum (XP), an autosomal recessive disease characterized by deficiency in the cellular mechanism responsible for repairing the pyrimidine dimers which inevitably form between adjacent pyrimidines of the same DNA strand following normal exposure to ultraviolet light.

In some of these disorders the precise molecular defect is not known, but, in each, distinctive cytogenetic features may permit antenatal diagnosis. Antenatal diagnosis of xeroderma pigmentosum has been accomplished by the diagnosis of decreased DNA repair capacity in amniotic fluid fibroblasts.[19]

Hemoglobinopathies

In sickle cell anemia, the thalassemias, and other disorders of hemoglobin biosynthesis the metabolic derangement is limited to one tissue—erythrocytes. Diagnosis can be made by measuring the capacity of fetal reticulocytes to synthesize normal hemoglobin, assayed through incorporation of radioactive leucine. Fetal blood may be obtained either by direct aspiration from the placenta or by aspiration from chorionic vessels under fetoscopic visualization. Hemoglobin assays are approximately 95% accurate.[1]

Unfortunately, the likelihood of abortion following fetoscopic or direct placental aspiration is 5–10%.[9] Nonetheless, the severity of the thalassemias and sickle cell anemia may justify the increased risk for many couples. Fetoscopic blood sampling for hemoglobinopathies may become obsolete, however, because of recent developments in molecular genetics that permit diagnosis of hemoglobinopathies using any nucleated cell, e.g., amniotic fluid fibroblasts.[2] These techniques allow diagnosis not on the basis of gene products (e.g., hemoglobin) but on the basis of the DNA that codes for the gene in question. DNA reannealing techniques can be used to diagnose α-thalassemia. Use of radioactive DNA probes, restriction endonucleases and DNA electrophoresis potentially permits diagnosis of 60–80% of fetuses with sickle cell anemia or β-thalassemias.[14, 15] With further advances it seems that it will be possible to diagnose almost all hemoglobinopathies on the basis of DNA studies.

Hemophilia and Other Disorders Detectable by Fetal Serum Assays

Many fetal disorders are potentially diagnosable by analysis of fetal sera. Hemophilia A appears reliably detectable on the basis of assays for factor VIII-related antigen and factor VIII-coagulant antigen, the latter but not the former of which is decreased in hemophiliac fetuses.[7] Hemophilia B (factor IX deficiency) can be detected by similar methodology,[16] as can homozygous von Willebrand disease.[13] However, the high risks involved (5–10% abortion rate) justify fetoscopic sampling only for serious disorders not detectable in other fashions.

Dermatologic Disorders Detectable by Fetal Skin Sampling

Mutant genes may produce life-threatening dermatologic abnormalities. Examples include several forms of epidermolysis bullosa and several forms of ichthyosis. As a generalization, both autosomal dominant and X-linked recessive forms of each exist, but usually it is the autosomal recessive forms that are severe enough to justify antenatal diagnosis. Because the metabolic basis of these disorders is not known, the only currently available method of antenatal diagnosis is fetal skin biopsy. The safety of this procedure is uncertain, but associated abortion is presumably at least the 5–10% observed following fetoscopic blood sampling. Diagnoses have been made for harlequin ichthyosis,[5] a lethal autosomal recessive disorder, for an autosomal dominant form of ichthyosis[8] and for epidermolysis bullosa.[20]

Diagnosis Based Exclusively on Ultrasonographic, Radiographic, or Fetoscopic Visualization

ROENTGENOGRAPHY

The skeletal dysphasias are one group of disorders in which roentgenographic diagnosis is potentially possible. For example, disorders characterized by an absent radius (thrombocytopenia-absent radius (TAR) syndrome) or polydactyly (e.g.,

Ellis-van Creveld syndrome) are potentially detectable. It may not be feasible to detect disproportionate dwarfism (e.g., achondroplasia) consistently because disproportionate growth may not be manifest by 20–24 weeks' gestation. In the future the skeletal dysplasia disorders may prove consistently detectable by ultrasonography.[10]

ULTRASONOGRAPHY

Some highly experienced ultrasonographers can diagnose neural tube defects, hydrocephalus, and certain renal anomalies.[10, 21] However, neural tube defects, usually inherited in polygenic/multifactorial fashion, can be detected with at least equal accuracy by assaying amniotic fluid α-fetoprotein. On the other hand, ultrasonography seems the only reasonable way to diagnose hydrocephalus or renal agenesis. Hydrocephalus is usually inherited in polygenic/multifactorial fashion, but X-linked recessive (aqueductal stenosis) and autosomal recessive forms (Dandy-Walker syndrome) exist. Diagnosis based solely on head size, i.e., biparietal diameter, is not definitive because the increased biparietal diameter may not become evident until too late in pregnancy to permit abortion; however, measurements of the lateral ventricles can identify affected fetuses by 20–24 weeks' gestation.

Bilateral renal agenesis, also more often a polygenic than a mendelian trait, can be detected by ultrasonography if one fails to visualize the fetal kidneys. Presence of fetal urine could exclude bilateral but not unilateral renal agenesis; however, absence of urine does not necessarily signify an affected fetus, for the fetus might have recently voided.

Great advances are being made in the ultrasonographic detection of skeletal dysplasias and cardiac anomalies, the latter of which are usually polygenic. Other disorders potentially diagnosable by ultrasonography include microcephaly, polycystic kidneys, and disorders characterized by intrauterine growth retardation.

In all these disorders, detection of an anomaly signifies diagnosis, but failure to detect an anomaly does not necessarily exclude the disorder because abnormalities may not become manifest until later in gestation. Indeed, late in gestation ultrasonography can demonstrate external genitalia, digits, facial profiles, and other anatomic details; however, detailed resolution cannot consistently be obtained early enough to allow termination of fetuses with abnormalities of these systems.

FETOSCOPY

Many caveats offered concerning fetal visualization by roentgenography or ultrasonography apply equally to fetoscopy. Use of fetoscopy to visualize anomalies in utero has been limited to disorders characterized by pronounced external abnormalities, e.g., polydactyly in Ellis-van Creveld syndrome. Experience suggests that it would be hazardous to attempt to exclude subtle anomalies by fetoscopic visualization, and probably ultrasound will soon supplant fetoscopic visualization.

Linkage Analysis: An Indirect Method for Prenatal Diagnosis

Every gene is located on a chromosome in definite linear relationship to other genes. A given gene is, therefore, closer to some genes than to others in the genome. Genes are said to be linked to one another if, after meiosis I, during which recombination can occur, the particular genes remain together more often than expected by chance, i.e., the genes are linked if they remain in the same gamete rather than segregate to the complementary gamete. The distance between loci can be determined by calculating the frequency with which alleles at different loci on the same chromosome become interchanged during meiosis I (recombination). If genes at different loci remain on the same chromosome with a frequency of 90%, they are said to be 10 map units apart. If the recombination frequency between two loci is 50% or greater, one cannot distinguish between loose linkage or absence of linkage; however, a common relationship between two loosely linked genes whose recombination frequency is greater than 50% can be recognized if both are linked to a third gene.

Linkage analysis can be used for antenatal diagnosis of disorders for which neither metabolic assays nor other diagnostic techniques are available. In such situations, one may test for a polymorphic gene which is tightly linked to the mutant gene in question. The presence or absence of the mutant gene is then inferred on the basis of analysis of the polymorphic gene. Figure 16.4 illustrates a situation in which linkage analysis might be useful. A female who is heterozygous for hemophilia and who has electrophoretic variants for G-6-PD of the A and B type has one son with hemophilia who is G-6-PD type A. The hemophilia gene and the G-6-PD gene are known to be tightly linked on the X-chromosome. This woman would like to know whether her current male fetus will have hemophilia. If the fetus is of G-6-PD type B, the mother can expect an unaffected child. Of course, as previously mentioned, hemophilia can also be diagnosed by testing fetal serum.

Diagnosis achieved by linkage analysis is never absolute because recombination can occur even between very closely linked loci. Nonetheless, linkage analysis will probably become increasingly useful in antenatal diagnosis as a more complete

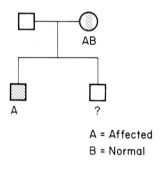

A = Affected

B = Normal

▨ Affected Male

◉ Heterozygous Female

Figure 16.4. Illustrative pedigree of a family which informative G-6-PD types could be utilized for antenatal diagnosis of hemophilia. (Reproduced with permission of the publisher from J.L. Simpson (23).)

map of the human genome becomes available. Linkage analysis should prove especially useful for autosomal dominant traits in which enzyme deficiencies have not been identified. Linkage relationships presently useful in antenatal diagnosis in addition to hemophilia and G-6-PD include myotonic dystrophy and the locus controlling secretion of ABO antigens into body fluids (secretor), the nail-patella syndrome and ABO, and HLA and adrenal 21-hydroxylase deficiency.

Fetal Sex Determination for X-Linked Recessive Disorders

Ordinarily in X-linked recessive or male-limited autosomal dominant traits, only males are affected. The Lesch-Nyhan syndrome, Fabry disease, G-6-PD deficiency and hemophilia are the only X-linked traits for which a definite diagnosis is possible. Affected infants with other X-linked disorders can be avoided by terminating all pregnancies in which the fetus is male; however, 50% of aborted males will be genetically normal.

POLYGENIC/MULTIFACTORIAL DISORDERS

In several common anomalies the recurrence risk for first-degree relatives is 2–5%. Such a recurrence risk suggests a polygenic/multifactorial etiology, although for no anomaly is this etiology proved.

Neural Tube Defects

Failure of embryonic neural tube closure leads to anencephaly, spina bifida (myelomeningocele or meningocele), or both. Anencephaly is incompatible with life, but spina bifida is not. Spina bifida may lead to hemiparesis, urinary incontinence, and, sometimes, hydrocephalus. Anencephaly and spina bifida represent different manifestations of the same pathogenic process—failure of neural tube closure. If the proband has anencephaly, the likelihood that a first-degree relative will have either anencephaly or spina bifida is 2% in the United States; if the proband has spina bifida, the total risks are also 2%, again for either anencephaly or spina bifida.[18] The risk is 5% in the United Kingdom, where neural tube defects are more common (1:200) than in the United States (1:500).

Couples who have had a child with either anencephaly or spina bifida should be informed that their subsequent offspring have approximately equal risks of having either disorder, irrespective of the specific neural tube defect in the proband. The clinical significance of this observation lies in the reality that the burden of caring for a liveborn child with spina bifida is much greater than the burden of bearing a stillborn anencephalic infant. Other suitable candidates for counseling include couples in which one or both parents have spina bifida.

Antenatal diagnosis of neural tube defects can theoretically be accomplished by either ultrasonography or assay of amniotic fluid α-fetoprotein (AFP). Ultrasonography by experienced investigators can reliably exclude anencephaly prior to 20 weeks' gestation, and some investigators are capable of detecting spina bifida through serial views of the vertebral column. By contrast, analysis of amniotic fluid AFP levels is available to any physician who performs amniocentesis and mails the specimen to an appropriate center. Thus, AFP assays seem likely to remain the preferable method for diagnosis of neural tube defects (see Chapter 17: Alpha-Fetoprotein).

Cardiac Anomalies

Many types of cardiac anomalies exist, and their patterns of inheritance differ. However, most carry recurrence risks of 1–4%. Echocardiographic or electrocardiographic techniques have detected anomalies late in the third trimester, but current techniques do not consistently allow diagnosis prior to 20–24 weeks' gestation. Further technical refinements seem necessary to permit routine diagnosis of cardiac anomalies in the second trimester.

Gastrointestinal Anomalies

Intestinal (duodenal, jejunal, or ileal) atresias can be diagnosed late in pregnancy by instilling radiopaque dyes into the amniotic cavity, which then outline the fetal gastrointestinal tract following fetal swallowing. Polyhydramnios is often associated. Diagnosis by 20–24 weeks' gestation seems feasible but cannot yet be considered routine. Moreover, fetal hypothyroidism has been reported in association with instillation of iodinated radiopaque dyes into the amniotic cavity. Also potentially amenable to ultrasonographic techniques are diaphragmatic hernias and omphaloceles.

Renal and Urologic Anomalies

Unilateral renal agenesis, bilateral renal agenesis, and ureteral obstructive anomalies, e.g., ureteropelvic junction obstruction, are usually polygenic/multifactorial in nature, although renal agenesis appears to be inherited in mendelian fashion in a few families. As alluded to previously, bilateral renal agenesis can be excluded by ultrasonographic visualization of kidneys or demonstration of fetal bladder containing urine. This approach is feasible prior to 20–24 weeks' gestation. Again, neither sensitivity nor specificity has been determined.

References

1. Alter, B.P. Prenatal diagnosis of hemoglobinopathies and other hematological diseases. *J. Pediatr.* 95:501, 1979.
2. Alter, B.P. Intrauterine diagnosis of hemoglobinopathies. *Semin. Perinatol.* 4:189, 1980.
3. Boué, A. Structural chromosome aberration in the parents. In *Prenatal Diagnosis*, edited by Murken, J.-D., Stengel-Rutkowski, S., and Schwinger, E. F. Enke, Stuttgart, 1979, p. 34.
4. Boué, J., Boué, A., and Lazar, P. Retrospective and prospective epidemiological studies of 1500 karyotyped spontaneous human abortuses. *Teratology* 12:11, 1975.
5. Elias, S., Mazur, M., Sabbagha, R., et al. The prenatal diagnosis of harlequin ichthyosis. *Clin. Genet.* 17:275, 1980.
6. Ferguson-Smith, M.A. Maternal age specific incidence of chromosome aberrations at amniocentesis. In *Prenatal Diagnosis*, edited by Murken, J.-D., Stengel-Rutkowski, S. and Schwinger, E. F. Enke, Stuttgart, 1979, p. 1.
7. Firshein, S.I., Hoyer, L.W., Lazarchick, J., et al. Prenatal diagnosis of classic hemophilia. *N. Engl. J. Med.* 300:937, 1979.
8. Golbus, M.S., Sagebiel, R.W., Filly, R.A., et al. Prenatal diagnosis of congenital bulous ichthyosiform erythroderma (epidermolytic hyperkeratosis) by fetal skin biopsy. *N. Engl. J. Med.* 302:93, 1980.

9. Hamerton, J.L. (Ed.) Prenatal Diagnosis of Genetic Disease: Past, Present, and Future. Summary of International Conference, Val David, Quebec, Canada, November 1979. Prenatal Diagnosis, 1980.

10. Hobbins, J., Grannum, P., Berkowitz, R., et al. Ultrasound in the diagnosis of congenital anomalies. *Am. J. Obstet. Gynecol. 134:*331, 1979.

11. Hook, E.B., and Chambers, G.M. Estimated rates of Down syndrome in live-births by one year maternal age intervals for mothers aged 20–29 in a New York State study: Implications of the risk figures for genetic counseling and cost-benefit analysis of prenatal diagnosis programs. *Birth Defects 13*(3A):124, 1977.

12. Hook, E.B., and Hamerton, J.L. The frequency of chromosome abnormalities detected in consecutive newborn studies—Differences between studies—Results by sex and by severity of phenotype. In *Population Cytogenetics*, Hook, E.B., and Porter, I.H. Academic Press, New York, 1978, p. 63.

13. Hoyer, L.W., Lindsten, J., Blombäck, M., et al. Prenatal evaluation of fetus at risk for severe von Willebrand disease. *Lancet 2:*191, 1979.

14. Kan, Y.W., and Dozy, A.M. Polymorphism of DNA sequence adjacent to human β-globin structural gene: Relationship to the sickle mutation. *Proc. Natl. Acad. Sci. U.S.A. 75:*5631, 1978.

15. Kan, Y.W., Lee, K.Y., Furbetta, M., et al. DNA polymorphism and prenatal diagnosis of β-thalassemia. *Blood 54*(suppl.):55a, 1979.

15a. Kuleshov, N.P. Chromosomal anomalies in infants dying during the prenatal period and in premature newborns. *Hum. Genet. 31:*151, 1976.

16. Mibashan, R.S., Rodeck, C.H., Thumpston, J.K., et al. Plasma assay of fetal factors: VIII-C and IX for prenatal diagnosis of haemophilia. *Lancet 1:* 1309, 1979.

17. Mikkelsen, M., and Stene, J. Previous child with Down syndrome and other chromosome aberration. In *Prenatal Diagnosis*, edited by Murken, J.-D., Stengel-Rutkowski, S., and Schwinger, E. F. Enke, Stuttgart, 1979, p. 22.

18. Milunsky, A. (Ed.) *Genetic Disorders and the Fetus.* Plenum, New York, 1979.

19. Ramsey, C.A. Prenatal diagnosis of xeroderma pigmentosum. *Lancet 2:*1109, 1974.

20. Rodeck, C.H., Eady, R.A., and Gosden, D.M. Prenatal diagnosis of epidermolysis bullosa fetalis. *Lancet 1:*949, 1980.

21. Sabbagha, R.E., and Shkolnik, A. Ultrasound diagnosis of fetal abnormalities. *Semin. Perinatal. 4:*213, 1980.

22. Schroeder, J. Transplacental passage of blood cells. *J. Med. Genet. 12:*230, 1975.

23. Simpson, J.L. Antenatal diagnosis of genetic disorders. In *Gynecology and Obstetrics*, edited by Sciarra, J.J. Harper & Row, Hagerstown, MD, 1979, chap 10.

24. Simpson, J.L. Antenatal monitoring of genetic disorders. *Clin. Obstet. Gynecol. 6:*259, 1979.

25. Simpson, J.L. Antenatal diagnosis of cytogenetic abnormalities. *Semin. Perinatol. 4:*165, 1980.

CHAPTER 17

Alpha-Fetoprotein

LARS L. CEDERQVIST, M.D.

Alpha-fetoprotein (AFP) is a glucoprotein with a molecular weight of around 64,000 daltons. It is synthesized mainly in the fetal liver and yolk sac and it can be recognized as early as 29 days after conception. AFP passes normally to the fetal blood and then reaches the amniotic fluid via the fetal urine; small amounts of AFP are transferred to the maternal blood. The concentration gradient of AFP between fetal serum and amniotic fluid is about 200:1 and between fetal and maternal serum is about 100,000:1.

Neural tube defects (NTDs) are associated with abnormally high concentrations of AFP in the amniotic fluid and maternal serum. The incidence of false-positive AFP elevations in maternal serum is high. Therefore if maternal serum is used as a tool for screening for NTDs, two sequential elevations in maternal AFP at least 1 week apart are required to consider a pregnancy at risk for NTD. High risk pregnancies will then be referred for amniocentesis. Approximately 1 of 13 pregnancies with persistent elevation of maternal serum AFP also has elevated amniotic fluid AFP due to NTD; the others have false-positive serum AFP.

Ninety percent of neural tube defects (the open lesions) can be diagnosed prenatally early in the second trimester, while the other 10% (the closed lesions) are not detectable.

It is now well established that the high amniotic fluid AFP levels found in pregnancies with open NTD are caused by AFP migrated through the serosa of the defect; fetal cerebrospinal fluid has significantly elevated levels when compared with those of amniotic fluid.

The optimal time for AFP screening is between 16 and 18 weeks' gestation. In most abnormalities the levels are substantially normal up to the 15th week of gestation: they then become elevated but frequently return to normal after weeks 26–28. If maternal serum AFP is elevated at weeks 16–18, there is time enough for retesting, amniocentesis and termination of a pregnancy with affected fetus if the patient so desires. The AFP levels are frequently measured by a radioimmunoassay (RIA) and the results can be available the day after the sample is obtained.

Ten percent of children with NTD are born to women who have previously given birth to such infants, while 90% of affected births are not foreseen. Thus a general screening of all pregnant women would have obvious benefits, although unnecessary anxiety would be caused in women with false-positive tests. Women who previously have given birth to an infant with NTD should undergo amniocentesis directly, without serum screening.

The AFP test is not specific for NTDs. Other conditions which have been associated with elevated levels of AFP include omphalocele, duodenal atresia, Turner's syndrome, congenital nephrosis, fetal distress and intrauterine death. The origin of the increased concentrations of AFP in amniotic fluid in these conditions is not well understood.

Multiple pregnancy, underestimated gestational age and intrauterine death are often noted in association with elevated

AFP in maternal serum. Demonstration of these conditions often eliminates the need for amniocentesis.

All pregnancies with increased AFP in amniotic fluid should be further evaluated with ultrasonography and/or amniography in an effort to determine the exact nature of the congenital defect. If only elevated AFP levels in amniotic fluid are used to diagnose NTD, a fetus with another malformation that is compatible with life

and is suitable for surgical repair might be aborted.

Suggested Reading

1. Haddow, J.E., and Macri, J.N. (Eds.) Screening for Neural Tube defects in the United States. Proceedings of the First Scarborough Conference, September 6–8, 1977.
2. Maternal serum-alpha-fetoprotein measurement in antenatal screening for anencephaly and spina bifida in early pregnancy. Report of U.K. collaborative study on alpha-fetoprotein in relation to neural-tube defects. *Lancet* 1:1323, 1977.

CHAPTER **18**

Stress Testing and Nonstress Testing

NIELS H. LAUERSEN, M.D.

Through antepartum electronic fetal heart rate (FHR) monitoring, the reserve of the fetus can be determined by FHR response either to the demands imposed on the fetal cardiac system by fetal movement or to the stress of induced or spontaneous contractions.

The inherent, spontaneous rhythmic contractions of fetal cardiac muscle can be altered by the cardiac autonomic nervous system. Activation of the parasympathetic division, the vagal influence, results in a rapid decrease in FHR followed by an equally rapid recovery. This parasympathetic component probably controls the FHR baseline variability.[24] On the other hand, sympathetic stimulation results in a more gradual change in FHR, an increase followed by a gradual return to baseline. The tissue of the central nervous system is perhaps the first tissue to be adversely influenced by fetal anoxia resulting from a decreased oxygen supply to the fetus. If anoxia is sufficient, severe brain damage and fetal death can occur. Since the FHR is under the control of the autonomic nervous system, it is the purpose of electronic FHR monitoring to detect subtle, deleterious effects of anoxia on the CNS long before irreparable damage by measuring the alteration in FHR.

It had long been observed that a drop in fetal heart rate as detected by auscultation was an indication of some problem with the fetus, but it was not until the advent of electronic FHR monitoring that patterns of FHR in relation to other events could be analyzed. The first report of successful continuous biophysical monitoring of the FHR was that of Hon in 1957.[11] In the same year, Southern[39] demonstrated a correlation between fetal anoxia and changes in the fetal electrocardiogram (FECG). Hon described the use of the FHR pattern as detected electronically during labor for the diagnosis of intrapartum fetal distress.[12] Electronic FHR monitoring was initially employed during labor as a means to identify a compromised fetus so that prompt corrective measures could be taken. Hammacher in 1966 was the first to suggest that FHR changes in response to either spontaneous or induced contractions during the antepartum period might serve as an index of fetal well-being in the weeks prior to labor.[9] If late decelerations occurred in response to uterine contractions, the test was considered positive and this was an indication of some compromise in the fetal environment.[10, 14] Ray and co-workers[31] were the first to report in the American literature on the clinical application of the oxytocin challenge test (OCT) in the management of the high risk patient. Their results confirmed earlier studies that a positive test, contractions associated with late decelerations, was an ominous sign that the fetus was at risk. The utility of the oxytocin challenge test, also called the contraction stress test (CST), as a measure of fetal well-being was confirmed by numerous studies.[1, 5, 8, 27, 38, 41]

It was Hammacher[9] whose work laid the foundation for the now widely used non-stress test (NST) for the evaluation of fetal well-being. It had been observed that certain fetal heart rate patterns, even in the absence of contractions, could be predictive of fetal outcome.[7, 19–21, 33] Indications of a good fetal result were fetal heart rate accelerations during fetal movement and fetal heart rate variability.

FETAL HEART RATE MONITORING TECHNIQUES

The value of any antepartum test of fetal well-being based on FHR is determined by the accuracy of the FHR recording. The most accurate technique for the measurement of FHR is a direct electrocardiogram (ECG) with the electrode attached to the fetus. However, this type of monitoring is impossible in the antepartum period, and the clinician must rely on one of the three available indirect monitoring methods. These three methods are abdominal fetal electrocardiogram (FECG), phonocardiography and ultrasonography.

Abdominal FECG

The major problem with this technique has been to separate and identify the comparatively weak fetal signal from the dominant maternal heart signal and from interfering background signals. It has only been the advances in electronic engineering over the past 2 decades that have resulted in the development of practical machinery for abdominal FECG. Two electrodes are placed on the maternal abdomen in the longitudinal axis of the fetus and secured either with the aid of a suction cup or with tape. The abdominal ECG signal, a mixed signal from both fetus and mother, is obtained, the maternal component is filtered out, and the fetal component is displayed and recorded. The major advantage of this technique is that it theoretically provides a beat-to-beat measurement of the fetal heart rate. Unfortunately, adequate readings are obtainable in only 30–75% of patients monitored.

Phonocardiography

In this technique, sensitive microphones placed on the maternal abdomen are employed to pick up the fetal heart sounds produced by valvular motion. In theory this technique is able to detect the interval between each heart beat and like the FECG provides a beat-to-beat recording. Unfortunately, the microphones pick up all noises, including pulsations from maternal vessels, bowel sounds and general background noise. The technique has a minimal chance of success in patients with obesity, polyhydramnios and prematurity.

Ultrasound

This is the most widely used noninvasive technique for the measurement of FHR in utero. It is based on ultrasound for the production and focusing of sound waves and on the Doppler theory of alteration of sound waves by movement. In this technique, a sound wave is transmitted into the uterus and the alteration in the sound wave as it reflects off the rhythmically contracting surfaces of the fetal heart valves is detected and recorded. Most commercially available Doppler ultrasound recording systems cannot detect each FHR event since, in order to obtain a clearer FHR record, they display the average of three beats. A ranged directional Doppler was developed in which the beam of sound was aimed more precisely toward the fetal heart, resulting in more reliable detection of the FHR pattern.[15, 17] The system was further modified by a separation of the Doppler signals to both detect and identify the movement of the fetal heart valve toward and away from the receiver. Once these independent movements could be specifically isolated, a beat-to-beat signal could be generated.[18] A good quality, detailed, clear-cut FHR is obtained 99% of the time with the Doppler.[16]

UTERINE ACTIVITY MONITORING TECHNIQUE

Uterine activity is most accurately recorded by direct measurement of intrauterine pressure changes achieved via an open-end catheter. However, the routine use of this invasive technique during the antepartum period is contraindicated. External monitoring of contractions by detection of tension changes which occur on the maternal abdomen during activity is the only means available for antepartum testing. The external technique is called *tocography*. This technique measures the frequency of contractions but cannot act as an index of their intensity.

MONITORING OF FETAL MOVEMENT

Fetal movements are recorded either by a slight alteration in the tocographic record of uterine activity or the mother can be given an opportunity to signal each time she feels a fetal movement.

OXYTOCIN CHALLENGE TEST

Indications

The OCT should be performed on antepartum high risk patients where there is suspicion of placental insufficiency or an increased risk of perinatal mortality. Conditions which indicate antepartum FHR monitoring are: diabetes mellitus, chronic hypertension, hypertensive disorders of pregnancy, suspected intrauterine growth retardation, hematological disorders such as Rh immunization and sickle cell anemia, a previous history of pregnancy wastage and postmaturity. The test would also be indicated if meconium was found on amniocentesis.

Contraindications

The test would be contraindicated in any clinical situation in which uterine stimulation would be contraindicated. Such situations would be a history of previous classical cesarean section, threatened premature labor, placenta previa, ruptured membranes, suspected abruptio placentae, incompetent cervix and multiple gestation.

Technique

The OCT can be performed as early as 28 weeks in very high risk patients but it is usually performed at 34 weeks, when termination of the pregnancy if clinically indicated would be feasible. An OCT should be performed either on or within easy accessibility to the labor floor. These precautions are needed since it is possible that the uterine stimulation could precipitate complications such as uterine hyperstimulation, fetal distress, placental separation or rupture of the membranes with prolapsed cord. The patient is given an intravenous infusion of 5% dextrose in water and is placed in a bed in the semi-Fowler position (a supine position tilted slightly to the left with the head elevated 30 degrees). Fetal heart sounds are located by auscultation, and the external FHR monitor is then placed on the mother's abdomen in the location of the best fetal heart sounds. The external tocograph is next placed and the patient is monitored for baseline activity for a period of 10 minutes to exclude any baseline FHR abnormality. If the patient is experiencing at least 3 regular uterine contractions per 10 minute interval, each contraction lasting from 40 to 60 seconds, further uterine stimulation is not required. In other cases, uterine activity is induced by intravenous infusion of oxytocin, administered via a constant rate infusion pump starting at a rate of 0.5 mU per minute. The dose is then doubled every 10 minutes until the patient experiences at least 3 regular contractions of 40–60 seconds duration every 10 minutes. The external tocograph cannot measure the absolute intensity of the contractions, and it is important that the clinician determine that the contractions are of sufficient intensity to stress the fetus. Once adequate uterine activity has been obtained, the oxytocin infusion is discontinued, but the patient should be carefully monitored until the uterine activity diminishes to pretesting levels.

Interpretation of Results

The baseline FHR is observed and noted. Normal FHR is between 120 and 160 BPM;

161 to 180 is moderate tachycardia and marked tachycardia is 181 BPM and higher. Bradycardia is defined as either moderate (100 to 119 BPM) or marked (99 BPM or less).[13] The occurrence of either condition can be indicative of a very seriously compromised fetus, and the etiology of either the tachycardia or the bradycardia should be thoroughly evaluated before the test is initiated by oxytocin infusion.

The pattern of FHR as influenced by uterine activity is then categorized.

POSITIVE

A positive OCT or CST is a test in which the majority of uterine contractions are accompanied by repeated, uniform, late FHR decelerations and evidence of a compromised fetal environment (Fig. 18.1).

Schifrin[36] offers a modified criterion for characterizing this antepartum FHR test. The author attempts to find a "10-minute window" in which each of at least 3 uterine contractions is accompanied by a late deceleration; this would be judged as a positive test. Only very rarely would positive and negative windows occur in the same recording, and in this case the positive would take precedence. In the late deceleration the FHR slowing begins at least 20–30 seconds after the onset of the contractions, reaches a low point well after the peak of the contractions, and does not begin to return to baseline until the contraction has completely subsided; this is one of the most ominous signs of fetal compromise. The degree of deceleration may be an indication of the severity of the

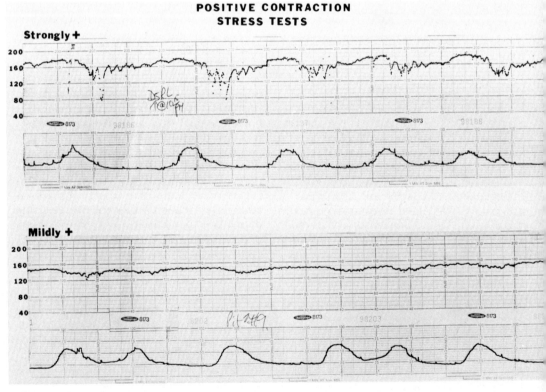

Figure 18.1. Positive oxytocin challenge tests (OCT) also called contraction stress test (CST). The tracings are from two patients. Both show consistent late FHR decelerations accompanying contractions. In the top tracing the FHR dropped 80 BPM, while the heart rate decrease in the lower tracing was only 20 BPM. However, both of these tracings are indicative of a deteriorating fetal status. Note particularly the diminished FHR variability in the lower tracing; this might be considered an ominous sign.

fetal distress; however, even very mild late decelerations, particularly when associated with loss of fetal heart rate variability, must be closely observed.

NEGATIVE

A negative OCT, a test in which uterine contractions are not accompanied by FHR decelerations, is an indication of fetal well-being.

SUSPICIOUS

A *suspicious* OCT is a test in which less than 50% of uterine contractions are associated with late decelerations, and this pattern of decelerations is neither uniform nor persistent. A suspicious test is not clearly predictive of fetal compromise but must be repeated within 24 hours.

HYPERSTIMULATION

The patient is considered to be hyperstimulated by the oxytocin infusion if the contractions are less than 2 minutes apart or have a duration longer than 90 seconds or if the baseline uterine tone remains elevated. The appearance of any of these symptoms would require that the oxytocin infusion be immediately stopped. If the FHR remains stable, it is interpreted as a *negative* test. If FHR deceleration does occur in response to the hyperstimulation, it is not considered a *positive* OCT because of the magnitude of the insult to the fetal environment. The test, however, should be repeated within 24 hours.

UNSATISFACTORY

In this test the quality of the recording of either uterine activity or FHR is too poor to interpret; the test should be repeated within 24 hours.

NONSTRESS TEST (NST)

Nonstress testing assesses fetal well-being by monitoring the degree of heart rate variability and the FHR changes induced by spontaneous fetal movements.

Indications

The indications for NST are the same as for OCT.

Contraindications

There are no contraindications for this procedure.

Technique

The NST like the OCT may be performed as early as 28 weeks' gestation but is usually done after the 34th week. The test may be performed either in the clinic or in the physician's office. The patient is placed in a semi-Fowler position, with a slight left lateral tilt to prevent maternal hypotension. The FHR monitor is applied in the most appropriate position for the best reading. Fetal movement (FM) can be recorded in one of three ways. The tocography belt can be placed on the mother, and the FMs directly record on the monitor as a short spike; the mother can be given a signal marker to press each time she feels a FM; or the trained personnel administering the test can keep his/her hand on the maternal abdomen to support the Doppler FHR monitor and then record on the strip each time a FM is felt. The recording is carried out for at least 20 minutes. If there are no fetal movements observed during this time, the possibility of the fetus being in a sleeping phase must be considered. At this point an attempt to rouse the fetus can be made by shaking the maternal abdomen from side to side or by sonic stimulation. If fetal movement still does not occur, it might be advisable to send the patient for a meal. The increase in blood sugar will usually wake the fetus. Some testing centers elect to have the patient imbibe a high sugar drink prior to testing to assure an adequate blood sugar level and fetal movement.

Interpretation of Results

As with OCT testing, the FHR baseline should be observed and significant deviations from normal should be immediately evaluated.

The patterns of FHR in NST are classified as follows.

REACTIVE

A *reactive* NST is an accurate indication of fetal well-being. The criterion for judg-

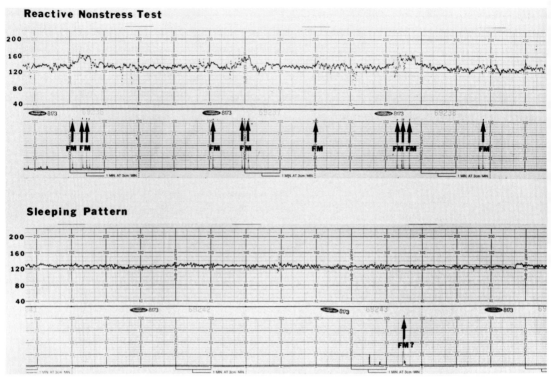

Figure 18.2. A reactive nonstress test is characterized by distinct FHR accelerations of at least 15 BPM accompanying each distinct fetal movement (*FM*). The FHR also shows good variability. These are signs of fetal well-being. The lower tracing is from the same patient and shows the ''sleeping pattern,'' with no fetal movements (FMs) and no accelerations. This pattern is at times mistakenly interpreted as a nonreactive NST; however, note that there is still good FHR variability, greater than 6 BPM, during this sleeping pattern even though it is less than during the aroused state.

ing reactivity varies in its particulars from institution to institution, but in general a reactive test is one in which fetal movements are accompanied by FHR accelerations of at least 15 beats per minute lasting 15–20 seconds. At least 3 fetal movements accompanied by FHR accelerations must be seen within a 20-minute window. The baseline FHR must demonstrate good ''variability,'' changes of greater than 6 BPM, 2 to 6 times per minute in order to consider the NST reactive (Fig. 18.2).

NONREACTIVE

A *nonreactive* NST could indicate a deteriorating fetal condition. In this instance, there will be no FHR acceleration in response to fetal movement or there will be occasional or inadequate accelerations of less than 15 beats per minute. Prospects of fetal jeopardy might be even greater if this is accompanied by FHR variability of less than 6 beats per minute.

SINUSOIDAL

A *sinusoidal* NST is a test in which the normal random FHR variability has been replaced by rhythmic oscillations with an amplitude of 5–10 beats per minute and a frequency of 2 or 3 per minute. FHR accelerations are also absent during fetal movements. This is a very ominous pattern and is usually seen only with severe fetal compromise such as in association with erythroblastosis fetalis[33] or severe fetal anemia.[25] A sinusoidal NST indicates that immediate therapy should be initiated. In cases of severe fetal anemia, the FHR pattern has improved after intrauterine fetal transfusion.

UNSATISFACTORY

An *unsatisfactory* NST is a test in which a clear FHR pattern has not been obtained or a test which was conducted under poor supervision with no indication of fetal movement. Such tests should not be acted on but should be repeated within 24 hours.

COMBINED NST/OCT TESTING

A *reactive* NST is a reliable indicator of fetal well-being. Schifrin[36] demonstrated that reactive NSTs were associated with low 5 minute Apgar scores in only 3.3% of deliveries and with an incidence of neonatal death of 1.3%. The NST will be reactive in approximately $\frac{2}{3}$ to $\frac{3}{4}$ of patients tested and can act as a screening technique. The *nonreactive* NST, observed in

the remaining $\frac{1}{4}$ to $\frac{1}{3}$, might suggest fetal jeopardy and would be an indication for OCT. This regimen would limit by at least $\frac{2}{3}$ the need for submitting patients to the more complex and hazardous OCT.

Indications for NST/OCT Testing

The same as for OCT.

Contraindications

The same as for the respective tests.

Technique

If the NST is reactive, the patient should be discharged and scheduled for retesting at weekly intervals. A patient with a *non-reactive* NST should be immediately admitted to the labor floor and the OCT performed. If the OCT is *negative*, it should be repeated within 24 to 48 hours. If the OCT is positive (Fig. 18.3), a partic-

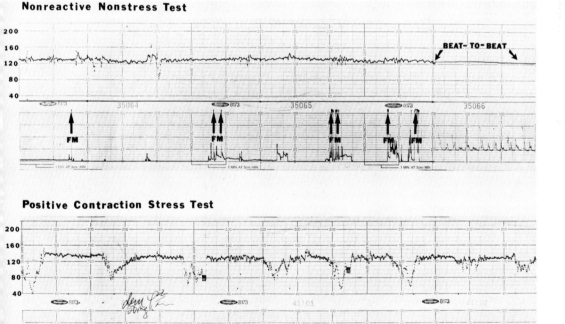

Figure 18.3. A nonreactive NST followed by a positive OCT in the same patient. In the upper tracing, distinct fetal movements were unaccompanied by FHR accelerations; when the monitor was placed in the "beat-to-beat" phase, FHR variability was absent. The patient was then submitted to an OCT and consistent late decelerations were present with each contraction.

ularly ominous sign of fetal compromise, immediate delivery should be considered if fetal lung maturity has been established.

OTHER INDICES OF FETAL WELL-BEING

Fetal response to environmental changes evidences fetal well-being. Fetal heart rate is at present the major parameter examined, but other parameters such as fetal breathing and fetal movements in relationship to fetal outcome are being investigated.

Fetal Breathing

Boddy and Robinson[3] applied an A-scan ultrasound to measure fetal breathing in 1971. This initial work was followed by a number of studies investigating the possibility of using fetal breathing as an index of fetal well-being.[22] Absence of fetal breathing movements was not found to significantly correlate with fetal distress.[32] Manning and co-workers[23] reported that fetal breathing movements were present in 88% of the *reactive* NSTs and in 67% of the *nonreactive* tests. A nonreactive NST without fetal breathing movements would be very suggestive of a compromised fetal environment.

Fetal Movement

The presence and degree of fetal movement is a well-established sign of fetal status; imminent intrauterine fetal death may often be first detected by the mother who notes diminished fetal movement. Attempts have been made to quantitate fetal movement so that it might be used as a simple index of fetal well-being. Sadovsky and co-workers[34] had women count and record fetal movements three times a day for 30 to 60 minutes. They reported that a decrease in fetal movement constituted a "movement alarm signal" which preceded the cessation of fetal heart beat. Timor-Tritsch et al.[40] classified fetal movement according to duration; movements lasting longer than 3 seconds, 1 to 3 seconds, less than 1 second, and respiratory movements. These authors emphasized the importance

of movement in relation to heart rate changes and stated that while movement changes can be a warning sign they cannot be used as the "sole parameter to determine maternal or fetal treatment."

Nonstress testing (NST) is gaining increasing popularity over the oxytocin challenge test (OCT) for the initial screening of high risk pregnancy. The ability of reactive NST to accurately reflect fetal well-being has been widely reported.[2, 19-21, 26, 29, 30, 33, 36, 37] Schifrin[36] found that a reactive NST was an even more reliable indicator of fetal well-being than was a negative OCT; there were 1.3% fetal deaths in a group of 308 reactive NST patients and 4.9% fetal deaths in 104 patients who had negative OCTs but nonreactive NSTs. Similar results were reported by Paul and Miller.[29] The prognostic value of the OCT has also been recently questioned by Parer and Afonso.[28] Fetal deaths can occur even after reactive NSTs, and it might be suggested that severely at risk patients have an NST at least twice a week.

While the presence of a reactive NST may be considered a reliable clinical indication of fetal well-being, a nonreactive NST is not so clearly an indication of fetal distress. Nonreactive NSTs can occur in a number of instances such as maternal ingestion of narcotics or tranquilizers. If the NST is not carefully performed, a tracing obtained during the fetus' sleep cycle might be mistakenly interpreted as a nonreactive test. Nonreactive NSTs may be obtained in $\frac{1}{4}$ to $\frac{1}{3}$ of patients tested, while the expected number of truly distressed fetuses is well below this number. The NST is therefore combined with the more hazardous but more discriminating OCT to afford a more reliable index of a deteriorating fetal environment.[19, 21, 26, 29, 30, 36]

Fox and co-workers[7] in 1976 and Braly and Freeman[4] in 1977 suggested the importance of evaluating FHR accelerations during OCT as supplementary evidence of fetal status. Pratt and co-workers[30] found that the incidence of fetal morbidity was 55% in nonreactive NST and 65% with positive OCTs, but when a patient had both a nonreactive NST and a positive OCT, the chance of predicting fetal morbidity rose to 83%. Similar results were reported by Schifrin and co-workers[37, 38] and Barrada et al.[2] The majority of institutions now use a combined regimen. The NST will be performed as a screening test and if the NST is nonreactive an OCT is indicated. If the subsequent OCT is negative the patient will be retested within 2 or 3 days and followed in an intensive high risk manner. A nonreactive NST followed by a positive OCT would be a strong indication for immediate delivery.

The ability of these antepartum tests to reflect the fetal environment was recently emphasized by the study of Scanlon and co-workers.[35] In a detailed prospective study, 54 infants with negative OCTs were compared to 13 infants with positive OCTs. The authors reported significant differences in 1 and 5 minute Apgar scores, in birth weights, and in two neonatal neurological behavioral screening tests. The results in infants with positive OCTs supported the hypothesis of some pathological placental insufficiency. Antepartum FHR monitoring is an established clinical tool for the assessment of the intrauterine fetal condition and in combination with other indices of placental function, such as biochemical tests, provides a more rational and informed basis for the management of the high risk pregnancy.

References

1. Barrada, M. I., Edwards, L. E., and Hakanson, E. Y. Antepartum fetal testing. *Am. J. Obstet. Gynecol.* 134:532, 1979.
2. Barrada, M. I., Edwards, L. E., and Hakanson, E. Y. Antepartum fetal testing: II. The acceleration/constant ratio: A nonstress test. *Am. J. Obstet. Gynecol.* 134:538, 1979.
3. Boddy, K., and Robinson, J. S. External method for detection of fetal breathing in utero. *Lancet*, pp. 1231–1233, December 4, 1971.
4. Braly, P., and Freeman, R. K. The significance of fetal heart rate reactivity with a positive oxytocin challenge test. *Obstet. Gynecol.* 50:689, 1977.
5. Cooper, J. M., Soffronoff, E. C., and Bolognese, R. J. Oxytocin challenge test in monitoring high-risk pregnancies. *Obstet. Gynecol.* 45:27, 1975.
6. Cremer, M. Direct derivation of action current of the human heart from the oesophagus and through the electrocardiogram of the fetus (German). *Muench. Med. Wochenschr.* 53:811, 1906.
7. Fox, H. E., Steinbrecher, M., and Ripton, B. Antepartum fetal heart rate and uterine activity studies. *Am. J. Obstet. Gynecol.* 126:61, 1976.
8. Freeman, R. K. The use of the oxytocin challenge test for antepartum clinical evaluation of utero-placental respiratory function. *Am. J. Obstet. Gynecol.* 121:481, 1975.
9. Hammacher, K. *Die Prophylaxe Fruhkindlicher Hirnschaden, edited by Elert, R., and Hüter, K. A. Georg Thieme Verlag, Stuggart, 1966.*
10. Hammacher, K., Hüter, K. A., Bokelmann, J., and Werners, P. H. Foetal heart frequency and perinatal condition of the foetus and newborn. *Gynaecologia* 166:349, 1968.
11. Hon, E. H. Instrumentation of fetal electrocardiography. *Science* 125:553, 1957.
12. Hon, E. H. The electronic evaluation of the fetal heart rate. *Am. J. Obstet. Gynecol.* 75:1215, 1958.
13. Hon, E. H., and Quilligan, E. J. The classification of fetal heart rate. *Conn. Med.* 31:779, 1967.
14. Kubli, F. W., Kesero, O., and Kinselmann, M. In *The Foetal-Placental Unit*, edited by Pecile, A., and Finzi, C. Excerpta Medica Foundation, Amsterdam, 1969.
15. Lauersen, N. H., Hochberg, H. M., and George, M. E. D. Evaluation of the accuracy of a new ultrasonic fetal heart rate monitor. *Am. J. Obstet. Gynecol.* 125:1125, 1976.
16. Lauersen, N. H., Hochberg, H. M., and George, M. E. D. Variable range directional doppler and abdominal ECG for FHR monitoring. *Int. J. Gynaecol. Obstet.* 15:507, 1978.
17. Lauersen, N. H., Hochberg, H. M., George, M. E. D., Tegge, C. S., and Meighan, J. J. A new technique for improving the doppler ultrasound signal for fetal heart rate monitoring. *Am. J. Obstet. Gynecol.* 128:300, 1977.
18. Lauersen, N. H., Hochberg, H. M., George, M. E. D., Tegge, C. S., and Meighan, J. J. Technical aspects of ranged directional doppler: A new doppler method of fetal heart rate monitoring. *J. Reprod. Med.* 20:77, 1978.
19. Lee, C. Y., DiLoreto, P. C., and Logrand, B. Fetal activity acceleration determination for the evaluation of fetal reserve. *Obstet. Gynecol.* 48:19, 1976.
20. Lee, C. Y., DiLoreto, P. C., and O'Lane, J. M. A study of fetal heart rate acceleration patterns. *Obstet. Gynecol.* 45:142, 1975.
21. Lee, C. Y., and Drukker, B. The nonstress test for the antepartum assessment of fetal reserve. *Am. J. Obstet. Gynecol.* 134:460, 1979.
22. Lewis, P., and Boylan, P. Fetal breathing: A review. *Am. J. Obstet. Gynecol.* 134:587, 1979.
23. Manning, F. A., Platt, L. D., Sipos, L., and Keegan, K. A. Fetal breathing movements and the nonstress test in high-risk pregnancies. *Am. J. Obstet. Gynecol.* 135:511, 1979.
24. Martin, C. B., Jr. Regulation of the fetal heart rate and genesis of FHR patterns. *Semin. Perinatol.* 2:131, 1978.
25. Modanlou, H. D., Freeman, R. K., Ortiz, O.,

Hinkes, P., and Pillsbury, G. Sinusoidal fetal heart rate pattern and severe fetal anemia. *Obstet. Gynecol. 49:*537, 1977.

26. Nochimson, D. J., Turbeville, J. S., Terry, J. E., Petrie, R. H., and Lundy, L. E. The nonstress test. *Obstet. Gynecol. 51:*419, 1978.

27. Odendaal, H. J. The fetal and labor outcome of 102 positive contraction stress tests. *Obstet. Gynecol. 54:*591, 1979.

28. Parer, J. T., and Afonso, J. F. Validity of the weekly intervals between oxytocin challenge tests. *Am. J. Obstet. Gynecol. 127:*204, 1977.

29. Paul, R. H., and Miller, F. C. Antepartum fetal heart rate monitoring. *Clin. Obstet. Gynecol. 21:* 375, 1978.

30. Pratt, D., Diamond, F., Yen, H., Bieniarz, J., and Burd, L. Fetal stress and nonstress tests: An analysis and comparison of their ability to identify fetal outcome. *Obstet. Gynecol. 54:*419, 1979.

31. Ray, M., Freeman, R., Pine, S., and Hesselgesser, R. Clinical experience with the oxytocin challenge test. *Am. J. Obstet. Gynecol. 114:*1, 1972.

32. Richardson, B., Natale, R., and Patrick, J. Human fetal breathing activity during electively induced labor at term. *Am. J. Obstet. Gynecol. 133:*247, 1979.

33. Rochard, F., Schifrin, B. S., Goupil, F., Legrand, H., Blottiere, J., and Sureau, C. Nonstressed fetal heart rate monitoring in the antepartum period. *Am. J. Obstet. Gynecol. 126:*699, 1976.

34. Sadovsky, E., Yaffe, H., and Polishuk, W. Z. Fetal movement monitoring in normal and pathologic pregnancy. *Int. J. Gynaecol. Obstet. 12:*75, 1974.

35. Scanlon, J. W., Suzuki, K., Shea, E., and Tronick, E. A prospective study of the oxytocin challenge test and newborn neurobehavioral outcome. *Obstet. Gynecol. 54:*6, 1979.

36. Schifrin, B. S. Antepartum fetal heart rate monitoring, In *Intrauterine Asphyxia and the Developing Fetal Brain,* edited by Gluck, L. Year Book Medical Publishers, Chicago, 1978, pp. 203–227.

37. Schifrin, B. S., Foye, G., Amato, J., Kates, R., and MacKenna, J. Routine fetal heart rate monitoring in the antepartum period. *Obstet. Gynecol. 54:*21, 1979.

38. Schifrin, B. S., Lapidus, M., Doctor, G. S., and Leviton, A. Contraction stress test for antepartum fetal evaluation. *Obstet. Gynecol. 45:*433, 1975.

39. Southern, E. M. Fetal anoxia and its possible relation to changes in the prenatal fetal electrocardiograms. *Am. J. Obstet. Gynecol. 73:*233, 1957.

40. Timor-Tritsch, I. E., Dierker, L. J., Jr., Hertz, R. H., and Rosen, M. G. Fetal movement: A brief review. *Clin. Obstet. Gynecol. 22:*583, 1979.

41. Weingold, A. B., DeJesus, T. P. S., and O'Keiffe, J. Oxytocin challenge test. *Am. J. Obstet. Gynecol. 123:*466, 1975.

CHAPTER 19

Determination of Fetal Age and Fetal Maturity

LARS L. CEDERQVIST, M.D.

The average duration of a pregnancy is 280 days or 40 weeks as computed from the first day of the last menstrual period (menstrual age) or 266 days from the conception (ovulation age). In determining the estimated date of confinement (EDC) it is customary to count back 3 months from the last menstruation and add 7 days (Nägele's rule). This method is correct in about 60% of the cases but can be used only if the date of the last period is known and if the periods are regular. Incorrect dating can result from irregular periods or from vaginal bleeding occurring during the pregnancy. Therefore, additional methods have been employed to determine the age of the fetus.

Palpation of the pregnant uterus gives only a rough estimate of fetal size. According to McDonald's rule the length of the uterus (in centimeters) divided by 3.5 gives the duration of the pregnancy in lunar months; this rule should be used only after the sixth month of pregnancy. McDonald's rule can be adversely influenced by a number of factors, such as: adiposity, tumors, full bladder, multiple pregnancy, hydramnios, intrauterine growth retardation and contracted pelvis.

The fetal heart should be heard by a head stethoscope by the 18th–20th week of gestation, although it often can be detected as early as the 16th week. The date when the mother first can feel the fetal movements (quickening) is also of some importance. The estimated date of confine-

ment is obtained by counting ahead 24 weeks in multigravidas and 22 weeks in primigravidas from the date of quickening.

Ossification centers of the skeleton appear early in the fetal life. This has made it possible to estimate fetal age by x-ray visualization of the fetal skeleton. Above the 16th week the fetal skeleton can be outlined by this method, although ossification centers have been demonstrated as early as the 6th week. The fetus has reached at least 35 weeks' gestational age if the distal ossification center of the femur is visible by x-ray examination, although this can appear as early as 32 weeks' gestation. The proximal tibial epiphysis is present in 50–75% of fetuses at term. This examination and measurement of the biparietal diameter of the vertex have been replaced by ultrasonographic methods.

The actual length of the fetus can be approximated according to Haase's rule. The length of the embryo or fetus in centimeters during the first 5 months may be estimated by squaring the number of lunar months of gestation. After the fifth month the lunar month should be multiplied by 5.

The fetus weighs approximately 100 gm at the end of the first trimester (12 weeks), 400 gm at 20 weeks, 800 gm at 28 weeks, 2500 gm at 36 weeks and 3200–3400 gm at 40 weeks.

With the advances in *in utero* evaluation of the fetus, high risk pregnancies are more commonly terminated electively. It is im-

153

portant to do this at a stage of gestation when the fetus is developed enough for extrauterine life. We are, therefore, for this purpose more interested in fetal maturity than in exact fetal age. Amniotic fluid lecithin/sphingomyelin (L/S) ratio, foam test, fat stained cells and creatinine concentrations have been used most often to estimate fetal maturity.

Respiratory distress syndrome (RDS) is the most important cause of death in the prematurely born infant. It is characterized by a progressive atelectasis due to lack of surface-active material in the lungs of the premature infant. Lecithin is the major constituent of the alveolar surfactant. It is produced in type II alveolar lining cells and keeps the alveoli expanded at low lung volumes. Infants dying of RDS have a significant decrease in lecithin in the lungs. The concentration of lecithin increases as the gestation progresses, while the sphingomyelin remains relatively stable.

The L/S ratio is the most valuable test for evaluating fetal maturity. It is usually determined by one-dimensional thin-layer chromatography on silica gel to separate lecithin from sphingomyelin. After these compounds are measured by reflectance densitometry, the L/S ratio is calculated. A ratio of 2.0 and greater indicates pulmonary maturity, a ratio of 1.5–1.9 is indeterminant, a ratio of 1.0–1.5 indicates immaturity and ratios of less than 1.0 indicate significant immaturity. Infants with an L/S ratio of less than 1.5 almost invariably develop RDS.

In normal pregnancies, the surfactant system matures at about 36 weeks' gestation. However, neither birth weight nor gestational age relates well with the L/S ratio. Accelerated fetal maturation has been found in maternal hypertension, chronic abruption of the placenta, advanced maternal diabetes, prolonged premature rupture of the membranes, maternal hemoglobinopathies, maternal heroin addiction and poor maternal nutrition. Hypertension is also associated with an earlier rise in the L/S ratio. A delayed fetal pulmonary maturation has been observed in maternal diabetes, Rh sensitization, intrinsic renal disease, hepatitis, collagen disease, hydrops fetalis, syphilis and toxoplasmosis. It is more striking in classes B through F diabetes than in class A diabetes. Careful metabolic control of the pregnant diabetic patient results in a normal L/S ratio, without increased risk of RDS. There is a more than 5 times greater risk of RDS in infants of diabetic mothers than in infants of normal mothers. A delayed fetal pulmonary maturation has also been observed in the smaller of identical twins.

The foam test, or shake test, is based on the formation of foam bubbles when different dilutions of amniotic fluid are mixed with ethanol. Usually 100% ethanol is mixed with the uncentrifuged amniotic fluid in a 1:1 ratio. This mixture is then shaken for 30 seconds. A tube is recorded as positive when the bubbles form a complete ring around the air-liquid interface of the tube. Different scoring systems have been used. At the New York Hospital-Cornell Medical Center the foam test has been used for several years and is considered to be as informative as the L/S ratio.

Nile blue staining of amniotic fluid cells is a simple, rapid and inexpensive method of determining fetal maturity. A drop of amniotic fluid is mixed with a drop of 0.1% aqueous solution of Nile blue hydrochloride on a coverslip. The majority of cells originate from the epidermis and appear blue. Cells with lipid material stain orange but may vary in color from pink to brown and are anuclear. These cells originate from fetal sebaceous glands. The proportion of these "fat cells" remains small until 36 weeks of gestation and rises sharply between 37 and 39 weeks. After 40 weeks' gestation the majority of the cells in the amniotic fluid stain orange. The fetus is considered mature or at a gestational age of greater than 36 weeks if the percentage of orange stained cells is greater than 10%. This method is unaffected by diabetes mellitus and severe toxemia which may affect the L/S ratio.

Creatinine values in amniotic fluid increase gradually late in pregnancy. The value of more than 2 mg/dl is considered to be indicative of fetal maturity. It is, however, more indicative of renal maturity than pulmonary maturity. The average value is 2 mg/dl at 37 weeks' gestation and 2.5 mg/dl at 39 weeks' gestation. It is unlikely to obtain a value of 2 mg/dl or more prior to 35 weeks of gestation. There is a great range of values and this test should not be used alone as an indicator of fetal maturity.

The disappearance of bilirubin as measured by spectrophotometer has also been used as an indicator of fetal maturity. Although the bilirubin peak usually disappears after the 36th week, the spread of data makes this test unreliable.

For the prediction of lung maturity prior to elective termination of pregnancy, the L/S ratio and foam test performed on amniotic fluid are the most reliable tests available. The results should, however, be used only as one useful parameter. The clinical findings throughout gestation and other tests such as ultrasonography should be taken into consideration before a particular pregnancy is terminated.

Complications of Pregnancy and Their Management

CHAPTER 20

Hypertensive Disorders of Pregnancy

RONALD M. CAPLAN, M.D.

TOXEMIA

The etiology of the toxemic state has eluded researchers in obstetrics to the present time. Indeed, this group of disease entities, better labelled the "hypertensive disorders or pregnancy," have separate causations and prognoses. True preeclampsia and eclampsia—that syndrome of hypertension, proteinuria, and edema, progressing in the eclamptic state to convulsions and coma—are seen most commonly in the primigravida of poor socioeconomic status. They occur in a previously normotensive patient and most commonly manifest themselves in the third trimester of pregnancy. Recently, more attention is being paid to the hypothesis that immunologic factors may be involved in the causation of this condition.[3, 5, 6]

CLASSIFICATION

In 1977 Friedman and Neff,[4] utilizing data of the Collaborative Perinatal Project, were able to define a high risk population in which there was an increased incidence of stillbirth, neonatal death, and abnormal neonatal development. Significant risk of these developments was noted in antepartum patients who developed a diastolic blood pressure reading of 95 mm of mercury or greater at anytime from the 28th week of pregnancy. Similarly, pregnant women who displayed "two-plus" proteinuria from the 28th week could be shown to have higher incidences of these sequelae. These two groups of patients were characterized as having "mild hypertensive disorder of pregnancy."

A synergistic effect was noted when

both conditions were present: the newborns of such patients were at the greatest risk. These patients were categorized as having "severe hypertensive disorder of pregnancy."

It was also noted that a diastolic blood pressure of 85 mm of mercury coupled with "one-plus" proteinuria was of significance.

Moreover, a new entity, "hypotensive disorder of pregnancy," was identified in which the diastolic blood pressure was less than 65 mm of mercury. This was significantly associated with a high fetal and neonatal loss as well as late neurologic and developmental abnormalities.

Townsend[9] has divided the hypertensive disorders of pregnancy into six categories. The first of these is *labile hypertension*, in which there is an elevation of blood pressure that returns to normal 2 weeks postpartum. *Preeclampsia* is classically defined when two of the three traditional signs, i.e., proteinuria, edema, and hypertension, are present. In *eclampsia*, convulsions and coma supervene. *Chronic hypertensive vascular disease* is diagnosed when a blood pressure of 140/90 is found prior to the 20th week of pregnancy. A separate classification is used for *chronic renal* disease with hypertension. A last category involves the *superimposition of preeclampsia and eclampsia* on one of the latter two disease states.

INCIDENCE

Worldwide, toxemia remains the third largest cause of maternal mortality, after hemorrhage and infection. It occurs in 7% of all pregnancies.[4] Four maternal deaths per 10,000 pregnant women occur because of toxemia. As well, its presence signifies an important danger to the fetus. The perinatal death rate is 6–10% and becomes much higher in the severe types. There is a significant incidence of prematurity associated with the condition. Friedman and Neff[4] observed that 10–25% of surviving infants had neurologic and developmental defects.

The Collaborative Perinatal Project[4] was able to identify significant predisposing factors and to develop a profile of the gravida at risk. Among these factors were nulliparity and the occurrence of genitourinary infection and glomerulonephritis.

ETIOLOGY AND PATHOGENESIS

A multiplicity of etiological factors have been invoked to explain the occurrence of preeclampsia and eclampsia, ranging from the presence of the disease states and environmental factors described under "Incidence" to the presence of local toxins in the uterus itself.[2] Much attention has been paid to hormonal and endocrine factors, including decreased uterine synthesis of prostaglandin E, and particularly the role of the renin—angiotensin system and various placental factors. The role of uterine ischemia has been stressed. In no case has definitive evidence been put forth to establish any of these as the primary cause of the condition.

It has long been known that the definitive treatment of the preeclamptic and eclamptic state involves termination of the pregnancy. As Willems[10] has pointed out the key factor in the maintenance of the condition is the presence of placental tissue, as uterine ischemia per se does not produce the syndrome in the nonpregnant state,[1] and the presence of a fetus is not critical, as can be seen by the development of toxemic symptoms in patients with trophoblastic disease. A description has been given elsewhere (see Chapter 8: "Immunology of Pregnancy") of the mechanisms which protect the fetus from "rejection." Prominent among these are the presence of the sialomucin barrier protecting the trophoblast and the immunologic enhancement secondary to the presence of maternal blocking antibodies.

Scott and Beer[8] have indicated that histoincompatibility between mother and fetus is more common in cases of preeclampsia. Willems[10] postulates that a failure of the immunologically protective mechanisms allows placental damage to occur.

This would be more common in the malnourished primigravida with her "untried" maternal immune system, where the placenta is large, and histoincompatibility between mother and fetus is significant. In such a patient, blocking antibody would not be present in sufficient quantity to protect the placenta.

The same maternal cytotoxic antibodies or "killer lymphocytes" that reject the placenta would attack the maternal kidney. Resultant decreased placental function could lead to decreased progesterone levels, thereby allowing aldosterone to act and resulting in sodium and water retention.

Moreover, the synthesis of prostaglandins E and A would be diminished. This would lead to a "vicious cycle," as these substances may allow low-resistance blood flow through the placenta via their relaxing effect on smooth muscle.

In addition, placental ischemia may cause uteroplacental renin production to become prominent. The role of the renin-angiotension system is summarized in Figures 20.1 and 20.2.

The etiology and pathogenesis of the preeclamptic and eclamptic states involve numerous modalities. However, it is an intriguing thought that the primary root incident may be a type of rejection phenomenon by the mother of the "foreign" (that is, partly paternal) trophoblastic tissue.

PATHOLOGICAL CHANGES IN PREECLAMPSIA AND ECLAMPSIA

Striking changes in major organ systems are the hallmark of the severely preeclamptic or eclamptic state. The most important of these is the change in the capillaries of the renal glomeruli, where the

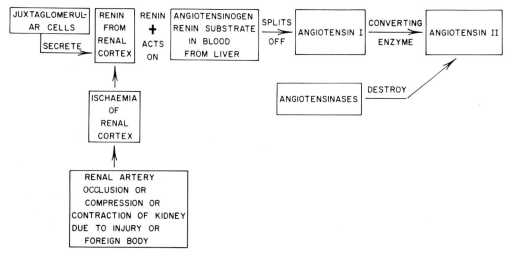

Figure 20.1. Renin-angiotensin pressor system. This is a mechanism of acute renal hypertension.

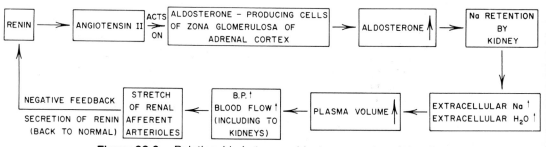

Figure 20.2. Relationship between aldosterone and angiotensin.

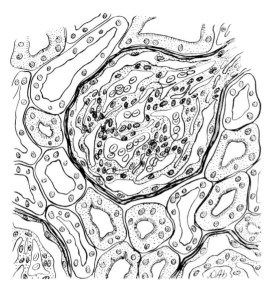

Figure 20.3. Renal glomerulus in preeclampsia.

characteristic lesion involves significant swelling of the capillary endothelial cells and thickening of the basement membrane (Fig. 20.3).[7] These changes are reminiscent of an acute rejection phenomenon seen in the transplanted kidney, where immunologic attack leads to a very similar picture.

Fibrin deposition in the kidney glomeruli is another prominent feature in preeclampsia and eclampsia.

In the brain, petechial hemorrhages are observed and edema is noted. Retinal edema and retinal arteriolar spasm are seen. In the liver, subcapsular swelling occurs and is responsible for the striking symptom of epigastric pain that is often a feature of severe preeclampsia.

The similarity of the changes in the placental arteries in preeclamptic patients to those vascular changes occurring in the rejection of a transplanted organ are notable.

SIGNS AND SYMPTOMS

The onset of preeclampsia, usually in the third trimester, is characterized by:

1. Rapid weight gain
2. Edema—notably in hands, feet, legs, and face. This is also evident in the presacral area in the patient at bed rest.
3. Proteinuria
4. Hypertension
   With increasing severity, *headache* and *visual changes* secondary to papilledema and arterial changes in the optic fundi are noted. *Hyperreflexia* can develop, and the patient may become *oliguric*.

Eclampsia is present when the patient develops

1. Convulsions
   and/or
2. Coma
   This condition is associated with a significant risk for both fetal and maternal mortality.

PREVENTION AND TREATMENT

Good **prenatal care** is essential to the diminution in incidence of preeclampsia and eclampsia. Adequate **nutrition**, characterized by a high protein diet is an integral part of proper prenatal care. Adequate **rest** is essential as well.

Various conditions may predispose the pregnant woman to preeclampsia. These include maternal diabetes, renal disease, multiple gestation, and hydatidiform mole.

If any one of the early signs of toxemia develops, a high protein diet should be utilized and the patient placed at bed rest. Hospitalization for observation is often required if two or more of the classical triad of symptoms are present.

Although antihypertensive medications such as hydralazine (hydrazinophthalazine) are useful in chronic hypertension in pregnancy, they are of equivocal value in preeclampsia and do not seem to significantly decrease the possibility of convulsions, although the blood pressure may be in the normal range. However, they are useful in diminishing the possibility of a cerebrovascular accident in the hypertensive, preeclamptic patient. Diuretics are contraindicated in the treatment of preeclampsia.

The pregnancy is carefully monitored (See Chapter 13: "Evaluation of Fetal Growth") as a gestation at high risk.

The classical treatment of fulminating

preeclampsia, still valid today, is twofold:

1. Magnesium sulfate to stabilize the condition. This is best utilized by slow intravenous drip via an infusion pump, at approximately 1 gm/hour, individualized to the patient. Intake, output, and vital signs are watched. The mother is carefully observed for signs of respiratory depression and depression of deep tendon reflexes. Serum magnesium levels can be followed and should be in the range of 4 to 6 mg/100 ml.
2. Deliver the baby.

Depending on the severity of the condition, delivery is opted for at a maximal time, ideally when the toxemia is temporarily stabilized and it has been ascertained that the fetus is mature. Labor may be carefully induced, depending on the circumstances, with monitoring of the fetus and uterine contractility. Cesarean section often becomes necessary. Remarkable improvement is often seen in the condition within 24 hours of delivery, but the patient is in danger of convulsing until significant diuresis has been achieved. This may occur as much as a week or more postpartum. It is essential, therefore, to carefully monitor intake and output of the patient as well as the blood pressure and other clinical signs of the resolving toxemia.

If the patient convulses, supportive measures must be undertaken in addition to magnesium sulphate therapy. The patient is kept in a quiet room, on her side, in some degree of Trendelenburg position, with constant medical attendance. Attention is given to maintaining an airway during convulsive episodes. Vital signs and intake and hourly output are monitored. If the patient becomes oliguric, steps may be taken to increase renal perfusion, with care that intake does not grossly exceed output.

When the patient is stabilized, the baby is delivered.

References

1. Cavanagh, D., Rao, P.S., Tung, K.S.K., et al. Eclamptogenic toxemia: The development of an experimental model in the subhuman primate. *Am. J. Obstet. Gynecol. 120*:183, 1974.
2. Dieckmann, W.J. *The Toxemias of Pregnancy.* C.V. Mosby, St. Louis, 1941.
3. Dimmette, J.E. Studies of human pregnancy: I. Immunoglobulins attached to the trophoblast. *Obstet. Gynecol. 47*:730, 1976.
4. Friedman, E.A., and Neff, R.K. *Pregnancy Hypertension.* PSG Publishing Co. Inc., Littleton, Mass., 1977.
5. Jenkins, D.M. Pre-eclampsia/eclampsia (gestosis) and other pregnancy complications with possible immunologic basis. In *Immunology of Human Reproduction,* edited by Scott, J.S., and Jones, W.R. Academic Press, London; Grune & Stratton, New York, 1976, pp. 297–348.
6. Kitzmiller, J.L. Immunologic approaches to the study of preeclampsia. In *Clinical Obstetrics and Gynecology,* Freedman, S.O., and Gold, P., guest editors. September 1977, vol. 20, no. 3, pp. 717–735.
7. Pollak, V.E., and Nettles, J.B. The kidney in toxemia of pregnancy: A clinical and pathologic study based on renal biopsies. In *Medicine.* December 1960, vol. 39, no. 4, pp. 469–522.
8. Scott, J.R., and Beer, A.E. Reproductive immunology. In *Obstetrics and Gynecology Annual,* ed. 3, edited by Wynn, R.M. Appleton-Century-Crofts, New York, 1974, pp. 101–136.
9. Townsend, L. Hypertensive disorders of pregnancy. In *Advances in Obstetrics and Gynecology,* edited by Caplan, R.M., and Sweeney, W.J. Williams & Wilkins, Baltimore, 1978, pp. 197–209.
10. Willems, J. The etiology of preeclampsia. In *Obstetrics and Gynecology.* October 1977, vol. 50, no. 4, pp. 495–499.

CHAPTER 21

Heart Disease

LUCIEN I. ARDITI, M.D.

DIAGNOSIS OF HEART DISEASE DURING PREGNANCY

History

It is important to establish whether the patient has heart disease antedating the pregnancy. A past history of rheumatic fever, the discovery of a heart murmur before the patient became pregnant, and a history of previous treatment for heart disease should be elicited. Symptoms that antedate pregnancy are most useful. The pregnant female often complains of dyspnea, pedal edema, limitations of physical activity in the absence of heart disease. Obtaining such a history in a patient is useful if it antedates the pregnancy. If the patient has been pregnant in the past, it is useful to seek information regarding cardiac complications which may have marred the previous pregnancy and regarding specific medical interventions deemed necessary in the past. If the patient has had a chest x-ray prior to her pregnancy, it is useful to review it; if she has undergone a cardiac catheterization or heart surgery, the detailed report of the cardiac catheterization, including pressures and cardiac output as well as the operative note, is of the utmost value. These data should be compiled during the initial interview and the specific reports obtained soon thereafter.

Physical Examination

The physical examination of the patient with heart disease in pregnancy offers many pitfalls. Pedal edema does not nec-essarily signify heart failure, because it normally develops during pregnancy. The hypervolemia of pregnancy is associated with a parasternal systolic murmur in a high percentage of patients. The murmur often radiates to the apex and has to be differentiated from the murmur of organic mitral regurgitation. The presence of an S3 gallop which usually signifies left ventricular failure cannot be similarly interpreted in the pregnant patient. More than 80% of women develop a third heart sound at some time during the gestational period. The frequency of an S3 during pregnancy parallels the increase in cardiac output.

Systolic flow murmurs, that is, innocent murmurs, may be hard to differentiate from hemodynamically significant murmurs if the patient is first examined during pregnancy. The loudness of the murmur, its transmission to the axilla or neck vessels, and its association with a palpable thrill are helpful in assessing its significance. The intensity of the murmur is conventionally graded I–VI. A grade I murmur can be heard with special effort, a grade II murmur is faint but easily recognizable, a grade III murmur is prominent but not loud, a grade IV murmur is loud, a grade V murmur is very loud, and a grade VI is loudest and can even be heard with the stethoscope barely in contact with the chest. In the absence of heart disease a pregnant patient should have no murmur louder than grade II. Flow murmurs associated with pregnancy are usually heard best along the left lateral sternal border and are present in over 90% of pregnant women. They do not usually radiate to the axilla, and they are not associated with thrills.

Systolic murmurs are intensified during pregnancy because of the flow across normal cardiovascular valves. This is particularly true of murmurs arising in the pulmonic and aortic areas. However, systolic murmurs of mitral regurgitation usually become softer during pregnancy, because of the fall in systemic arterial resistance. An exception to this occurs when mitral regurgitation is associated with hypertrophic subaortic stenosis: the regurgitation may then become more marked during pregnancy.[6] In hypertrophic disease, the fall in systemic arterial resistance may increase the outflow obstruction and thereby increase mitral regurgitation.

If a patient is found to have an apical systolic murmur that is delayed in onset and preceded by a midsystolic click, this patient most likely has a mitral valve prolapse syndrome and the diagnosis can be confirmed by echocardiography. The vast majority of patients with the mitral valve prolapse syndrome have a totally uneventful gestation. The importance of making the correct diagnosis in those patients lies in the fact that they are susceptible to subacute bacterial endocarditis and should be protected with antibiotics at delivery, or when subjected to procedures likely to be associated with transient bacteremia.

Diastolic murmurs of aortic regurgitation may become fainter, and sometimes inaudible, during pregnancy because of a drop in peripheral vascular resistance. Occasionally, the intensity of such a faint diastolic murmur can be increased if the physician has the patient squat or if he listens to the murmur while the patient performs a strenuous handgrip. Diastolic cardiac murmurs do not develop during pregnancy in the absence of heart disease. However, a loud S3 and its after vibrations could be mistaken for a diastolic murmur. Similarly, a diastolic bruit originating in the internal mammary artery may be misinterpreted as being cardiac in origin. A continuous murmur originating from the breast vasculature can be heard in 10% of pregnant women, especially during the third trimester. This murmur has been referred to as a *mammary souffle*. It can be obliterated by pressure on the breast proximal to the stethoscope and can be altered by pressing firmly on the stethoscope.

The X-Ray, the Electrocardiogram, and the Echocardiogram

A chest x-ray is useful to assess the presence of cardiomegaly, to determine selective chamber enlargement and to determine the presence of pulmonary overcirculation. It is, however, wisest not to expose the fetus to radiation, particularly during the first trimester. Abdominal shielding is necessary, and the number of x-ray exposures should be kept to a minimum. Preferably one should be satisfied with an x-ray taken within a few months prior to the onset of pregnancy. A chest x-ray recorded far along in pregnancy is less useful because often the diaphragm has been pushed up by the gravid uterus and the cardiac silhouette may have its axis shifted somewhat transversely, giving the appearance of cardiomegaly. During pregnancy, the mean QRS axis in the frontal plane of the electrocardiogram shifts slightly to the left. A Q wave may develop in lead 3, which often disappears with deep inspiration. The electrocardiogram is useful in assessing the presence or absence of ventricular hypertrophy as well as atrial enlargement. The echocardiogram is particularly useful in confirming the presence of the mitral valve prolapse syndrome, in assessing the degree of mitral stenosis, in excluding the presence of hypertrophic cardiomyopathy, in screening for aortic valve disease and in obtaining a reliable measurement of left atrial size.

MANAGEMENT OF CARDIAC COMPLICATIONS IN PREGNANCY

Dysrhythmias

Paroxysmal atrial tachycardias occur with greater frequency during pregnancy. Atrial premature beats, ventricular premature beats, ventricular bigeminy can appear de novo in pregnancy and do not necessarily implicate underlying heart disease. In a patient with heart disease, an episode of atrial fibrillation at a rapid ventricular rate can pose a serious problem. Direct current countershock conversion has been used in pregnancy with no evidence of deleterious effect on the fetus.[7] In patients with complete heart block with a slow ventricular rate, a temporary or permanent transvenous pacemaker can be inserted with no greater risk than in the nonpregnant state. The use of routine prophylactic digitalization in patients with heart disease is not advocated, except in the patient with moderate or tight mitral stenosis. If a pregnant patient with tight mitral stenosis goes from normal sinus rhythm into atrial fibrillation, the rapid ventricular rate may be lethal. Digitalization will reduce the chance of developing atrial fibrillation and, more important, it will control the ventricular rate in atrial fibrillation so as to allow an adequate period of ventricular filling and prevent the rapid development of pulmonary edema.

If either quinidine or procainamide is needed for the control of dysrhythmias during pregnancy, it can be safely used. There are no reports of untoward effects of these two drugs on the course of pregnancy. However, in the management of dysrhythmias during pregnancy, propranolol is best avoided. When administered during pregnancy it has been associated with postnatal bradycardia, hypoglycemia, and impaired responsiveness to anoxic stress. Propranolol administered to the mother does cross the placenta. The bradycardia it produces in the neonatal state may last up to 72 hours following the last dose administered to the mother, even though its half time is only 3 or 4 hours. The probable explanation for this protracted effect is based on the fact that propranolol is highly tissue and albumin bound and may continue to be released from such binding sites over a 3-day period. Severe hypoglycemia in the neonate has been reported, with blood sugar levels of 11–30 mg/dl persisting on the low side for about 8–24 hours.[3] Treatment consists of administering a 10% dextrose solution to the baby. Beta blockade impairs the ability of the fetus to develop a rebound tachycardia in response to transient anoxia. This is possibly the explanation for impaired responsiveness to anoxic stress due to propranolol. The depressed state of the fetus at birth, with delay in onset of sustained breathing, may require vigorous resuscitation and, possibly, administration of atropine and isoproterenol for the bradycardia. Babies born to mothers who have been on propranolol for such conditions as hypertrophic subaortic stenosis or dysrhythmias have been reported to be small for gestational age and to have a small placenta. It is of interest that even such small doses as 10 mg of propranolol four times a day have been associated with significant neonatal bradycardia, hypoglycemia, and respiratory distress. This finding suggests a cumulative effect of the drug. Hopefully, beta blockers which do not cross the placental barrier will become available.

Congestive Heart Failure

The diagnosis of congestive heart failure in pregnancy may at times be difficult. Rales audible at the bases may be atelectatic rales due to the elevated diaphragms pushed upward by the gravid uterus. Peripheral edema may be due to compression of the inferior vena cava by the gravid uterus, and heart size may be hard to assess clinically because of the lateral displacement of the apex by the elevated diaphragms. If one is convinced that the patient is in congestive failure, then the management should be digitalization, salt restriction, and judicious use of diuretics. The use of diuretics in pregnancy is not recommended unless they are definitely necessary. The continued use of diuretics in pregnancy can result in sodium depletion and hyponatremia, with ensuing hypotension. Potassium replacement should be a concomitant of diuretic therapy to avoid superimposing hypokalemia, especially in the presence of digitalis. Diuretics may cross the placental barrier and cause fetal electrolyte and water depletion. In the case of thiazide diuretics, neonatal jaundice and severe thrombocytopenia may result from their use late in pregnancy. Sodium restriction and diuretics do not prevent toxemia but may reduce plasma volume enough to accentuate maternal postural hypotension.

Prevention of Endocarditis

Patients with an organic heart murmur, a prosthetic patch, or a valve prosthesis are at risk of contracting subacute bacterial endocarditis from bacteremia. Since bacteremia can occur during delivery, it is imperative to cover the patient with antibiotics. An uncomplicated vaginal delivery may not be associated with bacteremia. However, the concern regarding such an event warrants the use of antibiotic prophylaxis. The recommended regimen is directed at the enterococcus *Streptococcus faecalis*, rather than at the broad spectrum of bacteria to which the patient is exposed and which do not usually cause bacterial endocarditis. One current regimen advocated is aqueous penicillin G 2,000,000 units intramuscularly or intravenously, or ampicillin, 1.0 gm intramuscularly or intravenously, *plus* gentamycin 1.5 mg/kg (not to exceed 80 mg) intramuscularly or intravenously, *or* streptomycin 1.0 gm intramuscularly. The initial dose should be given 30 minutes to 1 hour prior to delivery. If gentamycin is used, a similar dose of gentamycin and penicillin (or ampicillin) should be given every 8 hours for two additional doses. If streptomycin is used, then a similar dose of streptomycin and penicillin (or ampicillin) should be given every 12 hours for two additional doses.[1] Intravenous vancomycin (1.0 gm) should be substituted for penicillin if the patient is allergic to penicillin.

Thromboembolic Complications

Patients with prosthetic heart valves are usually on lifelong anticoagulation except in special situations, such as those of patients with porcine valves in the aortic position or porcine mitral valves in a heart with a small left atrium and normal sinus rhythm. Because patients who have to continue on anticoagulants throughout their pregnancy have only two out of three chances of their pregnancy having a normal outcome, they should be informed of the risk and encouraged not to get pregnant. If they do get pregnant, they should be encouraged to undergo a therapeutic abortion. However, if they understand the risks involved and still wish to carry their pregnancy to term, they will bear close watching. In the past, coumarin derivatives were used throughout the pregnancy. Because coumarin anticoagulants cross the placental barrier, they have been reported to be associated with fetal abnormalities. During the first trimester, the abnormalities which develop are referred to as warfarin embryopathy. The abnormalities include a hypoplastic saddle type nose and bone abnormalities, the most striking of which is stippling seen on x-rays of the newborn infants. Stippling may not be evident after the first year of life; however, calcific stippling is incorporated into epiphyses and may account for the scoliosis reported in some cases. Exposure to coumarin derivatives during the second and third trimester of pregnancy has been associated with such anomalies as mental retardation, blindness, deafness, seizures, scoliosis, and, occasionally, congenital heart disease.

Ueland[8] prefers to use low-dose subcutaneous heparin therapy throughout pregnancy, labor, and delivery. The heparin molecule (molecular weight 15,000–30,000) does not cross the placental barrier, and hence it is felt to be safer for the fetus. However, the effectiveness of low-dose subcutaneous heparin in the prevention of thromboembolic complications of valve prostheses has not been established. Chronic (over 6 months) heparin administration has led to the development of osteoporosis. Hall et al.[4] reviewed cases in which heparin was used during gestation, comparing the outcome of pregnancy in these cases with that of pregnancies in which coumarin derivatives were used. They note that although heparin does not cross the placental barrier, the likelihood of a normal outcome of the pregnancy is, at most, two thirds. This figure is amazingly similar to that in the group treated with coumarin anticoagulants. They calculate that when heparin is used during pregnancy, one eighth of the pregnancies will end in stillbirth and one fifth will be premature. They also point to the marked maternal complication rate with the use of heparin. They conclude that the overall likelihood of a relatively normal outcome of a pregnancy in which either coumarin derivatives or heparin is used is approximately two thirds. Because of difficulties in administration of heparin, they consider coumarin derivatives a reasonable alternative for anticoagulant therapy in pregnancy, if the patient understands the risks involved and does not wish to terminate the pregnancy.

In the New York Lying-In-Hospital obstetrical cardiac clinic a middle course is steered. During the first trimester of pregnancy, anticoagulation is switched from coumarin to heparin, administered subcutaneously in doses of 5,000 units every 12 hours. The coumarin anticoagulants are resumed during the second trimester and discontinued approximately 3 weeks prior to delivery. The 3 weeks of coumarin discontinuance prior to delivery are meant to allow enough time for the necessary coagulation factors in the fetus to return to normal. Substitution of heparin for coumarin during the 3 weeks prior to delivery should reduce the risk to the fetus. Postpartum coumarin anticoagulation can be resumed provided breast feeding is not planned. Because all oral anticoagulants are actively excreted in the breast milk, breast feeding should be prohibited when the mother is on oral anticoagulants. A major advantage of heparin administration in the puerperium is that it allows breast feeding. In patients who do not have prosthetic heart valves but who are at high risk for thromboembolic complications, prophylactic subcutaneous heparin administration should be continued for 2 or 3 weeks following delivery. Such patients would include those with a previous history of thrombophlebitis or with a past history of pulmonary embolization (Table 21.1).

Table 21.1   Selected Drugs Commonly used in Heart Disease. Features Pertinent to their use in Pregnancy

Name of Drug	Ability to Cross Placenta	Secretion in Breast Milk	Adverse Effect on Fetus or Neonate when used in Usual Doses
Digoxin	Yes	Yes	None if maternal levels do not exceed the therapeutic range.
Quinidine sulfate	*	*	None reported to date.
Procainamide	Yes	*	Has potential of accumulating in the fetus where it is much more slowly eliminated. Should be used with caution.
Propranolol	Yes	Yes	Postnatal bradycardia, hypoglycemia, impaired fetal responsiveness to anoxia. There are conflicting reports on safety of drug during breast feeding.
Phenytoin	*	Yes	10–30% incidence of multiple anomalies, neonatal hemorrhage.
Thiazide diuretics	Yes	Yes	Neonatal jaundice, electrolyte and water depletion, thrombocytopenia. Should also be avoided during lactation.
Hydralazine	*	*	Fetal anomalies reported, but this drug is considered the drug of choice in treatment of hypertension during labor and delivery.
Warfarin	Yes	Yes	Facial and skeletal anomalies, mental retardation, blindness and deafness. Avoid during lactation, although some data suggest only a very small amount crosses from plasma into milk.
Heparin	No	No	Stillbirths (12.5%), prematurity (20%). Mechanism of this effect not understood.
Sulfonamides	Yes	*	Enhance kernicterus. Contraindicated in 3rd trimester. Avoid also in patients with glucose-6-PO_4 dehydrogenase enzyme deficiency.

* No published data available.

Termination of Pregnancy

There are a few situations which warrant termination of pregnancy on the basis of underlying heart disease. In this category one should include patients with severe pulmonary arterial hypertension (Eisenmenger physiology).[2] These patients usually present with a history of hemoptysis, the finding of loud pulmonic second sound, left parasternal lift, and right ventricular hypertrophy on the electrocardiogram. They do poorly during the pregnancy and are at high risk during delivery and early postpartum. These patients are particularly vulnerable to a drop in systemic pressure. The diagnosis needs to be confirmed with right heart catheterization. In view of a mortality in the range of 27–50% even in women who are asymptomatic before pregnancy, one is justified in strongly urging termination of pregnancy.

Another group of patients who are at high risk during pregnancy and the puerperium includes those patients with Marfan's syndrome. The changes in the aorta which accompany pregnancy make such patients particularly vulnerable to aortic dissection, hence the need for early termination of pregnancy.

Patients with tight mitral stenosis are usually advised not to become pregnant. These patients should consider undergoing mitral valvotomy before entertaining pregnancy. However, if a patient with tight mitral stenosis is first seen early in the pregnancy and if evidence of congestive failure appears during the first trimester of pregnancy long before the peak burden is attained, a closed mitral valvotomy can usually be performed with impunity.[5] A similar statement cannot be made regarding cardiac surgery involving cardiopulmonary bypass, in which the risk to the fetus is significantly prohibitive.

Patients with a history of postpartum myocardiopathy constitute another category of patients who should be seriously offered termination of pregnancy during the first trimester. In this category are included those patients who gave no evidence of heart disease during pregnancy and delivery despite extensive cardiac evaluation and whose signs and symptoms of heart muscle disease first appeared 2–20 weeks postpartum. These patients present the constellation of a primary congestive cardiomyopathy. They have a proclivity for dysrhythmias and are exquisitely sensitive to digitalis. This diagnosis is most commonly made in black women over the age of 30. Such patients need to be on anticoagulation for the duration of the cardiomegaly. The diagnosis of postpartum myocardiopathy is associated with a high maternal mortality. These patients should be offered termination of their pregnancy. If cardiomegaly persists 6 months after the diagnosis has been made, the patient should be advised to avoid a subsequent pregnancy.

SPECIAL CONSIDERATIONS WITH REFERENCE TO LABOR AND DELIVERY

Vaginal delivery is favored over cesarean section for most patients with heart disease. Cesarean section involves anesthesia and a major surgical procedure, thereby adding to the risk. There are special situations in which the Valsalva maneuver is particularly noxious to the patient, and in those specific situations cesarean section is utilized. Included in this group are patients with coarctation of the aorta in whom death could occur from rupture of the aorta, patients with left ventricular aneurysms, and patients suspected of aortic dissection.

The majority of patients can be handled with regional anesthesia (pudendal or epidural block). Hypotension should be avoided, particularly in patients with septal defects and right-sided hypertension in whom a right-to-left shunt would suddenly perfuse the systemic circulation with unoxygenated blood and favor the development of dysrhythmias. Similarly, systemic hypotension in patients with tight aortic stenosis would result in decreased myocardial and coronary perfusion.

Shortening the second stage of labor by the use of forceps is favored. The maternal and fetal heart rate as well as the venous pressure should be monitored. Adequate analgesics, to relieve pain and thereby decrease the hemodynamic burden, are important. Sedatives are in order. Synthetic oxytocin is preferable to the natural product because it is less likely to be contaminated by pressor agents. Atropine should be used with caution because of its associated sinus tachycardia. Ergonovine and methylergonovine maleate tend to raise the venous pressure and should, therefore, be avoided in patients who are at risk of pulmonary congestion. Scopolamine is contraindicated.

Blood loss should be minimized, by prompt removal of the placenta and early bimanual compression of the uterus as well as with the use of synthetic oxytocin.

A careful history, meticulous physical examination, and close follow-up, together with adherence to the principles outlined above, have helped reduce drastically the maternal mortality and fetal loss previously attributed to heart disease during pregnancy. The close cooperation between the cardiologist and the obstetrician during pregnancy, delivery, and postpartum is essential for a successful outcome.

References

1. AHA Committee Report: Prevention of bacterial endocarditis. *Circulation 56*:139A–143A, 1976.
2. Gleicher, N., Midwall, J., Hochberger, D., and Jaffin, H. Eisenmenger's syndrome and pregnancy. *Obstet. Gynecol. Surv. 34*:721–741, 1979.
3. Habib, A., and McCarthy J.S. Effects on the neonate of propranolol administered during pregnancy. *J. Pediatr. 91*:808–811, 1977.
4. Hall, J.G., Pauli, R.M., and Wilson, K.M. Maternal and fetal sequelae of anticoagulation during pregnancy. *Am. J. Med. 68*:122–140, 1980.
5. Knapp, R.C., and Arditi, L.I. Closed mitral valvotomy in pregnancy. *Clin. Obstet. Gynecol. 11*:978–991, 1968.
6. Kolibash, A.J., Ruiz, D.E., and Lewis, R.P. Idiopathic hypertrophic subaortic stenosis in pregnancy. *Ann. Intern. Med. 82*:791–794, 1975.
7. Schroeder, J.S., and Harrison, D.C. Repeated cardioversion during pregnancy. *Am. J. Cardiol. 27*:445–446, 1971.
8. Ueland, K. Heart disease in pregnancy. In *Advances in Obstetrics and Gynecology*, edited by Caplan, R.M., and Sweeney, W.J. III. Williams & Wilkins, Baltimore, 1978, pp. 174–183.

CHAPTER 22

Diabetes and Pregnancy

LOIS JOVANOVIC, M.D.
CHARLES M. PETERSON, M.D.

Mortality of the infant of the diabetic woman has decreased markedly since the advent of insulin. Prior to 1922, the Joslin Clinic reported no ketotic-prone diabetic woman who delivered a live infant.[29] Subsequent to the commercial use of insulin there has been a decreasing incidence of infant mortality such that most centers report between 3.8 and 8% mortality[8, 16, 27] and one center recently reported no infant deaths in their small series.[2] The key to this improvement has been the realization that normalization of the maternal glucose was essential. This trend can be seen clearly if the major studies of infant mortality since 1922 are plotted against the mean blood glucose of the mother (Fig. 22.1).

However, the infant of the diabetic mother still suffers from a high incidence of morbidity (up to 80% in one series).[7] Perhaps with control of diabetics mellitus prior to conception and maintenance of control throughout pregnancy, morbidity of the infant whose mother has diabetes will decrease to levels seen in the general population.

DIABETOGENIC FACTORS OF PREGNANCY

Since elevated maternal blood glucose should be avoided at all times, a clear understanding of what is normal blood glucose is necessary. During early pregnancy, glucose crosses the placenta to the fetus by facilitated diffusion. Amino acids are actively transported, and of particular importance is the siphoning of the gluconeogenic amino acid alanine. The effect of maternal loss of glucose and gluconeogenic substrate to the fetus is a decrease in maternal fasting blood glucose to 55–65 mg/dl.[9]

As pregnancy progresses, three important factors work in concert to cause postprandial hyperglycemia: 1) the placenta produces increasing amounts of hormones which antagonize insulin; 2) maternal serum cortisol increases by threefold, and 3) the placenta itself contains enzymes which increase the degradation of maternal insulin.

Placental Hormones Which Antagonize Insulin

ESTROGENS AND PROGESTERONE

The literature on the glucose intolerance which emerges when predisposed women ingest oral contraceptives seems to point toward estrogens and progesterones as both direct and indirect contributors to hyperglycemia. However, the most convincing study[1] suggests the main cause of the alteration in carbohydrate metabolism with elevated serum estrogens and progesterones to be a large cortisol-mediated increase in hepatic gluconeogenesis and not the glucocorticoid-like action of these two hormones.

HUMAN PLACENTAL LACTOGEN (HPL)

The mechanism of action of HPL is still not clear despite years of vigorous research. It is known that HPL is a polypep-

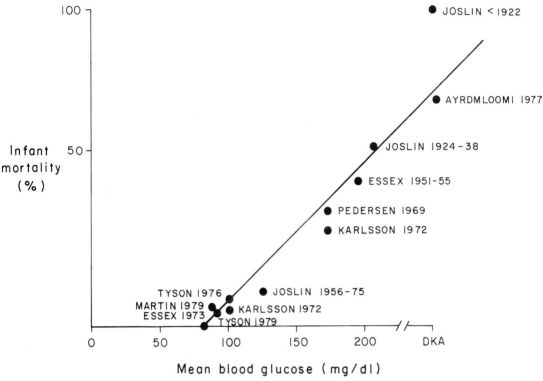

Figure 22.1. Mean maternal glucose versus infant mortality 1922–1979.

tide of placental origin and that circulating levels increase progressively with increasing placental size. Several groups[11, 18] reported that HPL leads to a deterioration in glucose tolerance, much like growth hormone and prolactin. HPL also promotes free fatty acid (FFA) production by stimulating lipolysis of triglycerides. FFA promotes peripheral tissue resistance to insulin, which leads to a high insulin concentration and a subsequent down regulation of the insulin receptors; this in turn results in hyperinsulinemia. Nevertheless, other investigators[23] find no correlation between HPL concentrations, glucose levels, and FFA. Therefore, the true effect of HPL on glucose tolerance remains to be shown.

Maternal Increase in Serum Cortisol

Total plasma cortisol levels are progressively increased in pregnancy. Also, transcortin (the cortisol-binding globulin) levels increase in plasma as a consequence of elevated serum estrogen levels. The free cortisol levels (the biologically active fraction of total cortisol) are also increased up to threefold and elevations of cortisol are known to unmask diabetes in a predisposed individual.

Degradation of Maternal Insulin

Insulin turnover is increased during pregnancy because of increased degradation of insulin by placental enzymes comparable to liver insulinase.[6] The placenta also has a membrane-associated insulin degrading activity.[24] This degradation of insulin may contribute to the diabetogenic factors of pregnancy.

Concomitant with the above hormonal changes of pregnancy, the rate of disposal of orally or intravenously administered glucose is slowed.[26] The normal pancreatic beta cells adapt to these alterations by potentiating the secretion of insulin. When the pancreas fails to respond adequately to these alterations, gestational diabetes mellitus emerges.

DEFINITIONS

Gestational Diabetes

Once the physiology of glucose metabolism during pregnancy is understood, then it becomes clear that fasting blood glucose in normal pregnancy is lower than in nonpregnant people and that postprandial glucose levels tend to be higher than those seen in age-matched nonpregnant people. In the normal pregnant state, fasting blood glucose is 55–60, mean blood glucose is 84 mg/dl and the 1 hour postprandial blood glucose is less than 140 mg/dl. The term "gestational diabetic" should be understood to include women who 1) have a normal blood glucose concentration in the fasting state but 2) show an abnormal glucose tolerance for the first time in their life from an oral glucose tolerance test (GTT) and 3) who show no glucose abnormality following delivery. Clearly, the diagnosis can only be made in retrospect. The glucose tolerance test is the tool which is used to make the diagnosis of glucose intolerance (Table 22.1). O'Sullivan[20] has reported that a simple screening test of all pregnant women uncovers more diabetic patients than does reliance on indicators such as family history, previous obstetrical history, or obesity. We employ the O'Sullivan screen of 50 gm of oral glucose and obtain a 1 hour plasma glucose. All patients who have a plasma glucose of ≥150 mg/dl are given a formal glucose tolerance test of 100 gm oral glucose. If the glucose tolerance test is abnormal, then the patient is referred for treatment (Fig. 22.2). The incidence of gestational diabetes in the Clinic population at the New York Hospital is 2% and is similar to the Boston City Study.[21]

Pregestational Diabetes

Since insulin-dependent diabetic women now live to the childbearing years, classifications of pregestational diabetes have emerged in an attempt to help the physician predict the outcome of pregnancy for both the mother and the child (Table 22.2). However, as the evidence mounts that maternal normoglycemia at the time of conception, organogenesis, and

Table 22.1.   Interpretation of Oral Glucose Tolerance Test

| | O'Sullivan and Mahan (21) | | USC (Seltzer (25)) | |
	Plasma (mg/dl)	Whole blood (mg/dl)	Plasma (mg/dl)	Whole blood (mg/dl)
Fasting	105	90	95	110
1 hour	190	165	170	200
2 hour	165	145	130	150
3 hour	140	125	110	130

throughout growth of the fetus until term is the major determinant of outcome, there need be only two classes of diabetes: good control and less than optimal control.

EFFECT OF HYPERGLYCEMIA ON PREGNANCY AND THE FETUS

When maternal diabetes mellitus is not well controlled, the fetus will be exposed to either sustained hyperglycemia or intermittent pulses of hyperglycemia. Both stimulate prematurely induced fetal insulin secretion. The Pedersen hypothesis[22] links this maternal hyperglycemia-induced fetal hyperinsulinemia to morbidity of the infant. Thus, fetal hyperinsulinemia may result in 1) increased fetal body fat (macrosomnia) and therefore difficult delivery, 2) inhibition of pulmonary maturation of surfactant, 3) decreased serum potassium which results in muscle weakness or cardiac arrhythmias, and 4) neonatal hypoglycemia which might result in permanent neurological damage. Hyperglycemia may also lead to maternal complications, such as polyhydramnios hypertension, urinary tract infections, monilial vaginitis, recurrent spontaneous abortions, and infertility. Therefore, a vigorous effort should be made to diagnose diabetes early and to achieve and maintain euglycemia throughout pregnancy.

TREATMENT DESIGNED TO ACHIEVE AND MAINTAIN NORMOGLYCEMIA

Diet Management

Once the diagnosis of diabetes is made, the patient should be referred for treat-

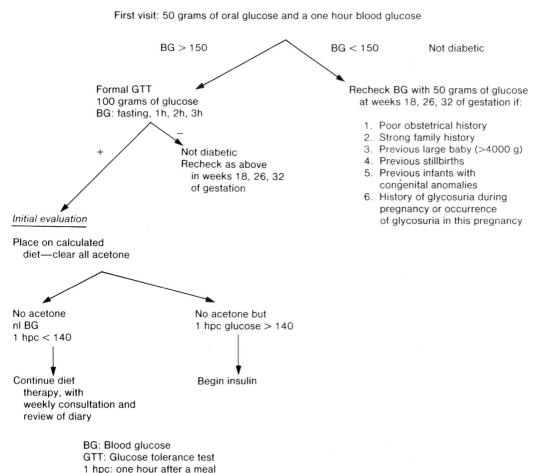

First visit: 50 grams of oral glucose and a one hour blood glucose

BG > 150

BG < 150   Not diabetic

Formal GTT
100 grams of glucose
BG: fasting, 1h, 2h, 3h

Recheck BG with 50 grams of glucose
at weeks 18, 26, 32 of gestation if:

1. Poor obstetrical history
2. Strong family history
3. Previous large baby (>4000 g)
4. Previous stillbirths
5. Previous infants with
   congenital anomalies
6. History of glycosuria during
   pregnancy or occurrence
   of glycosuria in this pregnancy

+

−
Not diabetic
Recheck as above
in weeks 18, 26, 32
of gestation

Initial evaluation

Place on calculated
diet—clear all acetone

No acetone
nl BG
1 hpc < 140

No acetone but
1 hpc glucose > 140

Continue diet
therapy, with
weekly consultation and
review of diary

Begin insulin

BG: Blood glucose
GTT: Glucose tolerance test
1 hpc: one hour after a meal

Figure 22.2. Screening during pregnancy and initiation of a treatment program.

ment. The initial history and physical examination is important for baseline data (see Table 22.3). In addition to the usual parameters measured during pregnancy, special attention should be given to the points listed in Table 22.3 which are pertinent to the pregnant woman who has diabetes.

The diet prescription should be calculated and taught to each patient with extreme patience because optimum nutrition is the main treatment of all pregnant women.

We have found the total caloric intake over 24 hours is equal to 30 Kcal/kg body weight. The calories are then divided into 3 meals and 4 snacks according to the "rule of eighteens" (Table 22.4). The breakfast must be very small for the highest blood glucose of the day is 1 hour after breakfast, perhaps due to the morning elevation in cortisol which deteriorates glucose tolerance. The calories should be proportioned such that 40% equals carbohydrate, 20% equals protein and 40% equals fat. A nutritionist should translate this prescription into food portions and instruct the patient how to use exchange lists. It is most important to monitor the patient's blood glucose after each meal and to insure that the patient does not have acetonuria of starvation. All too often a patient may fear to eat lest her blood glucose rise. Omission of meals only results in acetonuria of starvation. Until definitive studies show that this acetone is not harmful to the fetus,

Table 22.2. Classifications of Diabetic Pregnancies

White Classification
- A: Glucose tolerance test abnormal; no symptoms; euglycemia maintained with treatment by appropriate diet but without insulin
- B. Adult onset (age 20 or older) and short duration (less than 10 years)
- C. Relatively young onset (age 1–19) or relatively long duration (10–19 years)
- D: Very young onset (age less than 10) or very long duration (20 years or more) or evidence of background retinopathy
- E: Pelvic vascular disease (determined by x-ray)
- F: Renal disease
- R: Proliferative retinopathy
- RF: Both renal disease and proliferative retinopathy
- G: Multiple failure in pregnancy
- H: Arteriosclerotic heart disease
- T: Pregnancy after renal transplantation

Pyke Classification
Gestational diabetes
  That diabetes which starts during pregnancy and goes away after the pregnancy
Pregestational diabetes
  That diabetes which began before conception and continues after the pregnancy
Pregestational diabetes complicated by vascular disease
  Retinopathy, nephropathy, pelvic vessels or peripheral vascular disease

Prognostically Bad Signs During Pregnancy (PBSP)
1. Clinical pyelonephritis
   Urinary tract infection (culture positive) with acute temperature elevation (>39°C)
2. Precoma or severe acidosis
   Precoma: diabetic ketoacidosis with venous bicarbonate below 10 mEq/liter
   Severe acidosis: venous bicarbonate 10–17 mEq/liter
3. Pregnancy-induced hypertension
4. Neglectors
   Pregnant women who are in labor when first admitted, or who are psychopathic or of low intelligence, or who present less than 60 days before term

New Classification
1. Good diabetic control
   Fasting 55–65 mg/dl; average blood glucose (BG) 84 mg/dl; 1 hr postprandial <140 mg/dl
2. Less than optimal diabetic control
   a. Control not documented during pregnancy
   b. BG documented out of the ranges for good diabetic control

every attempt must be made to prevent acetone production. Therefore, the patient should be instructed to check her urine for acetone every time she voids. If acetone appears, the preceding meal or snack should be increased by 100 Kcal of carbohydrate. If adding calories clears acetonuria but causes the 1 hour postmeal blood glucose to be greater than 140 mg/dl, then insulin should be initiated and the diet held constant. This diet is designed to promote an average weight gain of 12.5 kg, which is in accord with the Committee on Maternal Nutrition of the National Research Council.[3]

Insulin Requirements and Adjustment

Once it has been determined that insulin is required for normalization of blood glucose, hospitalization of the pregnant woman is mandatory. This initial hospitalization is usually for about 1 week and is helpful in teaching the patient about diabetes and the requisite skills to manage her disease. In addition, the hospitalization time can be efficiently used to document gestational age, renal status, and ocular status.

Patients are taught to monitor their own blood glucose through the use of enzyme strips and a reflectance meter. Blood glucose is monitored before and after meals and at times of potential hypoglycemia so that insulin adjustment can be facilitated. We therefore have patients monitor their blood glucose at 7:30 AM, 10 AM, 12 noon (potential hypoglycemia), 2 PM, 4 PM, 6 PM, and 8 PM (potential hypoglycemia).

Table 22.3. Points of Special Attention in the Initial Evaluation of the Pregnant Woman with Diabetes

History	Documentation of menarche, period regularity, history of oral contraceptive use, previous pregnancies and outcome (note number of spontaneous abortions, difficulty in conceiving, number of stillbirths, number of infants >4000 gm or < 2500 gm, number of premature deliveries), history of glycosuria in pregnancy, previous pregnancy with an abnormal glucose tolerance test, history of polyhydramnios, urinary tract infections, or elevated blood pressure.
	Note family history of diabetes or other endocrinopathy.
	Note if patient smokes or drinks alcohol or takes medication.
	Note patient's own weight when she was born.
Physical examination	1. Blood pressure, pulse
	2. Weight
	3. Retinal examination with ophthalmoscopy
	4. Neck examination for thyroid size and character
	5. Heart examination: murmurs or gallops
	6. Pulmonary examination: wheezes or rhonchi
	7. Liver size
	8. Uterine size
	9. Pelvic examination: special attention for moniliasis
	10. Pedal edema
	11. Reflexes
	12. Vascular integrity of the extremities
Laboratory initial visit	1. Hemoglobin A_{1C}
	2. Complete blood count
	3. Creatinine clearance with total protein
	4. VDRL, toxoplasmosis, rubella
	5. Rh type

Table 22.4. Method to Calculate Diet

Time	Meal	Fraction Kcal/24 hours
8:00 AM	Breakfast	2/18 D*
10:30 AM	Snack	1/18 D
12:00 Noon	Lunch	5/18 D
3:00 PM	Snack	2/18 D
5:00 PM	Dinner	5/18 D
8:00 PM	Snack	2/18 D
11:00 PM	Snack	1/18 D

* D = 30 Kcal/kg body weight = total kilocalories over 24 hours.

One day is utilized in verifying the patient's results with simultaneous laboratory readings before insulin is calculated and adjusted. This day also allows the patient to document for herself her own level of control and provides increased motivation to adjust insulin in order to regulate her blood glucose.

Insulin requirements at the beginning of pregnancy are 0.7 units/kg body weight per 24 hours. This requirement will increase to 0.8 units/kg/24 hours at about 26 weeks and to 0.9 units/kg by 34 weeks. However, the insulin system must be continuously adjustable to provide for the continuous weight gain of pregnancy (total 12.5 kg in our series). Twenty-four hour insulin requirements (Table 22.5) are calculated therefore: total = 0.7 units/kg wt. This is given in divided doses so that intermediate acting insulin tends to cover basic metabolic needs and regular insulin covers course meals. Lunch is generally covered by slightly excess NPH in the morning overlapping with declining levels of regular. The total dose is divided in eighteenths and administered as documented in Table 22.5 with 2/3 being given in the morning (2:1 NPH: regular), 1/6 as regular before dinner and 1/6 as NPH before bedtime. It is noteworthy that the calculated bedtime NPH dose covers the fasting state for 8 hours and therefore can be used every 8 hours to cover fasting patients.

Although calculated insulin will markedly improve the patients' glucose profile, further titration is generally necessary in the hospital to achieve euglycemia with a range of 60–140 mg/dl (3.33–7.78 mM). Insulin titration is summarized in Table 22.6.

It is most efficient to normalize the fasting blood glucose first and at the same time eliminate morning ketosis. If there is morning ketosis, then the patient may require increased calories at 11 PM or an additional glass of milk at 3 AM. If the 7:30 AM blood glucose is greater than 100 mg/dl, the 10 PM insulin should be increased by 2 units until the fasting blood glucose is consistently below 100 mg/dl. Once the fasting blood glucose is "conquered," the rest of the blood glucose profile will stabilize relatively easily.

Hypoglycemia at given times can also be avoided by decreasing the appropriate insulin by 2 unit increments. Blood glucose monitoring at 12 noon allows one to detect hypoglycemia induced by regular insulin administered at 7:30 AM, and monitoring blood glucose at 8 PM allows the detection of hypoglycemia resulting from regular insulin administered at 4:30 PM.

Patients may wish to respond to momentary elevations of blood glucose by injecting extra insulin. This should be discouraged except at the usual injection times.

Table 22.7 details how a patient can respond to an elevated blood glucose "at the moment" so that she may cope with an increasing insulin requirement day by day. These extra doses of regular insulin should be incorporated into the appropriate NPH dose for the following day.

Monitoring Diabetic Control

In order to assure maintenance of normal blood glucose, each patient must be able to check her own blood glucose with a home glucose monitoring system. The physician should not only review the patient's diary but also confirm the control with a plasma glucose at each visit and measure hemoglobin A_{1c} every month.

Hemoglobin A_{1c} reflects control in the pregnant woman as accurately as it reflects control in other diabetic states.[15] Hemoglobin A binds glucose and as the glucose is increased in plasma more hemoglo-

Table 22.5.   Initial Calculation of Insulin*

	7:30 AM	4 PM	10 PM
NPH	8/18		3/18
Regular	4/18	3/18	
Total	2/3	1/6	1/6

* I = 0.7 units/kg = total dose of insulin over 24 hours.

Table 22.7.   Momentary Response to High Blood Glucose

1. If blood glucose is elevated at meal or snack time, do not eat until the blood glucose is <100 mg/dl.
2. If 7:30 AM or 4 PM blood glucose is:
   a. 100–140, add 2 units of regular insulin to calculated dose.
   b. >140, add 4 units of regular to calculated dose.
   c. Correct appropriate NPH dose for the following day (Table 22.6).

Table 22.6.   Insulin Titration

Time Insulin Administered	Insulin Type	Time of Monitoring Blood Glucose To Monitor Peak Action	Titration Procedure
10 PM	NPH	7:30 AM	If fasting glucose >100 mg/dl, add 2 units to 10 PM NPH. If fasting glucose <60 mg/dl, decrease 10 PM NPH by 2 units.
7:30 AM	Regular	10 AM	If postprandial glucose is >140 mg/dl, add 2 units regular to 7:30 AM dose the following day.
	NPH	4 PM	If 4 PM glucose is >100 mg/dl, add 2 units NPH to 7:30 AM dose. If 4 PM glucose is <60 mg/dl, decrease 7:30 AM NPH by 2 units.
4:30 PM	Regular	6 PM	If 6 PM blood glucose >140 mg/dl, add 2 units regular to 4:30 PM dose.

bin A becomes glycosylated to form Hb A$_{1c}$. Normally, hemoglobin A is glycosylated up to 5% in pregnancy; however, in diabetes out of control, hemoglobin A could be glycosylated up to 15%. Once hemoglobin A is glycosylated, it remains glycosylated for the life span of the red blood cell. The reaction is a postranslational, nonenzymatic reaction. The reaction is essentially irreversible because the glucose attaches to the N-terminal valine of the beta chain of hemoglobin A and spontaneously undergoes rearrangement such that the unstable aldimine becomes a stable ketamine (Fig. 22.3). As seen in Figure 22.4, hemoglobin A$_{1c}$ accurately reflected the elevated glucose of patients who entered into a program of tight control. Blood glucose, shown in the closed circles, normalized 1 week into the program and thereafter stayed in the normal range (hatched area) for the duration of the pregnancy. Hemoglobin A$_{1c}$, shown in the open circles, lagged behind blood glucose by 5 weeks, the time required to clear the old red cells. Thereafter, hemoglobin A$_{1c}$ accurately reflected the control.

Prevention of Hypoglycemia

Each patient is taught to respond to symptoms of hypoglycemia (tingling, diaphoresis, palpitations) by first checking her blood glucose (BG). If the BG is <70, then she may drink 240 ml of milk and

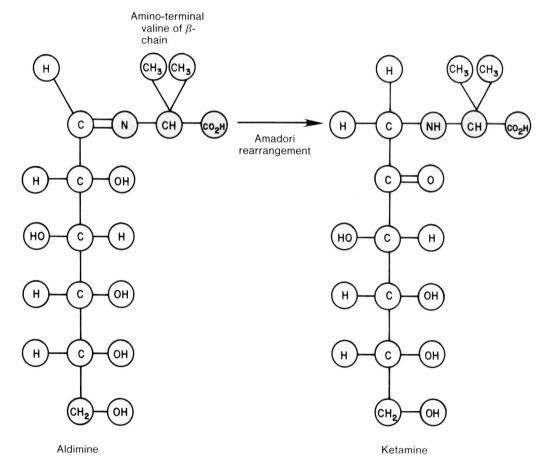

Figure 22.3. The nonenzymatic production of hemoglobin A$_{1c}$ requires the formation of a Schiff base between the aldehyde of the glucose and the amino-terminal valine of the beta chain, followed by an amadori rearrangement to the relatively more stable ketamine.

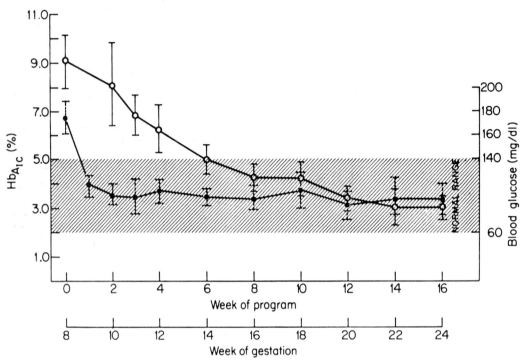

Figure 22.4. Time course for the normalization of hemoglobin A_{1c} and blood glucose for 10 insulin-dependent pregnant women. *Open circles*: mean hemoglobin A_{1c} plus or minus one standard deviation. Each point is based on the determinations obtained from all 10 patients at 2-week intervals. *Closed circles*: mean blood glucose plus or minus one standard deviation. Each point is based on 8–10 glucose determinations a day for the preceding 2 weeks for all 10 patients. The first point (week 0) is determined from plasma glucose values obtained in the hospital during a 24-hour glucose monitor. *Hatched area* is the normal range for both hemoglobin A_{1c} and for blood glucose in the third trimester.

recheck her BG in 15 minutes. If BG is still less than 70, she may drink another glass of milk and recheck her BG in another 15 minutes. This protocol is designed to bring the BG back up to normal without "over-shooting" the normal range.

TIMING OF DELIVERY

The risk of sudden intrauterine death increases as term is approached in the pregnancy complicated by overt diabetes mellitus.[29] In an attempt to decrease these losses, obstetricians have electively terminated such pregnancies between 35 and 38 weeks' gestation. However, this approach resulted in significant neonatal morbidity and mortality due to hyaline membrane disease (HMD).[4]

More recently it has been shown that the morbidity of HMD can be markedly reduced if delivery of the infant is delayed until pulmonary maturity is documented. In fact if one reviews the overall incidence of prenatal complications, neonatal morbidity correlates significantly with gestational age such that 80% of the preterm infants have some form of morbidity versus 40% in term infants.[7] Therefore, watchful waiting is judicious and should be maintained as long as maternal blood glucose is maintained in the normal range, fetal kick count is steadily rising, 24-hour urinary estriol excretion is rising, and contraction stress tests are critically reviewed and found to be negative.[5]

Fetal heart rate monitoring is probably the single best test to insure the clinician that watchful waiting may be continued.[10] Nonstress and oxytocin challenge tests can be utilized (see Chapter 18: "Stress Testing and Nonstress Testing"). A negative oxytocin challenge test remains a reassuring prognostic sign that the fetus is not in imminent jeopardy and, as long as maternal blood glucose is normal, delivery can be delayed (Table 22.8).

At 37–38 weeks' gestation the lecithin/sphingomyelin ratio (L/S) of the amniotic fluid should be assessed.[28] Decision for delivery should be based on:

1. Gestational age of fetus greater than 38 weeks and documented by accurate history, last menstrual period, serial sonography, heart sounds heard at 18–20 weeks, serial physical examinations, character of the cervix, and an L/S ratio of 2.5 or greater;

   or

2. A positive contraction stress test with mature L/S ratio or falling urinary estriol with mature L/S ratio;

   or

3. A positive contraction stress test and falling urinary estriol with an immature L/S ratio.

An attempt should be made to deliver vaginally if the cervix is favorable.[28] However, whether delivery is vaginal or by cesarean section, maintenance of normal blood glucose is critical for the well-being of the infant.

TREATMENT DURING LABOR AND DELIVERY

With improvement in antenatal care, it is becoming clear that intrapartum events may play a crucial role in the outcome of pregnancy.[17] The artificial beta cell may be used to maintain normoglycemia during labor and delivery. Figure 22.5 illustrates a representative profile of insulin and glucose requirements during this period. Of note is the fact that the last subcutaneous insulin-injection was NPH given at 2200 hours. Prior to active labor, insulin requirements are relatively high and glucose infusion is not necessary to maintain a blood glucose of 70–90 mg/dl. With the onset of active labor, insulin requirements decrease to zero and glucose requirements are relatively consistent at 2.55 mg/kg/min.[13]

Euglycemia may be maintained during

Table 22.8. Check List for Watchful Waiting

	Normal Blood Glucose (BG)	Rising Serum or Urinary Estriol (E₃)	Negative CST	Rising Fetal Kicks/hr.	L/S Ratio	Decision to Deliver
Frequency of test	6/Day	Daily	Weekly	3/Day	Weekly	
Gestational age (GA)						
34–37	+	+	+	+	NI	Wait
	−	+	+	+	NI	Correct BG; Wait
	+	+	+	−	<2.5	Wait; Do daily CST
	+	−	+	−	<2.5	Wait; Do daily CST
	+	−	+	−	>2.5	Deliver
	+	−	−	−	>2.5	Deliver
38–42	+	+	+	+	<2.5	Wait
	−	+	+	+	<2.5	Correct BG; Wait
	+	+	+	+	>2.5	Deliver if GA is documented by sonography
	+	+	+	−	>2.5	Deliver
	+	+	+	−	<2.5	Wait; Do daily CST
	+	−	+	−	<2.5	Wait; Do daily CST
	+	−	+	−	>2.5	Do phosphotydyl glycerol and if present, deliver

CST = contraction stress test; NI = not indicated.

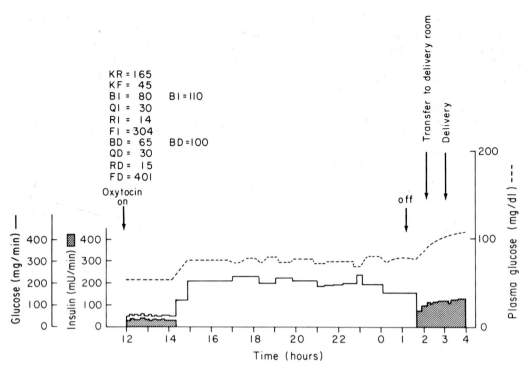

Figure 22.5. The graph of the infusion data of an insulin-dependent diabetic woman during induction of labor. The *dotted line* represents the maternal blood glucose (mg/ml) every minute. The *hatched area* represents the infusion of insulin (mU/min). The *solid line* represents the glucose infusion (mg/ml).

labor and delivery without an artificial pancreas, using the following protocol. The usual NPH dose is given at 2200 hours the evening prior to delivery. If labor is to be induced, insulin is withheld the day of induction. The morning of induction, an intravenous infusion is begun and blood glucose values are monitored every hour. The intravenous infusion rate is maintained at 100 ml/hour. If the blood glucose is >120 mg/dl, normal saline is infused. If blood glucose is 70–120, 5% dextrose is infused. If blood glucose is <70 mg/dl, 10% dextrose is infused.

POSTPARTUM CARE

Maternal

If intravenous infusion is required post delivery and the patient is NPO, then intravenous infusions may be maintained as described above with glucose monitoring every 2–4 hours. Insulin should be recal-

culated to account for weight changes of delivery at 0.6 units/kg and the standard 2200-hour NPH dose (1/6 of total) can be given every 8 hours.

Once the patient begins eating, the insulin and diet again can be recalculated according to weight. Insulin requirements will now total about 0.6 units/kg in those women who elect not to breast feed their infants.

Breast-feeding is not contraindicated in women with diabetes. However, diabetic women who breast feed have increased caloric requirements (27 Kcal/kg/day) and increased insulin requirement (0.7 units/kg/day) distributed as described under the section on insulin requirements above.

Infant

If blood glucose is normalized throughout pregnancy in a woman with diabetes, there is no evidence that excess attention need be paid to her offspring. However, if normal blood glucose has not been documented throughout pregnancy, then it is wise to monitor the baby in an intensive care situation for 24 hours postpartum. Blood glucose should be monitored hourly for 6 hours. If the baby shows no signs of respiratory distress, hypocalcemia or hyperbilirubinemia at 24 hours following delivery, then the infant may be discharged to the nursery. It should be noted that respiratory distress may occur up to 48 hours postpartum.

RELATIONSHIP OF GLUCOSE LEVELS TO OUTCOME OF PREGNANCY

As alluded to in the introduction, glucose control highly influences the outcome of pregnancy. Recent evidence indicates that congenital anomalies are higher in the offspring of women who have documented hypoglycemia at the time of conception and organogenesis.[19] Fetal mortality also correlates with hyperglycemia (Fig. 22.1). However, low levels of human chorionic gonadotropin, prolactin, and estradiol have been shown to be a prediction of intrauterine demise.[12] In hyperglycemic pregnant women these hormones are uniformly low and their levels correct to normal following the normalization of blood glucose.[15] As can be seen from Table 22.9,

diabetic women who are euglycemic throughout pregnancy have offspring with no increase in the incidence of hyperbilirubinemia, hypoglycemia, hypocalcemia, erythremia or respiratory distress.

In summary, the key to success in pregnancy and diabetes is to plan pregnancy and establish euglycemia prior to conception and throughout gestation, labor and delivery. Techniques are now becoming available to make this an increasingly feasible goal for all diabetic women.

References

1. Adams, P.W., and Oakley, N.W. Oralcontraceptives and carbohydrate metabolism. *Clin. Endocrinol. Metab.* 1:697, 1972.
2. Adashi, E.Y., Pinto, H., 2nd Tyson, J.E. Impact of maternal euglycemia on fetal outcome in diabetic pregnancy. *Am. J. Obstet. Gynecol.* 133:268, 1979.
3. Committee on Nutrition: *Nutrition in Maternal Health Care.* American College of Obstetricians and Gynecologists, Chicago, 1974.
4. Driscoll, S.G., Benirshke, K., and Curtis, G.W. Neonatal deaths among infants of diabetic mothers. *Am. J. Dis. Child.* 100:818–835, 1961.
5. Freeman, R.R. The use of the oxytocin challenge test for antepartum evaluation of uteroplacental respiratory function. *Am. J. Obstet. Gynecol.* 121: 481–489, 1975.
6. Freinkel, N. Effects of the conceptus on maternal metabolism during pregnancy. In *On the Nature and Treatment of Diabetes*, edited by Leibel, B.S., and Wrenshall, G.A. Excerpta Medica, Amsterdam, 1965, p. 679.
7. Gabbe, S.G., Lowensohn, R.I., Wu, P.Y., and Guerra, G. Current patterns of neonatal morbidity and mortality in infants of diabetic mothers. *Diabetes Care* 1:335–339, 1979.
8. Gabbe, S.G., Mestman, J.H., Frieman, R.I., Goebelsmann, U.T., Lowensohn, R.I., Nochimson, D., Cetrulo, C., and Quilligan, E.J. Management and outcome of pregnancy in diabetes mellitus, class B to R. *Am. J. Obstet. Gynecol.* 129:723, 1977.
9. Gilmer, M.D.G., Beard, R.W., Brooke, F.W., and Oakley, N.W. Carbohydrate metabolism in pregnancy: I. Diurnal plasma glucose profile in normal and diabetic women. *Br. Med. J.* 3:399, 1975.
10. Gluck, L., and Kulovich, M.V. Lecithin/sphingomyelin ratios in amniotic fluid in normal and abnormal pregnancy. *Am. J. Obstet. Gynecol.* 115: 534–546, 1973.
11. Grumback, M.M., Kaplan, S.L., Sciarra, J.J., and Burr, J.M. Chorionic growth hormone–prolactin (CGP): Secretion, disposition, biologic activity in man and postulated function as the 'growth hormone' of the second half of pregnancy, *Ann. N.Y. Acad. Sci.* 148:501, 1968.
12. Jovanovic, L., Dawood, Y., Landesman, R., and Saxena, B.B. The hormonal profile in early threatened abortion. *Am. J. Obstet. Gynecol.* 130: 274, 1978.

Table 22.9. Infant Morbidity (%)

	Literature Review* BS = 120 Mean G.A. = 38	New York Hospital Study† BS = 84 Mean G.A. = 38.8
Number	322	40
White classification	B–R	B–R
Hyperbilirubinemia (%)	37	0
Hypoglucose (%)	31	0
Hypocalcemia (%)	13	0
Erythremia (%)	8	0
Respiratory distress syndrome (%)	9	0
Congenital malformations (%)	6	0

* S.G. Gabbe, J.H. Mestman, R.I. Frieman, et al. (8).

† L. Jovanovic, C.M. Peterson, Y.M. Dawood, et al. (14).

13. Jovanovic, L., Forhan, S., and Peterson, C.M. Glucose and insulin requirements in labor and delivery in insulin dependent diabetic women. *Clin. Res.* 27:573A, 1979.

14. Jovanovic, L., Peterson, C.M., Dawood, Y.M., Saxena, B.B., and Saudek, C.D. The effect of normalization of blood glucose on the hormonal profile of insulin-dependent diabetic pregnant women. 39th Annual Meeting (abstract). *Diabetes* 28:348, 1979.

15. Jovanovic, L., Peterson, C.M., Saxena, B.B., Dawood, Y., and Saudek, C.D. Feasibility of maintaining euglycemia in insulin dependent pregnant women. *Am. J. Med.* 68:105–112, 1980.

16. Karlsson, J., and Kjellmer, I. The outcome of diabetic pregnancies in relation to the mother's blood sugar level. *Am. J. Obstet. Gynecol.* 112:213–220, 1972.

17. Kenny, J.D., Adams, J.M., Corbet, A.J.S., and Rudolph, A.J. The role of acidosis at birth in the development of hyaline membrane disease. *Pediatrics* 58:184, 1976.

18. Knopp, R.H., Saudek, C.D., Arky, P.A., and O'Sullivan, J.B. Two phases of adipose tissue metabolism in pregnancy: Maternal adaptations for fetal growth. *Endocrinology* 92:984, 1973.

19. Miller, E.H., Hare, J.W., Cloherty, J.P., Dunn, S.J., Soeldner, J.S., and Kitzmiller, J.L. Major congenital anomalies and elevated hemoglobin A_{1c} (Hgb A_{1c}) in early weeks of diabetic pregnancy. 39th Annual Meeting (abstract). *Diabetes* 28:347, 1979.

20. O'Sullivan, J.B., and Mahan, C.M. Criteria for the oral glucose tolerance test in pregnancy. *Diabetes* 13:278–285, 1964.

21. O'Sullivan, J.B., and Mahan, C.M. Glucose toler-

22. Pedersen, J. Diabetes and pregnancy. In *Blood Sugar of Newborn Infants*. Danish Science Press, Copenhagen, 1952.

23. Persson, B., and Lunell, N.O. Metabolic control in diabetic pregnancy: Variations in plasma concentrations of glucose, free fatty acids, glycerol, ketone bodies, insulin, and human chorionic somatomamotropin during the last trimester. *Am. J. Obstet. Gynecol.* 122:737, 1975.

24. Posner, B.I. Insulin-placental interactions. In *Early Diabetes in Early Life*, edited by Camerini-Davalos, R.A., and Cole, H.S. Academic Press, New York, 1975, p. 257.

25. Seltzer, H.S. Oral glucose tolerance tests. In *Diabetes Mellitus: Theory and Practice*, edited by Ellenberg, M., and Rifkin, H. McGraw-Hill, New York, 1970, p. 436–507.

26. Tyson, J.E., Fiedler, A.J., Austin, K.L., and Farinholt, J. Placental lactogen and prolactin secretion in human pregnancy. In *The Placenta: Biological and Clinical Aspects*, edited by Moghessi, K., and Hafez, E.S.E. Charles C Thomas, Springfield, IL, 1974, pp. 275–296.

27. Tyson, J.E., and Hack R.A. Gestational and pregestational diabetes: An approach to therapy. *Am. J. Obstet. Gynecol.* 125:100–109, 1976.

28. Usher, R.H., Allen, A.C., and McLean, F.H. Risk of respiratory distress syndrome related to gestational age, route of delivery and maternal diabetes. *Am. J. Obstet. Gynecol.* 11:826–832, 1971.

29. White, P. Infants of diabetic mothers. *Am. J. Med.* 7:609, 1949.

ance test: Variability in pregnant and nonpregnant women. *Am. J. Clin. Nutr.* 19:345–351, 1966.

CHAPTER 23

Hematologic Disorders During Pregnancy

NORTON M. LUGER, M.D.

ANEMIA

Anemia during pregnancy is the most common disorder affecting the mother. It is compounded by the physiologic changes in blood volume and composition which reduce the concentration of circulating red cells and hemoglobin: the so-called physiologic anemia of pregnancy. Hemoglobin levels of 10 gm/100 ml are not uncommon and may or may not be associated with symptoms. However, at their lower levels whether symptomatic or otherwise, it is wise to search for possible underlying disorders.

The extent of anemia in any group of pregnant women varies with the geography, race, and economics. In the United States, 56% of pregnant women are thought to be anemic.

The investigation of any anemia starts with a complete blood count, including the differential count. Since computerized electronic counters usually calculate the erythrocyte constants, i.e., mean corpuscular hemoglobin (MCH), mean corpuscular hemoglobin concentration (MCHC), and mean corpuscular volume (MCV), it is an easy matter to make preliminary conclusions as to whether the red cells are normocytic, macrocytic or microcytic as well as to assess their hemoglobin content. Examination of the peripheral blood smear will also permit accurate preliminary diagnoses as to the size, shape and pigment content.

The presence of abnormally shaped red cells or red cell inclusions such as Heinz bodies can lead to diagnoses of various hemoglobinopathic hemolytic states.

The reticulocyte count indicates whether the bone marrow is responding to the anemia. A reticulocyte count of more than 3% usually discloses marrow responsiveness. At acute higher levels it may reflect hemolysis or restitution following acute loss of blood, and at decreased levels it reflects a defective response to anemia, i.e., marrow suppression or a deficiency state.

Bone marrow examination completes the analysis of anemia. It provides information regarding iron deficiency, marrow responsiveness, quantity of marrow cells, and the presence of abnormal or tumor cells.

When anemia is encountered, a complete history and physical examination should be done. It is important to elucidate whether there is a personal history of anemia and the type, especially in relation to a previous pregnancy. A dietary history must be taken to establish whether food intake has been adequate in sources of iron, protein and folate. Any history of blood loss due to menorrhagia or bleeding from any other organ should be noted. A family history is important, especially in blacks, orientals and people of Mediterranean descent: people who may have hereditary disorders of hemoglobin, that is sickle disease or thalassemia. Other familial hemolytic anemias include those due to enzyme deficiency (G-6-PD) and congenital hemolytic anemia due to splenic sequestration.

Iron Deficiency Anemia

Many women are iron deficient during their reproductive years; 56% of pregnant women are truly anemic and iron deficiency is responsible in 77% of these.

The balance of iron in the body is a relationship of intake through food as opposed to loss via hair, skin, gastrointestinal and urinary epithelia and menstrual loss. Daily body loss of iron is equivalent roughly to 1 mg of elemental iron. If there is bleeding, 1 mg of iron is lost for each 2 cc of blood (0.5 mg/ml). Menstrual blood loss varies from 50 to 300 ml, carrying with it between 25 and 150 mg of iron.

The total body iron in a 50-K woman is estimated to be about 2 gm, of which 80% is in the red cells and 20% stored in liver, spleen, bone marrow and the reticuloendothelial system. A small amount is myoglobin, catalase, xanthine oxidase and transferrin. Approximately 200–400 mg of iron is storage iron, i.e., hemosiderin and ferritin.

The only source of iron to offset the losses must come from diet; while ordinarily about 10% of the dietary iron is absorbed, during pregnancy this increases to about 25% absorption. With the iron losses alluded to previously, it is clear that iron balance is precarious.

During pregnancy, additional needs for iron develop. The additional red cell mass requires about 440 mg; the fetus, cord and placenta, 370 mg; blood loss at delivery, 300 mg. If the daily obligatory loss of about 200 mg is added, this creates an additional need for 1310 mg of iron.

The diagnosis of iron deficiency anemia is made when there is a microcytic hypochromic anemia, and a bone marrow aspiration stained for iron shows absent iron stores. The marrow study eliminates other causes for microcytic and normocytic anemias. The serum iron and iron-binding capacity are not as reliable as the bone marrow study.

Treatment of this anemia requires iron supplementation. Ferrous sulfate is the least expensive supplement and is given in doses of 300 mg tid, preferably with food to minimize the gastrointestinal upset. If there is intolerance to ferrous sulfate, ferrous fumarate or gluconate can be substituted.

When none of the oral preparations are tolerated, then iron dextran can be given intravenously or intramuscularly. The intravenous route appears to be safe and easier since fewer injections are required. The entire dose can be given at one time.

The intramuscular route is more popular but has the disadvantage of requiring multiple injections and despite the use of a Z technique, the skin of the buttocks frequently stains brown.

Because most women will not absorb adequate iron from their diet for the needs of the pregnancy, it is common practice to routinely supplement the diet with ferrous compounds prophylactically. If left to normal diet alone without supplementation, it may take as long as 2 years to correct the iron deficiency. The exceptions to this rule are the patients carrying the gene for hemochromatosis and the patients with thalassemia who have been misdiagnosed as iron deficiency anemia. Here, iron supplementation is usually contraindicated unless there is an associated iron deficiency.

Macrocytic (Megaloblastic) Anemia

Macrocytic anemia can be caused by deficiency of vitamin B_{12} or folic acid. B_{12} deficiency causes pernicious anemia, which usually develops later in life and is rare during pregnancy. On the other hand, folic acid deficiency is commonly encountered in obstetrical practice.

Folic acid and folate are used interchangeably but differ in that folic acid is pteroylglutamic acid and is a pharmacologic compound with one glutamic acid residue. Folates are groups of similar compounds found in leafy vegetables, organ meats, yeast and peanuts which are polyglutamic acids. The polyglutamates are split by intestinal conjugase and absorbed in the upper third of the small intestine and transported to the liver.

Folic acid is essential for the production

of DNA in all cells of the body. Folate deficiency therefore results in widespread cellular changes that are most apparent in blood. Macrocytosis is the peripheral manifestation of disordered red cell production. Multisegmented neutrophiles are present and thrombocytopenia may also be present and may contribute to postpartum hemorrhage.

Folate deficiency occurs in a variety of settings:

1. Dietary deficiency resulting from malnutrition, food fadism and restrictive weight reduction diets. Depletion of folate reserves can occur within 3 weeks on a severely restricted diet.
2. Malabsorption of folate associated with sprue, enteritis, gastric and small intestinal resection, granulomatous enteritis, multiple fistulae, intestinal blind loops and jejunal bypass for obesity.
3. Folate deficiency in the third trimester when the fetal demand is maximal and maternal folate is preempted by the fetus.
4. Use of specific medications such as oral contraceptives, phenytoin (Dilantin) taken for epilepsy, nitrofurantoin for urinary infections and antifolics for leukemia and cancer chemotherapy.
5. Increased requirement for folic acid in all hemolytic anemias, thalassemia, sickle diseases and other hemoglobinopathies, in which marrow activity is increased and increased production of DNA is required.
6. Multiparity and multiple pregnancy.

Diagnosis is made on the basis of a dietary history suggestive of possible folate deficiency. Physical evidence of glossitis and stomatitis and laboratory evidence of macrocytic anemia alone or associated with thrombocytopenia and hypersegmented neutrophiles are looked for. Confirmation requires demonstration of decreased folate levels in serum or erythrocytes. Bone marrow examination will demonstrate megaloblasts. When the marrow is stained for iron, the presence or absence of concurrent iron deficiency is confirmed. When folic acid is given therapeutically, reticulocytosis should be sought from the fourth to the eighth day as confirmatory evidence. Absence of reticulocytosis suggests the presence of simultaneous B_{12} deficiency or another medical disorder.

Therapy for proven folate deficiency consists of oral folic acid in doses of 1 mg daily, with observation of reticulocyte response. Routine prenatal therapy with folic acid is questioned by those who do not believe folic acid should be given to those not deficient. Nevertheless it is widely prescribed prophylactically and is not harmful.

While there is disagreement among authorities as to whether there is an increase in placental abruption associated with folate deficiency, there is a risk of postpartum hemorrhage due to the associated thrombocytopenia.

Thalassemia

In the thalassemia syndrome, the abnormal hemoglobin is secondary to a defect in the rate of synthesis of the alpha or beta polypeptide chains. The specific title, alpha or beta thalassemia, denotes the specific globin chain that is decreased.

In beta thalassemia the deficiency of beta chains leads to overproduction of alpha chains. These in turn form tetrameres of alpha chains, or 2 alpha and 2 delta chains, which comprise Hb A2, or 2 alpha and 2 gamma chains forming Hbf (fetal hemoglobin). Tetrameres of alpha chains are unstable, precipitating in the red cells as Heinz bodies, which weaken the cell membranes and result in premature destruction by the spleen.

BETA THALASSEMIA

Beta thalassemia is most commonly encountered in Mediterranean countries, southern Europe, North Africa, and Asia Minor and in the western hemisphere. It was originally described as Cooley's anemia—a severe progressive hemolytic anemia found in the children of parents of Mediterranean derivation, which resulted in death during the first 2 decades of life.

There are rare reports of cases in children without Mediterranean ancestry.

Cooley's anemia is homozygous beta thalassemia. The clinical severity is related to the extent of beta-chain deficiency. In utero the fetus is protected by hemoglobin F, but this protection disappears and the anemia usually becomes manifest within the first year.

The physiologic response to ineffective erythropoiesis is further expansion of erythropoietic tissue. The bone marrow becomes hyperplastic and extramedullary centers develop in the liver and spleen. The anemia cannot be overcome because there is increased destruction of abnormal blood cells by the reticuloendothelial system. Frequent transfusion therapy is necessary and widespread hemosiderosis and hemochromatosis result, involving the liver, spleen, pancreas and heart. Diabetes, cirrhosis and myocardial insufficiency result and death usually occurs within the first 2 decades.

The removal of iron by chelation has offered some hope to these patients. Long-term studies are currently being done to determine whether this therapy can prolong life.

Only occasional survivors come to their reproductive years and infertility is usual. When pregnancy does occur it is rarely successful and the course if complicated, requiring multiple transfusions. Congestive heart failure is common. The diagnosis is usually made clinically. The routine blood counts show anemia, microcytosis, hypochromia, nucleated red cells, reticulocytosis, Heinz bodies, and many bizarre red cells. Hemoglobin F comprises 40–70% of the total hemoglobin, hemoglobin A2 is elevated and hemoglobin A is reduced or absent.

HETEROZYGOUS THALASSEMIA B (THALASSEMIA MINOR)

This is usually a mild disorder that is frequently overlooked and frequently misdiagnosed as iron deficiency anemia. When iron therapy fails, suspicion should be aroused and further study can reveal the diagnosis. Hemoglobin electrophoresis discloses that Hgb A2 is increased above 3.5% and Hb F is slightly increased. In contrast to iron deficiency anemia, the serum iron and ferritin are elevated and the iron-binding capacity shows greater saturation.

Once the diagnosis is established, the only therapy required is the use of folate. In some women with heterozygous thalassemia B, iron stores may not be adequate and iron supplementation may be required in addition to folate. This need can be ascertained by staining bone marrow for iron or by noting decreased serum iron-binding capacity.

An intermediate form of heterozygous thalassemia B occurs, in which the anemia is of greater severity and may require transfusion, especially during pregnancy. In thalassemia minor patients, pregnancy is usually uncomplicated despite the presence of anemia. These women frequently have hemoglobin concentrations of 8–10 gm in the last half of pregnancy.

ALPHA THALASSEMIA

Alpha thalassemia is found in Southeast Asia and, with increased immigration from that area, it may assume more than theoretical importance in the future for American practitioners.

In homozygous thalassemia with all four genes absent and no alpha chains being made, the fetus manufactures a tetramere of four gamma chains (Hb Bart's). Oxygen is released slowly from the hemoglobin. This condition is incompatible with life, and hydrops fetalis and intrauterine death result.

Heterozygous alpha thalassemia is very difficult to diagnose since all hemoglobins are decreased. Family studies and studies of the infant's blood may show some elevation of Hb Bart's (Hb H). The usual microcytic anemia is seen but the severity is variable. The management is the same as for other hemoglobinopathies.

Hemoglobin H disease is a variety of alpha thalassemia, characterized by a moderately severe hemolytic anemia with splenomegaly. Hemoglobin H, consisting of four beta chains, is present in 4–30%,

Hb Bart's in 2-5% and the remainder is Hb A. Pregnancy may be associated with increased severity of anemia and transfusions may be needed.

SICKLE THALASSEMIA B DISEASE

In this condition there is double heterozygosity, resulting in one gene for thalassemia from one parent and one for sickle disease. Clinically this results in a condition similar to Hb S C disease. A chronic hypochromic anemia is present and is unresponsive to iron therapy. The exact frequency is not known and this disorder is probably underdiagnosed. The physical appearance is normal. Chronic hemolysis may occur, with resultant hepatosplenomegaly. Crises, increased susceptibility to infection, bone changes and renal problems do occur but with lower incidence than in sickle disease.

Hemoglobin electrophoresis is similar to Hgb AS disease, with 60-75% HB S, 5-15% AB f, 3-5% Hb A2 and 5-15% HbA. The red cells are microcytic and hypochromic but the sickle test is positive.

Family analysis of hemoglobin patterns is used to help make the diagnosis.

The clinical course during pregnancy is milder than in sickle disease or Hb SC disease but is more severe than sickle trait. The severity is related to the amount of Hg S present in erythrocytes. Maternal mortality figures vary greatly in various studies, but there is a definite increase in maternal morbidity. Infant morbidity and mortality are increased but not to the extent found in sickle or sickle C disease.

Treatment in general follows that for sickle C disease, with careful observation, transfusion as needed and folic acid.

Sickle Cell Anemia

HOMOZYGOUS (HB SS) SICKLE DISEASE

Sickle cell anemia is a hereditary hemolytic anemia affecting blacks, characterized by the presence of a sickle shaped deformity of erythrocytes, episodic crises due to hemolysis, vascular (both arterial and venous) thrombosis and an increased susceptibility to infection. About 9% of American blacks are heterozygous carriers and one in each 600 pregnancies is homozygous. Sickle cell anemia is transmitted as an autosomal recessive factor.

The disease is due to the substitution of valine for glutamic acid on the 6th position of the beta chain of the globin molecule. The resultant abnormal hemoglobin (Hb S) in the deoxygenated state forms microstrands which coalesce, forming microtubules and the larger polymers which are responsible for the typical sickle deformity. These cells are rigid and do not easily pass through smaller vessels, resulting in agglutination and red cell thromboses.

The sickling process is reversible early in the reduced state. However, after a period of deoxygenation, potassium and water are lost and these cells can no longer be restored by oxygenation. The typical red cells in the homozygous state are short-lived and the bone marrow becomes hyperplastic. As a result of this chronic hemolysis, pigment gall stones are frequent. The anemia leads to stunted growth and delayed development.

Another problem also derives from the nature of the sickle cell in that thrombosis is frequent and widespread, causing painful abdominal crises, bone pain, myocardial and valvular disease of the heart and urinary problems frequently associated with papillary necroses and hyposthenuria. Urinary tract infections are also common both in homozygous (Hb SS) and in heterozygous patients (Hb SA).

Infection is the third major inciting factor in these patients. The increased susceptibility to infection (especially pneumonia, urinary tract infection and osteomyelitis) is probably due to decreased splenic activity as a result of destruction by thrombosis. While affected children may have enlarged spleens, these soon become atrophic and even in childhood infection is common.

Hypoxia and acidosis both predispose to sickling and, once the process starts, the typical painful crisis results in further hemolysis or further acidosis. Infection also provokes the process in the same fashion.

The diagnosis of the underlying disease

is usually not difficult when suspected. Sickled red cells may be seen under the microscope either on routine smear or with special suspensions of red cells in a reducing agent such as sodium metabisulfite. Confirmation is made by hemoglobin electrophoresis demonstrating HbS.

Once the diagnosis is established, there are no definitive treatments available other than maintaining the patients general health, avoiding infections, correcting anemia, folic acid supplementation and prompt medical intervention when symptoms occur. While sickle crises are easy to diagnose, it must be remembered that these patients can have other diseases that nonsickle patients get. Affected sickle patients should be monitored, for these ordinary disorders may provoke a sickle crisis.

OBSTETRICAL ASPECTS

Sickle cell anemia impairs fertility and the reproductive experience is poor. There is a high rate of prematurity, spontaneous abortion, intrauterine and perinatal death, and low weight infants.

When sickle patients do become pregnant they must be carefully observed. Those women who had crises in the past are more likely to have crises during pregnancy. They are especially susceptible to toxemia, urinary tract infections, venous thrombosis and pulmonary embolism.

Monthly visits to the physician may suffice for the first 24 weeks. Thereafter, visits should be weekly. On each visit, symptoms or signs should be checked, nutrition reviewed and folic acid 1 mg bid given. Iron deficiency can occur with Hb SS disease, but iron should not be prescribed routinely since iron overload may be present if transfusions have been given in the past.

If the hematocrit is below 15–20% or hemoglobin is less than 6 gm, transfusion of red cells should be given. Partial exchange transfusions have been used to reduce the concentration of Hb SS. Transfusions not only increase the amount of Hb A erythrocytes but also suppress the production of Hb SS red cells. Partial exchange transfusions are currently being studied. The goal is to keep the hematocrit between 30 and 35% and the Hb A concentration between 40 and 90%. The effects of an exchange last about 6–8 weeks. Retransfusion is done if the Hb A level falls below 20% or within 4–6 weeks prior to delivery to permit labor to proceed in a good hematologic state.

Postpartum care includes careful observation for blood loss, endometritis, and phlebitis.

It must be remembered that sickle patients can have other complications of pregnancy that can cause abdominal pain.

SICKLE TRAIT (HETEROZYGOUS HB SA)

This condition causes no anemia or hemolytic state per se. The only morbidity related to this condition is increased incidence of urinary tract infection, bleeding, and decreased ability to concentrate urine. Under extreme hypoxia, sickling may occur. Careful monitoring for urinary infections is necessary; if urinary infection occurs, treatment is best done with antibiotics since there may be coexistent G-6-PD deficiency contraindicating sulfonamides and nitrofurantoins.

HEMOGLOBIN SC DISEASE

Hemoglobin SC disease is a severe disorder resembling sickle cell anemia in many ways, including decreased fertility, susceptibility to infection, crises, pulmonary infarction, toxemia, and increased fetal wastage. A unique feature of this disease is bone marrow infarction with resulting pulmonary embolism. The treatment is the same as for Hb SS disease.

Hemoglobin CC and hemoglobin AC diseases are mild disorders, with little reproductive consequence. Target cells are usually seen on blood examination.

PRENATAL DIAGNOSIS OF HEMOGLOBINOPATHY

In the prenatal diagnosis of hemoglobinopathy, it is important to determine whether the fetus has homozygous disease. Two methods are available. In one, fetal blood is sampled and hemoglobin analysis is done. The second technique is DNA analysis using cultured fetal fibroblasts obtained by amniocentesis. (See Chapter 16: Prenatal Diagnosis of Genetic Disorders.)

Fetal blood sampling has enjoyed the widest use and, in centers with high incidence of thalassemia such as Sardinia and Greece, intrauterine diagnosis has achieved a high degree of accuracy. The new DNA technology is currently evolving and is helpful especially in alpha thalassemia.

OTHER HEMOLYTIC ANEMIAS

The hemolytic anemias may complicate pregnancy but are not caused by pregnancy. Hemolysis should be suspected when the anemia is normocytic and the reticulocyte count is above 5%. Much diagnostic information can be obtained from examining the Wright stained blood films and some of this can prove to be specific. For example, the observation of microspherocytosis may pinpoint the diagnosis of hereditary spherocytosis. Similarly the presence of burr cells or helmet cells can help in the diagnosis of microangiopathic hemolytic anemia (intravascular hemolysis).

HEREDITARY DEFECTS

Hereditary Spherocytosis

This is an autosomal dominant disorder affecting the cell membranes. Instead of being biconcave the erythrocytes are spherical and, because of this, more fragile. The trauma of traversing the microcirculation, especially the spleen, shortens cell life. Pigment stones in the gall bladder result from excess pigment produced by the chronic hemolysis. Mild acholuric jaundice may occur and splenomegaly is frequent. Serious aplastic crises can occur due to viral infections.

The diagnosis is made on the basis of the family history, laboratory proof of hemolysis, microspherocytosis and demonstration of increased osmotic fragility. Splenectomy should be done prior to conception since the procedure is curative and

the unpredictable aplastic crises can be lethal.

Hereditary Enzyme Defects

Glucose-6-phosphate dehydrogenase (G-6-PD) deficiency results in hemolytic anemia with exposure to oxidant chemicals and medications. Pyogenic infections and hepatitis virus infections similarly provoke hemolysis.

Two susceptible populations exist. A milder form occurs among blacks and a more severe form in Mediterranean nonblacks and in Asians. It is estimated that approximately 100,000,000 people worldwide have this deficiency. Approximately 40 medications are sufficiently oxidant to provoke the oxidation of hemoglobin to methemoglobin, resulting in hemolysis. Sulfonamides and sulfones, aspirin, phenacetin, nitrofurantoin, chloramphenicol, para-aminosalicylic acid, probenicid, and water soluble vitamin K analogs are medications most frequently at fault.

The diagnosis is confirmed by the determination of enzyme levels in lysed erythrocytes. Immediately during or after a hemolytic crisis, the levels of G-6-PD may be normal. This paradoxical finding, which is uncommon, is explained by the destruction of the older deficient cells. The remaining young erythrocytes may have normal enzyme content.

Women with G-6-PD deficiency have an increased incidence of urinary tract infection during pregnancy.

There is no specific therapy for this deficiency except prevention of exposure to oxidant medication or chemicals in the environment.

Pyruvate kinase deficiency is a hereditary deficiency resulting in hemolytic anemia appearing during childhood. It is usually well compensated. Pigment gallstones and splenomegaly are usually present and may lead to confusion with hereditary spherocytosis.

Autoimmune Hemolytic Anemia

This is associated with a positive Coombs test. This immune state is usually a manifestation of another concurrent disease. Lymphoproliferative disorders such as chronic lymphocytic leukemia, lymphoma and Hodgkin's disease as well as collagen vascular disease exemplified by disseminated lupus erythematosus produce warm reacting antibodies of the IgG type.

Cold agglutinins are of the IgM variety and are associated with mycoplasmal pneumonia, infectious mononucleosis, and solid tumors such as lymphoma. The Coombs test may be only weakly positive, but specific antibodies will demonstrate strong reaction to complement which remains attached to the red cell. There is a type of autoimmune hemolytic anemia which is not associated with any apparent underlying disease.

Drug-related autoimmune hemolytic anemias are Coombs positive and result from antibodies to a drug-cell complex, a drug-protein complex or a drug-induced antibody to red cell components such as the Rh antigens.

Stopping the drug should eventually cure the hemolytic state. Steroids, splenectomy, or immunosuppressive drugs may be required.

Drugs commonly involved in provoking this variety are penicillin, sulfonamides, quinines and quinidine, p-aminosalicylic acid, phenacetin, α-methyldopa and dopamine.

THROMBOTIC THROMBOCYTOPENIC PURPURA

This disease affects young adults and especially young women. The syndrome consists of hemolytic anemia with jaundice, petechiae, thrombocytopenia, encephalopathy and nephropathy. It is a serious disease with high mortality. Recent work advises steroid treatment and splenectomy.

Microangiopathic hemolytic anemia results from physical trauma to the red cell either by prosthetic heart valves or the presence of fibrin in small blood vessels or severe hypertension, eclampsia, carcinoma, or large hemangiomas. It is commonly found in disseminated intravascular coagulation.

DISORDERS OF HEMOSTASIS

Bleeding Disorders

Hemostasis is essential for the successful completion of the pregnancy. A bleeding state jeopardizes both mother and fetus, and hemorrhage prior to or during labor and delivery can be catastrophic.

Every pregnant patient should be asked about previous hemorrhage (especially with childbirth or surgery) and bleeding tendencies, including epistaxis, gastrointestinal bleeding, and a tendency to bruise easily.

A family history of bleeding disorder should be carefully sought. Medication taken may cause bleeding tendencies by impairing platelet function.

In general, deficiencies of platelet numbers or function are reflected in purpura, petechiae, mucosal and dental bleeding, while hemarthrosis and hematomas are associated with clotting factor deficiencies.

The laboratory investigation encompasses the bleeding time, prothrombin time, partial thromboplastin time, and a complete blood count including examination of the stained blood smear for platelets. A platelet count below 100,000 represents thrombocytopenia.

The routine screening tests noted above uncover clotting deficiencies of all factors other than I and XIII. The most important of the factor deficiencies are those of factor VIII including von Willebrand's disease and hemophilia A (carrier).

Von Willebrand's Disease (Factor VIII Deficiency)

Factor VIII is identified as the antihemophilic globulin (AHG). Since hemophilia A is sex-linked, women rarely present with this disorder. However, von Willebrand's disease is inherited in an autosomal fashion (both dominant and recessive forms have been described) and women are involved.

Clinically, these patients present with evidence of mucosal or cutaneous bleeding, and menometrorrhagia. Testing reveals abnormal bleeding time (unlike hemophilia A) as well as prolonged partial thromboplastin time (PTT). The prolonged bleeding time is due to an AHG-related effect inhibiting platelet adhesiveness. This effect is found when testing platelet adhesiveness on glass beads or on exposure to ristocetin and is corrected with administration of AHG. AHG also is measured by its coagulant activity and by a radioimmunoassay using prepared antisera. However, the coagulant and antigenic activity of AHG do not correspond and cannot be used interchangeably. All three tests should be done to establish the diagnosis.

During pregnancy, levels of AHG usually increase and at times may approach normal. With lower levels, bleeding may occur at delivery. When AHG coagulant levels are close to normal, treatment may not be needed. This is most important since frozen plasma or cryoprecipitates which come from pooled plasma may transmit hepatitis. It must be remembered that bleeding may occur several weeks postpartum when AHG levels fall.

Replacement treatment is given when the factor VIII coagulant levels fall below 50% or if abnormal bleeding occurs. If cesarean section is required, preparation with cryoprecipitate will correct the deficiency and permit surgery. Frequent testing for the adequacy of treatment is necessary.

Thrombocytopenic Purpura

Decrease in the platelet count normally occurs during pregnancy, due to dilution associated with blood volume expansion. The nadir is reached in the mid third trimester. The platelet count is not reduced below 100,000/cu mm. When the platelet count falls below this level, bone marrow examination is necessary. Decrease in megakaryocytes signifies production failure, while hyperplasia of megakaryocytes reflects peripheral destruction with appropriate marrow response. In addition the marrow examination will help identify failure due to destruction by tumor or leukemia.

Decreased production is usually associated with infections (both viral and bacterial), deficiency of folic acid and vitamin B_{12}, excessive alcohol, tumor invasion and a wide variety of drugs. Platelet destruction is mediated by immune and nonimmune toxic reactions associated with drugs, infections, disseminated intravascular coagulation, transfusion reactions associated with hemolysis or may follow massive transfusions. The latter is due to antiplatelet antibodies associated with mismatched platelet antigens.

Idiopathic Thrombocytopenic Purpura

ITP is an immune process in which an antibody attaches to and impairs platelet membranes, leading to early destruction in the spleen. Production increases may compensate for the shortened life span of the platelets. Bleeding does not occur unless the peripheral count falls below 30,000–40,000.

ITP, the most common disorder of bleeding in children and young adults, may start as a flulike syndrome. Although the acute phase is short-lived, antibody production persists and chronicity is usual. If splenomegaly or lymphadenopathy is present, the diagnosis is not likely to be ITP. Careful review of the history is necessary to eliminate medicinal or chemical toxic cause of the thrombocytopenia. Marrow aspiration shows normal or increased megakaryocytes. Treatment requires immunosuppression with steroids which usually are effective. Should this fail to bring the platelets above the "safe" level of 40,000–50,000, splenectomy is necessary. Splenectomy in the pregnant woman is a complicated feat and in one series had a 30% fetal mortality. Cyclophosphamide or azathioprine may also be used, but the effect on the pregnancy is not currently established. Platelet transfusions may be helpful as a temporary adjunct to protect the patient during surgery or during delivery, but these transfusions cannot be considered for maintenance therapy because of the risk of hepatitis and development of platelet antibodies rendering the treatment ineffective.

ITP OBSTETRICAL CONSIDERATIONS

Maternal

Steroid therapy in pregnancy can be associated with hypertension, toxemia, psychosis and adrenal suppression in the fetus.

Fetal

The placental barrier is traversed by maternal antibodies resulting in fetal thrombocytopenia. Spontaneous abortions are significantly increased and mortality from vaginal delivery is as high as 20% due to intracranial hemorrhage. The infant's platelet count must be observed carefully for at least 1 week postpartum.

Method of Delivery

Normal vaginal delivery poses little threat to the mother since uterine bleeding is controlled by muscular action of the uterus. No maternal death associated with ITP has been reported since 1950. However, lacerations or episiotomies may bleed profusely.

The fetal problem is the major issue in choosing the mode of delivery. Fetal thrombocytopenia predisposes to intracranial hemorrhage. Authorities are divided on whether to permit vaginal delivery with the risk to the fetus or to resort to cesarean section with the attendant risks to the mother.

Recommendations have been made that cesarean delivery should be done if the maternal platelet count is below 100,000 or if the mother had been previously splenectomized, regardless of the platelet count.

Thrombotic Thrombocytopenic Purpura

Thrombotic thrombocytopenic purpura is an acute, rapidly progressive, highly fatal febrile illness of unknown cause. It is manifested by thrombocytopenia, cerebral symptoms, microangiopathic hemolytic anemia with mild jaundice and progressive renal failure. At autopsy, disseminated hyaline intravascular thromboses are found. The mortality rate is approximately 90%. Therapy with steroids and splenectomy has successfully stopped the process in a few cases. Fortunately this disease, which may be difficult to differentiate from severe toxemia, is rare.

Disseminated Lupus Erythematosus

Disseminated lupus erythematosus may be associated with thrombocytopenia and in fact it may be the first manifestation. The diagnosis relies on the presence of antinuclear or anti-DNA antibodies and changes in serum complement. The management of the thrombocytopenia would be that of lupus. Lupus frequently remits during pregnancy but flares up early in the postpartum state.

Disseminated Intravascular Coagulopathy

Disseminated intravascular coagulopathy refers to bleeding associated with defibrination. It can occur in placental abruption, amniotic fluid embolism, retention of a dead fetus or retention of placental fragments, septic abortion, shock and toxemia of pregnancy.

Liberation of thromboplastic material into the maternal circulation results in intravascular coagulation, fibrinolysis, and consumption coagulopathy with thrombocytopenia, microangiopathic hemolytic anemia, vascular injury and bleeding ranging from purpura to massive hemorrhage.

The diagnosis of the syndrome is based mainly on the clinical findings, decreased fibrinogen and increase in fibrin split products. Abnormalities of multiple clotting factors reflected in the PT and PTT, thrombocytopenia and red cell fragments are usually seen.

Treatment requires prompt, accurate diagnosis of the immediate cause. In most of the obstetrical situations, evacuation of the uterus will end the process. General supportive measures to correct shock, maintenance of blood volume, respiratory support and combatting infection when present are necessary. Under some circumstances, heparin will stop the process by inhibiting clotting and the resulting consumption coagulopathy. Replacement of blood factors with fresh frozen plasma may be required in selected situations.

Bibliography

1. Alter, B.P. Intra-uterine diagnosis of hemoglobinopathies. *Semin. Perinatol.* 4:189–198, 1980.
2. Bell, W.R. Hematologic abnormality in pregnancy. *Med. Clin. North Am.* 61:165, 1977.
3. Bloom, A.H. Physiology of factor VIII. In *Recent Advances in Blood Coagulation*, ed. 2, edited by Poller, L. Churchill Livingston, Edinburgh, London, 1977, pp. 141–181.
4. Carloss, H.W., McMillan, R., and Crosby, W.H. Management of pregnancy in women with immune thrombocytopenia purpura. *J.A.M.A. 244:* 2756–2758, 1980.
5. Freedman, W.L., and Shashaty, G.G. Hemoglobinopathies and pregnancy. In *Advances in Obstetrics and Gynecology*, edited by Caplan, R.M., and Sweeney, W.J. III. Williams & Wilkens, Baltimore, 1978, pp. 184–196.
6. Herbert, V. The nutritional anemias. *Hosp. Prac.* 15:65–89, 1980.
7. Horger, G.O. III, and Keane, M.W.D. Platelet disorders in pregnancy. *Clin. Obstet. Gynecol. 22:* 843, 1979.
8. Morrison, J.C. Hemoglobinopathies and pregnancy. *Clin. Obstet. Gynecol.* 22:819–842, 1979.

CHAPTER 24

Rh Isoimmunization

RONALD M. CAPLAN, M.D.

DEFINITION

Rh isoimmunization is the immunologic reaction of an Rh-negative mother to her Rh-positive fetus, resulting in destruction of fetal erythrocytes.

PATHOGENESIS

The homozygous Rh-positive father will transmit the Rh factor (D) to the fetus. With a heterozygous father and an Rh-negative mother, there is a 50% chance that the fetus will be Rh positive, as D is dominant.

As fetal and maternal circulatory systems do not communicate, no fetal antigen (D) enters tbe maternal circulation until a break occurs in the integrity of the systems. Such a break ordinarily will not occur until delivery, when a fetal-maternal transfusion of 0.1 ml of fetal blood or less can cause the elucidation of maternal 7S γ-globulin G (antibody).[19] These antibodies tend to appear 2–3 months after delivery.[10, 21]

With a subsequent pregnancy, an anamnestic response can occur, and the antibody, with a molecular weight of 160,000 can cross the placenta (see Figure 24.1) and coat the fetal erythrocytes. These coated erythrocytes are bound to phagocytic cells of the fetal reticuloendothelial system.[11, 16] The process is maximal at birth.

The end result is fetal hemolytic anemia and high levels of circulating indirect bilirubin, which can cause kernicterus postpartum. As a result of hepatic failure,[3] the fetus may become hydropic. Fetal death ensues (Fig. 24.2).

INCIDENCE

Thirteen percent of all Caucasians are Rh negative. Of all deliveries, 1.4% will result in hemolytic disease of the newborn, of which 57% will be ABO incompatible, 41% will be Rh incompatible (approximately 1/200 births), and 2% will be due to other factors: C, K, E, etc.[21]

By the end of the second Rh-positive pregnancy, 17% of Rh-negative women are immunized. This is not true of women who have had Rh immune globulin.

Untreated, 15–30% of fetuses affected die in utero between 17 and 40 weeks of gestation.

THE INITIAL WORKUP

The history is taken and examination is performed.

Blood type and Rh determination are carried out, as well as screening for Rh and atypical antibodies. This is done regardless of whether the patient is Rh negative or Rh positive.[18]

If antibodies are present, the zygosity of the father is studied. As no antibody to "D" is known, heterozygosity can only be surmised statistically on the basis of the relative frequency of various CDE/CDE patterns.[14] It may be helpful to determine the zygosity of the other children (if any) and of the husband's parents.

Ideally, patients with discovered Rh isoimmunization should be followed in a medical center that has a functioning Rh committee, high-risk clinic, intensive care labor and delivery suite, intensive care nursery, necessary laboratory facilities in-

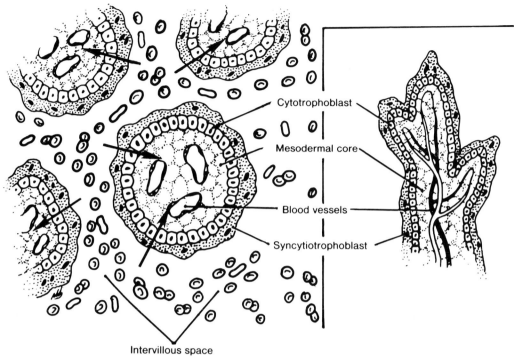

Figure 24.1. Low molecular weight maternal antibody (IgG) can cross into fetal circulation (*arrows*).

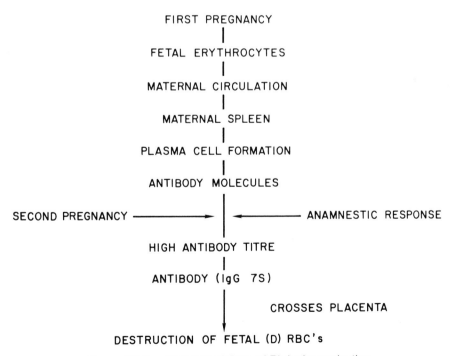

Figure 24.2. Pathophysiology of Rh isoimmunization.

cluding spectrophotometry and its interpretation, and individuals familiar with
the mechanics of intrauterine transfusion.

PREDICTING THE SEVERITY OF SENSITIZATION

The available modes of predicting the
severity of isoimmunization are history,
titer, and amniocentesis.

History

The patient's history is an important
index in predicting the severity of erythroblastosis fetalis.

There are important differences between a first affected, or first sensitized
pregnancy and later sensitized pregnancies. A first affected pregnancy is that
pregnancy in which antibodies are first
detectable: for previously described reasons (see "Pathogenesis") this does not
usually occur in the primigravida. More
commonly, the first affected pregnancy
would be the mother's second actual pregnancy.

The risk of Rh death or severe anemia
in the neonate (8 gm% of hemoglobin or
less) is negligible before 34 weeks in a first
affected pregnancy.[20] Even after 33 weeks,
a low titer will result in a 4% risk of death
or severe anemia in the first affected infant. However, higher titers are associated
with a 27% risk.

In later sensitized (subsequent sensitized) pregnancies, fetal loss can occur at
all stages of the pregnancy: as early as 20
weeks, or even earlier. If previously affected fetuses had no anemia (Hgb over 15
gm%) and survived, the risk of fetal death
or severe anemia in the present pregnancy
is probably low, irrespective of the present
peak titer.

However, with a history of moderate
anemia and a presently high titer, the risk
rises to 29%. With previous fetal death or
severe anemia and a presently low titer,
the risk is 50%; with previous fetal death
or severe anemia and a presently high titer,
the risk rises to 92%.

The overall accuracy of such prognostication on the basis of history and titer

alone is probably in the range of 62%, most
obviously because it is impossible on this
basis alone to decide which of the specific
fetuses in a given risk group are actually
in danger.

The use of history for prognostication
may become somewhat more important in
the case of an immunized multiple pregnancy, when the multiplicity of amniotic
sacs detracts from the value of amniocentesis.[7]

Titer

The titers discussed above are measurements of indirect antiglobulin (Coombs')
titer, which measures the level of 7S γ-
globulin G ("albumin" antibody).

It should be noted that the critical level
of the titer varies from laboratory to laboratory, and all interpretations must be
made within that context. In the absence
of specific data, a titer of 1:8 should be
considered the minimum critical level: that
level of antibody titer below which severe
involvement of infants does not occur.

Titer levels are of limited prognostic
value, as previously discussed.

In severely sensitized mothers, although
the fetus may become progressively affected, the titer may stay at one level,
although such a phenomenon may be seen
with an Rh-negative (therefore unaffected)
fetus.[9]

Thus it may be seen that, although history and titer must be considered, their
primary present usage is to select those
cases in which it is necessary to proceed
to the next step: amniocentesis.

It has been pointed out that other blood
group antibody titers should be tested for
as well. Pools of human red blood cells
covering all the important blood group antigens are commercially available. If agglutination occurs with such a mixture, then
the specific antibody responsible can be
determined.

TIMING OF TITERS

Titer determination should be done on
every patient at the initial antepartum visit
and again at 28 weeks[2] and 36 weeks.[1] If

titers are positive, they are obtained every 4 weeks.

If values rise above the minimal critical level, then amniocentesis is resorted to. Six week's and 6 month's postpartum antibody testing has been advocated.[1]

Amniocentesis

Amniotic fluid should be obtained for examination as early as 20 weeks of gestation in any woman in whom the antibody titer exceeds or is equal to the minimal critical level.[2] In subsequent isoimmunized pregnancies, amniocentesis may be indicated even if the titer is below the critical level.

The timing of the initial tap depends on history and titer, as previously described.[19] With a previous hydropic infant or perinatal death, initial amniocentesis is performed early, as intrauterine transfusion may become necessary as early as 24 weeks.

At the opposite extreme, in a first affected pregnancy, initial amniocentesis may be delayed to approximately 30 weeks.

TECHNIQUE

Prior to amniocentesis, a sonogram should be obtained for placental localization. Penetration of the placenta by the trochar is best avoided because of the possible complications of enhanced immunization and fetal hemorrhage.

The fetus is avoided by inserting the trochar on the uterine side containing the fetal limbs or posterior to the fetal neck.[19] Alternatively, in early pregnancy the presenting part may be elevated and a suprapubic tap performed.[19] Approximately 10 ml of fluid is collected in a dark bottle to prevent the action of light.

ASSAY

The amniotic fluid obtained is subjected to spectrophotometric analysis. The important factor is a deviation (difference) in optical density at 450 mμ wavelength. It is at this wavelength of light that bilirubinoid pigments become evident.

INTERPRETATION

It is important that the physician concerned with management should inspect the optical density curves and not simply deal with the optical density difference (Δ O.D.) figures obtained.

Among the possible causes of artifacts are oxyhemoglobin and meconium. Maternal jaundice, drug addiction, and usage of hepatotoxic drugs can cause elevated Δ O.D.

The optical density differences obtained are plotted on a Liley[15] curve or similar graph (Fig. 24.3). This is a prognostic table based on observations of fetal outcome in cases of varying optical density difference. Thus, a Δ O.D. of 0.350 at 28 weeks of gestation falls into zone 3, signifying that previous experience has shown the fetus to be in imminent danger of death.

The trend of serial Δ O.D.s is more significant than are single observations. If Δ O.D. is in zone 2, then amniocentesis should be repeated weekly (prior experience shows that such fetuses can safely be watched for up to 2 weeks prior to repeat tap).

A zone 1 Δ O.D. signifies minimal fetal involvement.

Alternatively, the method of Freda can be used.[8] The range of Δ O.D. is used for predicting the current status of the infant, rather than for predicting the eventual outcome at delivery.

TREATMENT

The goal of antenatal treatment is to deliver a viable, nonhydropic infant with as high a hemoglobin level as possible. The main modalities presently used are early delivery and intrauterine transfusion.

Early Delivery

The major drawback to this mode of action is the possibility of death of the premature infant. Since the major cause of death in premature infants is the respiratory distress syndrome (RDS), this method of treatment is the one of choice at 36 weeks or thereafter; in major premature nurseries, the death rate from RDS after 36

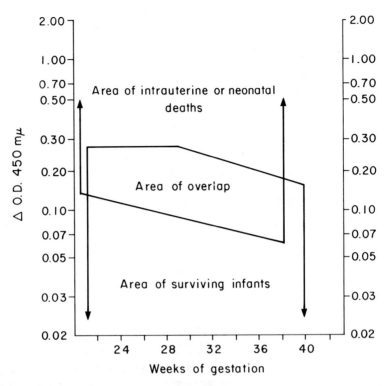

Figure 24.3.   Method of correlating optical density difference readings with clinical status of the fetus at various ages of gestation (after Queenan).

weeks is negligible. Amniocentesis should not be done, therefore, at 36 weeks or beyond; if doubt exists, the infant should be delivered.

Moreover, after 34 weeks, the death rate from RDS is low enough that delivery is the treatment of choice.

It is possible that, at a given age of gestation, there is a difference in RDS incidence between babies born by the vaginal versus the abdominal route. Nonetheless, induction of vaginal delivery in such cases may prove hazardous, due to a floating presenting part, an uneffaced cervix, and the general well-being of the fetus, as evidenced by the Δ O.D. and by serum or urinary estriol determinations.

Prior to 32 weeks, the accepted mode of treatment for the fetus in imminent danger of death is intrauterine transfusion. Usually, intrauterine transfusion is the method of choice in these cases up to 34 weeks. In any isoimmunized pregnancy, delivery should occur no later than 38 weeks of gestation.

It should be emphasized that early delivery presupposes the knowledge of exact fetal age and lung maturity: in that regard, the use of history of last menstrual period, progressive physical signs, sonography, and amniotic fluid criteria such as LS ratio, creatinine, and foam test must not be overlooked.

Intrauterine Transfusion

INDICATIONS

Less than 10% of Rh-sensitized pregnancies should require fetal transfusion in utero. This hazardous procedure should be strictly reserved for those fetuses which, on repeated amniocentesis fall into zone 3: that is, fetal death is imminent.

As previously pointed out, at 34 weeks' gestation or beyond, delivery should be utilized in preference to intrauterine transfusion. Ideally, candidates for intrauterine transfusion will be discovered prior to the onset of hydrops fetalis, which carries a grave prognosis.

TECHNIQUE OF INTRAUTERINE TRANSFUSION

Real time, gray scale ultrasonography is used to visualize the fetal peritoneal cavity. Alternately, 20 cc of a water-soluble radiopaque material (Hypaque) can be injected into the amniotic sac after amniocentesis.[17] The contrast medium outlines the fetus and is swallowed by the fetus. Thus, the fetal intestine becomes visualized, locating the fetal peritoneal cavity. If the fluid is not swallowed by the fetus or if scalp edema, abdominal distention, or limb flaccidity is noted, prognosis is poor.

With the aid of lead markers on the maternal abdomen and under fluoroscopic vision, the needle is placed into the fetal abdominal cavity. After contrast material is injected to ensure proper placement, a polyethylene catheter is advanced.

Loosely packed Rh-negative group blood cells cross-matched against the mother's blood are introduced in small amounts (35–120 cc).[17] The procedure is repeated every 2 weeks until delivery is feasible.

COMPLICATIONS

Complications of intrauterine transfusion include the puncture of the fetus in practically every organ. Inguinal and umbilical hernias are more common.[18] Fetal hemorrhage may occur. Premature onset of labor occurs in one third of cases.[18]

Maternal complications include hemorrhage and infection, including *Clostridium welchii* infection. Maternal structures may be injected. Amniotic fluid embolus is a possibility. Serum hepatitis has been reported.

RESULTS

The risk of fetal death due to trauma at first transfusion is 10%. This risk falls to 3–5% in subsequent transfusions.

Even if the fetus has ascites (hydrops fetalis), by the use of intrauterine transfusion and adjunctive therapy it is now possible to salvage a significant percentage.[3, 4]

The overall survival rate after intrauterine transfusion ranges between 21 and 78%, depending on the series considered[4, 19] and whether or not fetal ascites is present.

The overall perinatal mortality from Rh isoimmunization should presently be in the range of 1.5%.[4]

Other Modes of Therapy

Phenobarbital has been used[19] both in the mother 2–3 weeks prior to delivery and in the infant after birth. The aim is to induce hepatic microsomal glucuronyltransferase activity, increasing hepatic uptake and excretion of bilirubin.[19] Suggested dosage for the mother is 30–60 mg/day.

Promethazine hydrochloride has recently been suggested as a possible therapy, although results to date are inconclusive. The drug inhibits the ability of fetal macrophages to bind Rh-positive red blood cells.[11, 12]

Instillation of digoxin into the fetal peritoneal cavity and administration of digoxin and a diuretic to the mother are accepted therapy in the case of hydrops fetalis.[3]

Plasmapheresis (removal of maternal plasma and replacement with plasma substitute) may be a promising adjunctive therapy in Rh isoimmunized patients.[13]

In affected infants, the umbilical cord should be clamped promptly at birth.

Postnatal therapy, including exchange transfusion and phototherapy, is utilized in the neonatal intensive care unit.

PREVENTION OF RH ISOIMMUNIZATION

Anti-D immunoglobulin G (Rhogam) is administered to the nonimmunized Rh-negative mother.

Mechanism of Action and Dosage

Anti-D immunoglobulin G is obtained from immunized human donors.[10] Three hundred micrograms[3] are administered intramuscularly within 72 hours of delivery or abortion to the Rh-negative, nonimmunized mother who delivers an Rh-positive,

Coombs negative baby. A preparation that may be given intravenously has been tested.[6]

As most fetomaternal transfusion occurs at the time of delivery, this passive antibody binds the antigen sites on the fetal red cells prior to the development of a maternal immunologic response.[19]

However, 1.5–2% of Rh-negative women with Rh-positive babies are immunized prior to delivery.[3] Moreover, if more than 30 cc of Rh-positive cells have entered the maternal circulation, higher dosage of immunoglobulin is needed.[5] Detection of large fetomaternal transfusions is accomplished by screening Rh-negative women postpartum by the Kleihauer technique.

Alternate Method

Antenatal administration of the Rh immune globulin can overcome the problem of antenatal immunization. This technique is especially useful when invasive procedures, such as diagnostic amniocentesis, which may increase the risk of isoimmunization are used.

Ancillary Modes of Prevention

Acts which can increase fetomaternal transfusion at delivery, such as manual removal of the placenta, should be avoided when possible.

References

1. Beck, R.P. Management of the Rh-negative mother. *Can. Med. Assoc. J.* 109:903–904, 1973.
2. Bishop, E.H. and Brown, T.E., Jr. *ACOG Technical Bulletin.* Number 17, July 1972.
3. Bowman, J.M. Hemolytic disease of the newborn. *Can. Med. Assoc. J.* vol. III, September 7, 1974.
4. Bowman, J.M. The management of Rh-isoimmunization. *Obstet. Gynecol.* 52:1–16, 1978.
5. Bowman, J.M. Suppression of Rh-isoimmunization. *Obstet. Gynecol.* 52:385–393, 1978.
6. Bowman, J.M., et al. WinRho: Rh immune globulin prepared by ion exchange for intravenous use. *Can. Med. Assoc. J.* 123:1121–1124, 1980.
7. Desjardins, P.D., et al. Rh-D isoimmunization in A triplet pregnancy. *Can. Med. Assoc. J.* 106:1000, 1972.
8. Freda, V.J. Antepartum management of the Rh problem. In *Progress in Hematology*, edited by Brown, E.B., and Moore, C.V. 1971, pp. 266–296.
9. Freda, V.J. and Bowe, E.T. Hemolytic disease due to Rh sensitization. In *Current Therapy*, edited by Conn, H. Saunders, Philadelphia, 1969.
10. Gorman, J.G., Freda, V.J., et al. Protection from immunization in Rh-incompatible pregnancies: A progress report. *Bull. N.Y. Acad. Med.* 42:458–473, 1966.
11. Gusdon, J.P., Jr., et al. Possible ameliorating effects of erythroblastosis by promethazine hydrochloride. *Am. J. Obstet. Gynecol.* 117:1101, 1973.
12. Gusdon, J.P., Jr., et al. Modification of the human fetal phagocytic response by promethazine hydrochloride. *Am. J. Obstet. Gynecol.* 119:543, 1974.
13. Hauth, J.C., et al. Plasmapheresis as an adjunct to management of Rh isoimmunization. *Obstet. Gynecol.* 57:132–135, 1981.
14. Hellman, L.M., and Pritchard, J.A. *Williams Obstetrics*, ed. 14. Appleton-Century-Crofts, 1971, pp. 1036–1051.
15. Liley, A.W. The administration of blood transfusions to the foetus in utero. *Triangle* 7:184–189, 1966.
16. Ota, H., et al. Enhanced uptake of anti-Rh. coated red cells by cultured human monocytes. *Acta Haematol. (Basel)* 51:270–274, 1974.
17. Queenan, J.T. Amniocentesis and transamniotic fetal transfusion for Rh disease. *Clin. Obstet. Gynecol.* 9:491–507, 1966.
18. Queenan, J.T. *Modern Management of the Rh Problem.* Harper & Row, New York, 1967.
19. Queenan, J.T. (ed.) The Rh problem. *Clin. Obstet. Gynecol.* 14:491–646, 1971.
20. Usher, R., and MacLeish, H. A Re-evaluation of History and Titer as Indices of Severity in Rh Erythroblastosis (abstract). Program and Abstracts of 76th Annual Meeting of The American Pediatric Society, Atlantic City, May 1966, p. 67.
21. Walker, R.H. (ed.) *Hemolytic Disease of The Newborn.* American Society of Clinical Pathologists Commission on Continuing Education, Chicago, 1971.

CHAPTER 25

Infectious Disease

WILLIAM LEDGER, M.D.

Infections in obstetric patients pose serious problems for the clinician. The physician is constantly besieged by a barrage of new microbiologic concepts, a seemingly unending parade of new antibiotic agents, and the knowledge that improper therapy may contribute to the future loss of reproductive function. Because of this, it is important to evaluate problems of infection from the view of an assessment of a rapidly changing science and not one in which all principles of therapy have been established.

In the past decade, there has been a significant change in our understanding of soft tissue pelvic infections. In the past, we have viewed these problems with the microbiologic theory that one pathogen yields a clinical infection. The major focus of concern was the aerobes, particularly organisms like the coagulase positive staphylococcus or *Escherichia coli*. Identify the pathogen and treat with a specific antibiotic. This is not reality. Pelvic infections are polymicrobial, and anaerobes are important causative factors. These anaerobic bacteria can be recovered from the infection site in over 70% of the patients sampled,[40] from the bloodstream in at least 25% of women with bacteremia,[25] and one species, *Bacteroides fragilis*, is frequently isolated from those patients with the most serious of all areas of infections, the pelvic abscess.[17] New organisms, such as *Mycoplasma*[9] and *Chlamydia*,[31] with unfamiliar antibiotic susceptibilities have been found in a number of clinical states. All of these changes in our microbiologic understand-ing of disease have had an impact upon therapeutic strategies.

Keeping pace with the increased understanding of microbiology of soft tissue pelvic infections has been the proliferation of new antibiotics. New agents effective against anaerobes have been introduced, including clindamycin, cefoxitin, and metronidazole. Each of these agents has had great clinical effectiveness, as well as unique toxicities. A second and third generation of cephalosporins have been introduced.

The question of the impact of antibiotics upon future patient fertility has not been resolved. With the exception of a few studies, evaluations of the treatment of salpingitis have been limited to the immediate response to therapy. Not enough attention has been paid to the question of the effect of specific antibiotic agents upon the long-term fertility of the patient. There is a wide variety of response of the human host to various types of pelvic infection.

COMMUNITY ACQUIRED INFECTIONS

Infected Abortion

Today there are fewer problems with patients with infected abortion. The frequency of these infections has decreased. This is probably related to the more widespread availability of effective contraceptive techniques as well as the ability of women to get pregnancy terminations from physicians. In addition to this decrease in frequency, there has been a lessening of the severity of the infections seen in this population of women. The reason for this decrease in serious infection is not known, but the ready availability of pregnancy termination has made it easier for women to have their pregnancy terminated earlier, decreasing the risk of the procedure.

The treatment of the patient with an infected abortion is straightforward. She is given systemic antibiotics and a curettage is performed to remove the infected products of conception. The best antibiotic to employ in these patients is not known, because few prospective comparative studies have been done. In one evaluation of a small population of women using penicillin-chloramphenicol or cephalothin-kanamycin, no difference in the treatment results were noted.[32] Anaerobes seem to be an important consideration in the therapeutic strategy for these women; Rotheram and Schick showed anaerobes to be the most frequent bloodstream isolates in women with this diagnosis.[35] Gram-negative aerobic bacteria are also important; in a comparative study of clindamycin alone versus penicillin-chloramphenicol, there were more treatment failures in the clindamycin group.[21] Because of these results, prospective antibiotic coverage of gram-negative aerobes and most anaerobes is favored. Since most of these patients are not seriously ill, single antibiotic coverage with a drug like cefoxitin would be a satisfactory choice, followed by a curettage after systemic levels of antibiotic have been achieved. The old admonition to avoid curettage until the patient becomes afebrile no longer is held to. For the patient allergic to penicillin or cephalosporins, a combination of clindamycin and an aminoglycoside could be used. An alternative to clindamycin is metronidazole.

The patient with an extrauterine mass may have a pelvic abscess or a uterine perforation with intraperitoneal bleeding that has subsequently become infected. In these women, the antibiotic coverage should be with clindamycin and gentamicin from the beginning, with operative intervention in the form of laparotomy to be used in those patients who continue to have a spiking temperature course after 48–72 hours. When laparotomy is deemed necessary, the surgical strategy should be to drain or remove grossly infected material. There is no need to do a total abdominal hysterectomy and bilateral salpingo-oophorectomy on these women unless these organs are specifically involved in the infection.

Salpingo-oophoritis

There is no other entity of pelvic infection in which our understanding has expanded so much in the past decade. For years, the focus on the clinical teaching in patients with pelvic pain was to avoid the situation of the physician prescribing antibiotics for "PID" in the patient subsequently discovered to have an ectopic pregnancy. Because of this, there were rigid clinical criteria that had to be met before the clinical diagnosis of a pelvic infection could be made. In the nonpregnant woman, the most important clinical criteria were the presence of an elevated temperature and bilateral adnexal finding. The widespread utilization of laparoscopy in women admitted to the hospital with a clinical diagnosis of salpingitis has demonstrated that 40% or more of women with a visual diagnosis of salpingitis are afebrile.[13] Additional confusion has come in the past decade with the awareness that salpingitis in the nonpregnant patient is not always a bilateral process. Unilateral tubo-ovarian abscess has been reported, and this is an entity seen more frequently in women who are using an intrauterine contraceptive device.[11] For the physician caring for a sexually active woman, salpingitis should be considered in the patient with adnexal pain and pain on cervical motion. In patients in whom the clinical diagnosis is in doubt, a pregnancy test, culdocentesis, and/or laparoscopy will help to clarify the situation and direct subsequent therapy.

In the patient with a clinical diagnosis of salpingo-oophoritis, there is a biologic marker that may be helpful in establishing a prognosis. This is the presence of a pelvic mass at the time of the pelvic examination, prior to the administration of antibiotics. Patients with a pelvic mass do not respond as well to antibiotic therapy[38] and frequently require some form of operative intervention, either the drainage or removal of a pelvic abscess for cure. A wide variety of clinical response to systemic antibiotics is noted in patients with salpingo-oophoritis and a pelvic mass. It is likely that many but not all of the patients with a pelvic mass who respond to antibiotics have a tubo-ovarian complex and not an abscess. Some women with a pelvic abscess may be cured with systemic antibiotics alone. There are investigations using ultrasonography currently being carried out to see if this differentiation can be made.

Laboratory findings indicate that one population of women at a lower risk is the group in whom *Neisseria gonorrhea* is recovered from the endocervical canal at the time of pelvic examination, just prior to treatment. Investigations in Sweden suggest this population of women usually responds well to therapy and has a better chance of remaining fertile with open tubes after antibiotic treatment is completed.[6]

There are no good guidelines for the antibiotic therapy of patients with clinical evidence of salpingitis. Comparative studies have been limited to date and the critical question of the impact of any specific therapy upon the eventual fertility of the patient has not been addressed. An important question, whether or not these women should be treated as inpatients with parenteral antibiotics, has not been evaluated and the role of laparoscopy has not been established in this country. With this in mind, there are a number of therapeutic strategies available to the clinician treating the woman with salpingitis. An evaluation of the outpatient treatment of salpingitis with either ampicillin or tetracycline showed no difference in the treatment results.[39] The most important lesson of that study is the unacceptable high failure rate of both forms of therapy. Cefoxitin[38] and cefamandole[10] have been effectively used

in the patient with salpingitis, but these parenteral antibiotic forms required hospitalization for the patient. The patient with a pelvic mass is in a higher risk category. There is no question that she should be hospitalized and treated with drugs effective against anaerobes and gram-negative aerobic bacteria. Presently, the combination of clindamycin and gentamicin is favored, although metronidazole with either cefamandole, cefoxitin or an aminoglycoside may be an acceptable alternative treatment. The best systemic antibiotic therapy awaits future prospective study that includes follow-up to determine patency of the tubes.

Some patients with salpingo-oophoritis will need operative intervention for cure. The worst gynecologic emergency, because of its life-threatening aspect, is the woman with a ruptured tubo-ovarian abscess. This diagnosis should be suspected in the patient with clinical evidence of diffuse peritonitis and a pulse rate far in excess of the temperature elevation. Free-flowing purulent material from the culdocentesis helps to confirm the diagnosis. Immediate laparotomy is indicated, with bilateral removal of tubes and ovaries.[4] Traditionally, the uterus has been removed in these women, but recent experience indicates good results occur when the uterus is left or a subtotal hysterectomy is performed.[19] Operations are also performed in women when it is not such an emergency situation. In women who remain febrile despite the use of appropriate antibiotics, an operation may be necessary for a cure. The least amount of surgery compatible with a cure should be done. If the patient has a mass protruding into the posterior cul-de-sac, colpotomy drainage can be done.[36] If the mass is not accessible to extraperitoneal drainage, then laparotomy should be carried out with the removal of the minimal amount of tissue consistent with a clinical cure. If the patient has a unilateral tubo-ovarian abscess, only the involved side needs to be removed.[14] A small percentage of these patients, who have recovered from the colpotomy drainage of a pelvic abscess or the operative removal of a unilateral tubo-ovarian abscess, have become pregnant and have carried the pregnancy to term.

Urinary Tract Infections

Physicians caring for women of child-bearing age should bear in mind that many bacterial infections will be limited to the urinary tract. The diagnosis of infection is based upon quantitative urine cultures, with a colony count of 10^5 or greater of the same organism on two voided specimens, correlated with significant bacterial colonization in more than 95% of the cases.[15]

Asymptomatic bacteriuria, present in 5–10% of adult women, has great significance for the obstetrician. Screening for bacteriuria identifies a population of women at high risk for developing pyelonephritis later in pregnancy.[16] Intensive therapeutic efforts should be carried out to eliminate bacteriuria in these patients. There seems to be an association of the delivery of low birth weight infants and the finding of bacteriuria in pregnancy.[8] Whether this relationship can be altered by appropriate antibiotic therapy has not been established by prospective study.[41] The antibiotic therapy in these women with bacterial colonization of the urinary tract is much less complicated than is the treatment of the multibacterial pelvic infections. Usually only one organism is involved and in more than 90% of cases these are gram-negative aerobes, with E. coli the most common isolate. Good success has been achieved with sulfas and the nitrofurantoins in these women. Treatment failures should have the subsequent course of antibiotic therapy based upon culture and susceptibility data.

Many women are seen with burning on urination and frequency. Since these symptoms are seen so frequently in patients with cystitis, a frequent response is to order a sulfa drug without any sort of a workup. This is a mistake. Approximately 50% of these women will have cystitis and this will be acceptable therapy. The other 50% will have a variety of conditions, ranging from a urethritis from N. gonorrhea to a vaginitis with a variety of organisms. Clearly, sulfa drugs for this population will not be helpful. These women require an examination and appropriate laboratory studies so that an accurate diagnosis can be made prior to the prescription of therapy.

Pylonephritis is a serious clinical entity and is particularly important in the pregnant patient. In the past, there was associated premature labor in a small number of women, and there has been diminished renal function in a small percentage of women with pyelonephritis.[18] This is a clinical area in which total focus upon antibiotic therapy may be detrimental to the patient. Many of these women are seriously dehydrated at the time of admission to the hospital. They need careful evaluation of their blood electrolytes and sufficient intravenous fluids to insure a urinary output of 50–100 cc/hour. Clinical observation of these women demands careful monitoring of renal function. Antibiotics are important, but the fluid and electrolyte needs of these women must be a prime focus of therapy.

HOSPITAL ACQUIRED INFECTIONS

Hospital acquired infections are underreported. On many occasions, a wound requiring drainage is not cultured and the progress notes include references to a "seroma." Accurate clinical statistics require some sort of a surveillance system run by a person not directly involved in patient care on the obstetric service.[28]

There is a large number of postoperative infections that can be recognized. There are a number of hints on the site of infection based upon clinical signs. These are important for the clinician for the various infections require a wide variety of antibiotic therapies. The most recognizable clinical sign is a febrile response and this frequently is the first clinical hint of infection. Since most of the first temperature elevations in patients with a proven pelvic infection occur in the late afternoon or early evening,[29, 37] it is important that rounds to detect patient morbidity are done during these hours. The timing of onset of infection is important for the clinician, for it suggests possible sites of infection.

There is no reason for the clinician to be sanguine about temperature elevations in the first 48 hours after operation. These infections that manifest first symptomatology at this early time may be life-threatening for the patient. These women require careful observation, and the height of the temperature response may be an important sign of the potential severity of the infection. For women with a temperature below 101°F orally, the most common site of difficulty is the respiratory tract, with atelectasis the most common problem. Efforts to improve deep inspiration of the patient help prevent further progression of the condition and the problem is usually self-limited. There are a number of major concerns in the patient who presents with an oral temperature above 101°F in the first 48 hours. The most dangerous entity is the fever related to the infusion of contaminated intravenous fluids.[1] In these women with no other apparent cause of fever, the intravenous bottle and line should be changed and a portion of the fluid submitted for culture. The discontinuation of the IV infusion may be lifesaving if contamination has occurred. Serious respiratory infection from aspiration of gastric contents can occur. This may not occur in or be recognized in the operating room, and the diagnosis requires careful auscultation and the use of roentgen examination of the lungs. The best treatment of these women has not been established by prospective study, but systemic steroids may be helpful in this situation.[22] The most common cause of these early temperature elevations is a bacteremia, sometimes with a group A β-hemolytic streptococcus. Other organisms, both aerobic and anaerobic, may be involved. These patients should not be observed but should be treated with first-line antibiotics that cover the broad spectra of potential bacterial pathogens. These include clindamycin or metronidazole in combination with an aminoglycoside or a cephalosporin. This aggressive antibiotic approach

must be stressed. These women seldom have localizing signs and too many women with sepsis are observed on clinical services for 24 hours or more because they have a "viral" syndrome or the "flu."

Those women that develop a fever after the first 48 hours during the initial hospitalization may have a variety of sites of infection. A common source is the urinary tract. This is related in part to the use of an indwelling foley catheter. When these indwelling urinary lines are kept in place for more than 24 hours, there is a rise in the number of urinary tract infections. The diagnosis is made by a colony count of urine either obtained from the indwelling catheter or a clean voided specimen. In postoperative women with a urinary tract infection, drugs like sulfas and nitrofurantoins, with their major activity limited to the urinary tract, should be prescribed.

Another large group of postoperative infections occur in those women who have undergone pelvic surgery. These patients are febrile, often complain of a feeling of fullness in the lower abdomen or pelvis, and have a rapid defervescence of their fever and loss of symptoms when the purulent material is drained. In the majority of these patients, no masses can be palpated in the pelvis. They are diagnosed as having pelvic cellulitis and should be treated with systemic antibiotics effective against gram-negative aerobes and all anaerobes. Cefoxitin alone is an effective agent, while a combination of clindamycin and an aminoglycoside or metronidazole and an aminoglycoside or a cephalosporin can be used. The patient who continues to have elevated temperatures on these regimens should have a repeat pelvic examination. If a collection is found, it can be drained. If there are no masses, the diagnosis of septic pelvic thrombophlebitis can be entertained. These women should be treated with antibiotics and have a continuous infusion of heparin until the partial thromboplastin time (PTT) reaches 2–$2\frac{1}{2}$ times normal.[5] In women with septic thrombophlebitis, the temperature returns to normal within 36–48 hours. If these women remain febrile, the physician should be concerned that the patient has a pelvic abscess and a laparotomy is indicated. Another source of fever in these women may be an infection of an abdominal wound. Any draining wound should be opened in its full extent to be sure that the fascia is intact and the drainage is not due to a dehiscence or an evisceration. Drainage alone usually suffices for cure; if there is evidence of spreading inflammation on the skin, systemic antibiotics that are effective against the coagulase positive staphylococcus should be prescribed. Debridement should be performed in the operating room if the inflammation continues to spread. Although the treatment of an infected abdominal wound is straightforward, the goal of care should be prevention. The work of Cruse and Foord suggests a number of preventive measures can be employed.[5] Patients should have as short a preoperative stay in the hospital as possible. The skin should be prepped with an iodine solution and not green soap. Cutting with a coagulation knife should not be done, adhesive wound drapes should not be used, and drains that exit in the wound should not be employed. All of these techniques have been associated with an increased wound infection rate.

Another serious group of postoperative infectious complications are seen in women after they have been discharged from the hospital. The major possibility of a pelvic abscess with anaerobes present must be considered in such cases.[3] These patients should be treated with antibiotics effective against anaerobes, particularly *B. fragilis* and gram-negative aerobes. In seriously ill patients, many physicians favor the use of three antibiotics, penicillin, clindamycin, and an aminoglycoside.[24] Despite this broad spectrum of antibiotic coverage, these women with a well-established infection have a poor prognosis. Approximately half of them will require some form of operative intervention for cure.[24]

A recent therapeutic innovation has been the employment of prophylactic antibiotics to reduce the incidence of postoperative infections. This has been a remarkable development, because of the strong feelings against this antibiotic strategy, engendered by studies in patients in whom prophylactic antibiotics were ineffective.[33] The animal studies of Burke et al.[3] demonstrated the importance of the timing of administration of systemic antibiotics in attempts to eliminate local lesions caused by contaminating bacteria. Systemic antibiotics were most effective in this experimental model when administered before the local bacterial contamination occurred. These observations were followed by the excellent clinical study of bowel surgery by Polk and Lopez-Mayer[34] in which the preoperative administration of systemic antibiotics markedly reduced the incidence of postoperative abdominal wound infection. With their protocol of three doses of a prophylactic antibiotic as a guide, similarly good results were noted in the prophylaxis of premenopausal women undergoing vaginal hysterectomy.[30] Since this report, a number of studies have provided good detailed information on the role of prophylactic antibiotics. With the exception of intramuscular chloramphenicol,[12] which usually provides inadequate serum levels, all of the antibiotics reported to date have been effective. These successful prophylactic agents include the penicillins, cephalosporins, and tetracyclines. One evaluation of short-term versus long-term prophylaxis showed equivalent clinical results when the two regimens were compared.[20] Since the most serious toxicity from prophylactic antibiotics, death from pseudomembranous enterocolitis, has been associated with prolonged prophylaxis,[27] it is advisable for physicians to continue to use short-term prophylaxis. The role of systemic antibiotic prophylaxis in operations other than the vaginal hysterectomy has not been as well established.

There has been a revolution in obstetrical practices in the past decade and this has influenced the frequency and types of infections mothers acquire within the hospital. The major influence upon obstetrical practice has been a change in philosophy which has put greater emphasis upon the fetus than the mother. This was influenced by the development of intrapartum fetal monitoring, which made it possible for the obstetrician to make second-to-second evaluations of fetal well-being. This intrapartum monitoring involved an increase in the number of invasive diagnostic techniques, including the use of an indwelling intrauterine catheter, a fetal scalp electrode, and repetitive incisions of the fetal scalp in labor to evaluate blood pH. All of these techniques increased our knowledge of the status of the fetus, but all were invasive and carried out in an area heavily contaminated by bacteria. Better awareness of the health of the fetus was followed by attempts to diminish the trauma of delivery. Difficult vaginal deliveries, the patient requiring a mid-forceps rotation, or the delivery of a breech were replaced with primary cesarean section. As a result, the incidence of mid-forceps rotation and the vaginal delivery of a breech markedly decreased, while the percentage of women undergoing cesarean section increased. All of these events influenced the rates and the types of postdelivery infections seen in the 1980s.

There are a few observations that universally seem to pinpoint obstetrical patients at high risk for infection. Women from lower socioeconomic populations have a higher frequency of and more severe infections. There is also a vast difference in the risk of infection following the two modes of delivery. Those women who delivery vaginally have less frequent as well as less severe infections than do those who delivery by cesarean section. Of interest in the evaluation of traditional risk factors such as length of labor, the duration of ruptured membranes, the frequency of vaginal examination and the use of internal monitoring is the fact that there is no uniform finding of increased risk in every study.

There is a logical diagnostic approach to the febrile postpartum patient. The physician's first responsibility is to do a complete physical examination in order to determine the site of infection. This may be difficult, particularly in the patient who becomes febrile in the first 48 hours after delivery, for she may have few localizing signs. The examination is helpful to determine the extent of a pelvic infection and it is important in determining that there is adequate uterine drainage. Since urinary tract infections commonly occur in the postpartum period, an uncontaminated urine specimen should be evaluated microscopically for the presence of bacteria and a portion should subsequently be sent for culture. Cultures should be obtained for aerobes, particularly the group A β-hemolytic streptococcus, and blood cultures should be performed prior to the prescription of systemic antibiotics. This workup should be repeated in the patient who fails to respond to systemic antibiotics, and particular care should be given to the abdominal wound.

There is a logic to the therapy of postpartum infection. Patients with evidence of a urinary tract infection should be treated with single agents that are most effective against urinary tract pathogens. If the patient has a lower urinary tract infection, then a sulfa or a nitrofurantoin can be employed. If the patient develops a postpartum pyelonephritis, ampicillin or a cephalosporin can be used. If the pyelonephritis occurs after a cesarean section or in a woman with an extensive sulcus laceration following vaginal delivery, an intravenous pyelogram should be done to be certain there is no ureteral blockage. For those patients who develop an endomyometritis following vaginal delivery, a single antibiotic is usually appropriate, either ampicillin or a cephalosporin. For the woman who develops an endomyometritis following cesarean section, the choice of antibiotics is much more critical. Di Zerega et al.[7] found a combination of clindamycin-gentamicin to be superior to the frequently employed penicillin-gentamicin regimen. There is concern about the routine use of clindamycin in these women, because of the potential toxicity of this antibiotic. There is much interest in the newer cephalosporin, cefamandole,[26] and the cephamycin, cefoxitin.[2] Preliminary studies indicate that these agents are effective, but comparative studies with the clindamycin-gentamicin regimen have not been reported.

Some patients will develop late postpartum infection. In view of the animal model proposed by Gorbach et al., the major concern should be abscess formation with anaerobes as the major pathogens. Because of this, antibiotics should be used that are effective against anaerobes, particularly *B. fragilis*, including clindamycin or metronidazole, plus coverage against gram-negative aerobes, either aminoglycosides or the newer cephalosporins. The most important therapeutic maneuver is to search for an abscess. If this is the abdominal wound, the wound should be opened and drained in the operating room so that fascial integrity can be checked. If the abdominal wound is free of any signs of infection, a careful examination should be followed by an ultrasound evaluation for the presence of a pelvic abscess. If the patient remains febrile and there is evidence of a pelvic abscess, laparotomy is indicated to remove infected material. If the uterus is grossly infected, then hysterectomy is indicated. A subtotal hysterectomy can be performed in some women and there seems to be no difference in the postoperative morbidity. A small number of patients may have septic pelvic thrombophlebitis. These women have a persistent spiking fever despite the use of acceptable antibiotics and no evidence of a pelvic abscess on examination. In these patients, the infusion of intravenous heparin may be associated with a dramatic defervescence of the maternal fever. The most appropriate technique of heparin administration is by continuous intravenous infusion by pump, until the partial thromboplastin time is between 2 and $2\frac{1}{2}$ times normal. In the past, it has been assumed that the rapid temperature response was due to the heparin therapy of the septic pelvic thrombophlebitis. Heparin may increase the amount of active antibiotic at the site of infection. The mechanism may be clarified by future prospective studies. Venacaval ligation is reserved for the patient who continues to have repeated pulmonary emboli despite heparinization. This operative approach is rarely necessary.

References

1. Bosomworth, P.P., and Hamelberg, W. The etiologic and therapeutic aspects of aspiration pneumonia. *Surg. Forum 13*:158, 1962.
2. Bryant, R.F., and Hammond, D. Interaction of purulent material with antibiotics used to treat *Pseudomonas* infections. *Antimicrob. Agents Chemother. 6*:702, 1974.
3. Burke, J.F. The effective period of preventive antibiotic action in experimental infections and dermal lesions. *Surgery 50*:161, 1961.
4. Collins, G.C., Nix, F.G., and Cerha, H.T. Ruptured tubo-ovarian abscess. *Am. J. Obstet. Gynecol. 72*:820, 1956.
5. Cruse, P.J.E., and Foord, R. A five-year prospective study of 23,649 surgical wounds. *Arch. Surg. 107*:206, 1973.
6. Cunningham, F.G., Hauth, J.C., Strong, J.D., et al. Evaluation of tetracycline or penicillin and ampicillin for treatment of acute pelvic inflammatory disease. *N. Engl. J. Med. 296*:1380, 1977.
7. Di Zerega, G. Yonekura, L., Roy, S., et al. A comparison of clindamycin-gentamicin and penicillin-gentamicin in the treatment of post cesarean section endomyometritis. *Am. J. Obstet. Gynecol. 134*:238, 1979.
8. Elder, H.A., Santamarina, B.A.G., Smith, S., et al. The natural history of asymptomatic bacteriuria during pregnancy: The effect of tetracycline on the clinical course and the outcome of pregnancy. *Am. J. Obstet. Gynecol. 111*:441, 1971.
9. Eschenbach, D.A., Duchanan, T.M., Pollock, H.M., et al. Polymicrobial etiology of acute pelvic inflammatory disease. *N. Engl. J. Med. 293*:166, 1975.
10. Gibbs, R. Personal communication.
11. Golde, S.H., Israel, R., and Ledger, W.J. Unilateral tuboovarian abscess: A distinct entity. *Am. J. Obstet. Gynecol. 127*:807, 1977.
12. Goosenberg, J., Emich, J.P., and Schwarz, R.H. Prophylactic antibiotics in vaginal hysterectomy. *Am. J. Obstet. Gynecol. 105*:503, 1969.
13. Jacobson, L., and Westrom, L. Objectivized diagnosis of acute pelvic inflammatory disease. *Am. J. Obstet. Gynecol. 105*:1088, 1969.
14. Kass, E.H. Asymptomatic infection of urinary tract. *Trans. Assoc. Am. Physicians 69*:56, 1956.
15. Kass, E.H. Bacteriuria and pyelonephritis of pregnancy. *Arch. Intern. Med. 105*:194, 1960.
16. Kincaid-Smith, P., and Bullen, M. Bacteriuria in pregnancy. *Lancet 1*:395, 1965.
17. Ledger, W.J. Anaerobic infections. *Am. J. Obstet. Gynecol. 125*:111, 1975.
18. Ledger, W.J., and Child, M. The hospital care of patients undergoing hysterectomy: An analysis of 12,026 patients from the professional activity study. *Am. J. Obstet. Gynecol. 117*:423, 1973.
19. Ledger, W.J., Gassner, C.B., and Gee, C. Operative care of infections in obstetrics-gynecology. *J. Reprod. Med. 13*:128, 1974.
20. Ledger, W.J., Gee, C., and Lewis, W.P. Guidelines for antibiotic prophylaxis in gynecology. *Am. J. Obstet. Gynecol. 128*:1038, 1975.

21. Ledger, W.J., Gee, C.L., Lewis, W.P., et al. Comparison of clindamycin and chloramphenicol in treatment of serious infections of the female genital tract. *J. Infect. Dis. 135:*530, 1977.
22. Ledger, W.J., and Headington, J.T. Group A beta hemolytic streptococcus: An important cause of serious infections in Obstetrics and Gynecology. *Obstet. Gynecol. 39:*474, 1972.
23. Ledger, W.J., Kriewall, T.J., and Gee, C. The fever index: A technique for evaluating the clinical response to bacteremia. *Obstet. Gynecol. 45:*603, 1975.
24. Ledger, W.J., Moore, D.E., Lowensohn, R.I., et al. A fever index evaluation of chloramphenicol or clindamycin in patients with serious pelvic infections. *Obstet. Gynecol. 50:*53, 1977.
25. Ledger, W.J., Norman, M., Gee, C., et al. Bacteremia on an Obstetric-Gynecologic service. *Am. J. Obstet. Gynecol. 121:*205, 1975.
26. Ledger, W.J., and Peterson, E.P. The use of heparin in the management of pelvic thrombophlebitis. *Surg. Gynecol. Obstet. 131:*1115, 1970.
27. Ledger, W.J., and Puttler, O.L. Death from pseudomembranous enterocolitis. *Obstet. Gynecol. 45:*609, 1975.
28. Ledger, W.J., Reite, A.M., and Headington, J.T. A system for infectious disease surveillance on an obstetric service. *Obstet. Gynecol. 37:*769, 1971.
29. Ledger, W.J., Reite, A.M., and Headington, J.T. The surveillance of infection on an inpatient gynecologic service. *Am. J. Obstet. Gynecol. 113:*662, 1972.
30. Ledger, W.J., Sweet, R.L., and Headington, J.T. The prophylactic use of cephaloridine in the prevention of pelvic infections in pre-menopausal women undergoing vaginal hysterectomy. *Am. J. Obstet. Gynecol. 115:*766, 1973.
31. Mårdh, P.A., Ripa, T., Svensson, L., et al. *Chlamydia trachomatis* infection in patients with acute salpingitis. *N. Engl. J. Med. 296:*1377, 1977.
32. Ostergard, D.R. Comparison of two antibiotic regimens in the treatment of septic abortion. *Obstet. Gynecol. 36:*473, 1970.
33. Petersdorf, R.G., Gustin, J.H., Hoeprick, P.D., et al. A study of antibiotic prophylaxis in unconscious patients. *N. Engl. J. Med. 257:*1001, 1957.
34. Polk, H.C., and Lopez-Mayer, I.F. Postoperative wound infection: Prospective study of determinant factors and prevention. *Surgery 66:*97, 1969.
35. Rotheram, E.B., and Schick, S.F. Non clostridial anaerobic bacteria in septic abortion. *Am. J. Obstet. Gynecol. 46:*80, 1969.
36. Rubenstein, P.R., Mishell, D.R., Jr., and Ledger, W.J. Colpotomy drainage of pelvic abscess. *Obstet. Gynecol. 48:*142, 1976.
37. Sack, R.A. Epidemic of gram negative organism septicemia subsequent to elective operation. *Am. J. Obstet. Gynecol. 107:*394, 1976.
38. Svensson, L., Westrom, L., Ripa, T., et al. Differences in some clinical and laboratory parameters in acute salpingitis related to culture and serologic findings. *Am. J. Obstet. Gynecol. 138:*1017, 1980.
39. Sweet, R.L., and Ledger, W.J. Cefoxitin: Single agent treatment of mixed aerobic anaerobic pelvic infections. *Obstet. Gynecol. 54:*193, 1979.
40. Swenson, R.M., Michaelson, T.C., Daly, M.J., et al. Anaerobic bacterial infections of the female genital tract. *Obstet. Gynecol. 42:*538, 1973.
41. Whalley, P.H., Cunningham, F.G., and Martin, F.G. Transient renal dysfunction associated with acute pyelonephritis of pregnancy. *Obstet. Gynecol. 46:*174, 1975.

CHAPTER 26

Preterm Birth

FRITZ FUCHS, M.D.
OLAVI YLIKORKALA, M.D.

In terms of mortality and morbidity of the infant, preterm birth is by far the most important problem in modern obstetrics. During the third quarter of the 20th century, the concern of the obstetrician shifted from the mother to her offspring. In the Western world, the maternal mortality rate almost reached the irreducible minimum, but the perinatal mortality, although it has been greatly reduced, is still too high. The dominant cause of perinatal death is prematurity, and while the mortality rate of premature infants has been reduced by improved care, the incidence of prematurity has not been reduced. On the contrary, it seems to be rising. This rise may well be due both to socioeconomic factors, such as the continuous shift of population from rural to urban environment, and to medical factors, such as the increasing incidence of induced abortion, whether legal or illegal.

The incidence of preterm birth varies between 5 and 10% of the number of live births; it varies from country to country and also from one geographical region to another within countries. If 8% can be taken as an average figure, these 8% account for about 75% of the total perinatal deaths. A reduction of the incidence of prematurity from 8 to 6% would reduce the perinatal mortality by about 18%. Such a reduction would require both preventive and therapeutic measures, but it is not an unrealistic goal for modern obstetrics.

A reduction of the incidence of preterm birth would lead not only to a decrease in the perinatal mortality but also to a reduction in the neonatal and infant morbidity. It is well documented that the incidence of physical and behavioral sequelae is considerably higher in premature infants than in infants born at term. Expert care often can reduce but cannot eliminate these sequelae, and the prevention of preterm birth must therefore be given the highest priority.

DEFINITIONS

A widely accepted definition of premature or preterm birth is delivery before completion of 36 weeks of gestation, calculated from the first day of the last menstrual period. Since the interval between the first day of the menstrual cycle and the time of ovulation varies considerably, this can cause an error which can only be corrected with approximation on the basis of the usual length of the cycle in the particular individual.

The classical definition based upon birth weight, according to which infants weighing less than 2500 gm at birth were classified as premature, had to be discarded when it was realized that infants of 37 weeks or more could have birth weights below this limit. Such "small-for-dates" infants are now known to constitute a considerable fraction of the infants with low birth weights, particularly, but not exclusively, in the group weighing 2000–2499 gm. On the other hand, infants who are premature in regard to gestation age may weigh 2500 gm or over, as seen for instance in infants of diabetic mothers.

Although infants born between 20 and 28 weeks of gestation are considered "immature" rather than "premature," the term *premature labor* is used to describe labor occurring between 20 and 36 completed weeks of gestation. A better terminology, which avoids any reference to the maturity of the fetus, is *preterm labor*.

Another problem is the distinction between "premature labor" and "false labor." Premature labor may be defined as rhythmic uterine contractions before the completion of 36 gestational weeks, leading to progressive effacement and dilation of the cervix, while false labor could be defined as uterine activity which, although it may be fairly strong and regular, does not affect the cervix and eventually stops without any other treatment than bed rest.

The term *threatened premature labor* is ambiguous and should not be used. *Threatened preterm birth* is more precise and should be used for the situation which applies when premature labor has set in. Since premature labor can often be arrested by pharmacological means, it is important that the differential diagnosis *false labor* is ruled out by careful observation of the pregnant woman, to avoid unnecessary treatment.

FACTORS DETERMINING THE LENGTH OF GESTATION

The length of gestation and the degree of development of the newborn vary greatly from species to species. While not the only important factor, the degree of development of the offspring at birth is certainly an essential factor for the survival of the species. The uterus provides excellent protection for the embryo but, except for the very early phase, intrauterine existence depends on the development of a special organ for the supply of oxygen and nutrients to the growing conceptus, namely the placenta. Where such an organ is missing, as in the marsupials, the embryo can be sustained in utero for only a brief period.

Just as the number of cells increases exponentially from a single fertilized ovum to a fully developed newborn, the supply of nutrients from mother to fetus must increase exponentially. In most species, the demands of the fetus put the mother under considerable strain. Obviously, there are limits to how long the maternal organism can sustain exponential growth of the fetus. Is it unreasonable to assume that when approaching the limit for one or more crucial factors, the fetus reacts by sending a signal that other means are now required? The crucial factor may not be oxygen, in spite of the fact that a deficiency of oxygen will have the most rapid effects. It could be calcium and/or phosphate, the two inorganic substances of which the largest amounts are required. Both calcium and phosphate are crucial for the function of every single cell. It is possible that during evolution the length of gestation has become genetically controlled; that the signal for parturition no longer requires that a functional limit in the maternal supply of a vital component should be reached but is given while a safety margin still exists. Nevertheless, these considerations point to the fetus as the source of the signal.

Observations in women show that certain stress situations may precipitate parturition before the physiological or genetic end point of human gestation. It is well-known that multiple pregnancies often end prematurely. In fact, with three or more fetuses, the pregnancy almost never goes to term. Although the uterine volume per se has been implicated as a crucial factor in the onset of labor, it is probably more reasonable to ascribe the premature onset of labor to an inability of the maternal organism to supply the requirements of more than one fetus. After all, the presence of even a single fetus increases the cardiac output of the mother by almost 50%.

The hypothesis that the signal for parturition comes from the fetus rather than the mother is not based upon theoretical considerations alone, it is supported by a growing body of evidence. Nor is the hypothesis new, it was proposed by Hippocrates.

PREDISPOSING FACTORS

Epidemiological studies have identified a number of conditions which are associated with an increased incidence of preterm delivery. Although the cause-relationship is far from clear in all instances, such conditions may be considered as predisposing factors. As shown in Table 26.1, it is practical to divide them into maternal, placental, fetal, and iatrogenic factors. In some cases, more than a single such predisposing factor may be present. However, in about half of the cases, no predisposing factor can be identified. In such instances, one has to assume that the timing mechanism, which normally prevents the initiation of labor before fetal maturity, either is not functioning or is overruled by a strong, although unidentifiable, stimulus.

Table 26.1.   Predisposing Factors in Preterm Labor

Maternal factors
   Age below 20 or over 35 years at first delivery
   Primiparity
   Small stature
   Low socioeconomic status
   Cigarette smoking
   Small heart volume
   Congenital cardiac disease
   Chronic debilitating disease
   Anatomical defects of the uterus
      Congenital uterine malformations
      Uterine synechia
      Fibromyomas
      Incompetent cervix
   Pregnancy complications
      Urinary tract infection
      Intercurrent febrile infections
      Accidental traumas
      Mental and physical stress
Placental factors
   Abruptio placentae
   Placenta previa
   Placental insufficiency
Fetal factors
   Multiple gestation
   Anencephaly
   Adrenal hyperplasia
   Anomalies associated with polyhydramnios and oligohydramnios
Iatrogenic factors
   Induction of labor for pregnancy complications
      Preeclampsia
      Rh isoimmunization
      Diabetes mellitus
   Elective induction of labor
   Intrauterine contraceptive device in situ

Many studies have documented the association of premature birth with maternal age below 20 or above 35 years at the time of the first birth, with primiparity, with small stature of the mother, and with socioeconomic deprivation. The association of low birth weight with maternal cigarette smoking is also well documented. While the causal relationship to the demographic and constitutional factors is unclear, the relationship between maternal smoking and low birth weight is thought to be due to the increased uptake of carbon monoxide in smokers.

The increased incidence of premature birth in mothers with congenital heart diseases and other severe cardiovascular disorders is probably due to a relative insufficiency of the transport of nutrients to the fetus. The same explanation must pertain to the relationship between small heart volume relative to body size and increased incidence of prematurity which was first reported by Finnish workers.

The relationship of urinary tract infection and prematurity is well documented, and it has been shown that even asymptomatic bacteriuria is a predisposing factor. The relationship between febrile conditions and prematurity is presumably due to the increased motility of the myometrium at high body temperatures.

Anatomic defects of the uterus as causes of preterm labor are not very common but are easily understood. Malformations due to incomplete fusion of the Müllerian ducts may prevent the normal growth of the uterus or interfere with placental development. The same mechanism applies to excessive scarring of the uterus, including the formation of synechiae, and to submucous fibromyomas. The incompetent cervix, resulting in mid trimester abortion or premature birth, may be due to a congenital defect or to a traumatic lesion inflicted in connection with induction of abortion. Thus, it may occasionally belong in the category of iatrogenic factors.

The placental factors are obvious. Placental insufficiency may be due to malformations or infarcts or may be purely functional without any anatomical defects.

The association of fetal factors and prematurity are easy to understand. In multiple gestation the transport system may become insufficient for the adequate supply of the fetus. This occurs frequently in twin gestation, and if there are three or more fetuses the pregnancy is practically never carried to term. However, this does not preclude pharmacological treatment of threatened preterm birth, which is often successful. The high incidence of prematurity in association with anencephaly and other severe malformations of the fetal central nervous system supports the assumption that the center controlling the length of gestation is located in the fetal brain. The anomalies associated with hydramnios probably cause premature labor indirectly, by rapid distention of the uterus. Potter's syndrome, with oligohydramnios, is also associated with an increased incidence of prematurity, for unknown reasons.

Induction of labor before term is indicated in a number of pregnancy complications, and the risk of the fetus remaining in utero must be balanced against the risk of prematurity in each individual case. Induction for the convenience of the patient or the obstetrician should probably not be done at all, or at least not without ascertaining fetal maturity by amniocentesis or other means.

The increased risk of prematurity in pregnancies with an intrauterine contraceptive device (IUD) has recently been documented. Because of this and the increased risk of abortion, occasionally septic, the general opinion is that when pregnancy occurs with an IUD in situ, the IUD should be removed.

PREVENTIVE MEASURES

From the list of predisposing factors it is evident that in some instances preterm birth may be prevented by proper management of the pregnancy. Thus, mothers should be warned against the harmful effects of heavy smoking. If they have congenital heart disease, or for that matter any heart disease, they should be advised to rest as much as possible and avoid all sources of infection. Urinary tract infection should be treated vigorously in pregnancy, and febrile conditions should be treated with antipyretics to avoid activation of the myometrium.

Anatomical defects of the uterus may require operative correction. Cervical incompetence which is the most common reason for operative prevention of preterm birth should be diagnosed before the start of pregnancy, as a part of evaluation of previous pregnancy failure. The previous obstetric history and a hysterogram are the most important tools in the diagnosis. The Shirodkar and McDonald cerclage operations to reinforce the cervix are best performed at 12–16 weeks' gestation, when the presence of a living fetus can be confirmed by ultrasound. Bleeding, contractions, or rupture of the membranes are contraindications to the operation. In over 75% of the cases, such patients deliver healthy infants after operative treatment.

Multiple gestation should be diagnosed as early as possible; the increased use of ultrasonography is very helpful in this regard. Most obstetricians advocate increased bed rest to mothers with twin pregnancies, although the opinions are divided as to whether this will improve the outcome. If there are three or more fetuses, discontinuation of work and increased rest become mandatory.

As mentioned above, elective induction of labor or cesarean section cannot be justified unless fetal maturity can be documented. Whether the use of amniocentesis is acceptable for this purpose is debatable. The risks are small but definite; they must be balanced against the advantage of being able to induce labor or operate upon a subject who has an empty stomach, who is in the hospital and who is mentally and physically prepared for the procedure.

DIAGNOSIS

To determine whether labor is premature or not, it is essential to know the length of gestation. Obvious as this may seem, it often is the cause of confusion. The history must include not only the date of the last menstrual period but also the length of previous cycles, as well as any abortion, miscarriage or delivery with or without lactation shortly before the conception. Discontinuation of oral or intrauterine contraception is also relevant. The history should include signs and symptoms from the early part of the current pregnancy, growth of the uterus, time of quickening, etc. The immediate history must include a description of the uterine activity, passage of amniotic fluid, bleeding from the vagina, etc.

The examination of the patient suspected to be in preterm labor should include a palpation of the uterus to determine contractions, weight of the fetus, and fetal lie. The fetal heart rate must be determined. Unless there are signs of premature rupture of the membranes or vaginal bleeding, a vaginal examination is necessary to determine the degree of cervical effacement and dilatation and verify the fetal presentation.

As a rule, a period of observation is necessary to determine whether a patient is in false labor which will stop by itself after a period of bed rest or is in true preterm labor. Pharmacological inhibition of labor is applied if the uterine activity consists of contractions of 30–60 seconds' duration at least once every 10 minutes, and the cervix shows signs of effacement and dilatation. The estimated fetal weight must not exceed 2500 gm, and the fetus must be alive. Although multiple gestation is by no means a contraindication for treatment of preterm labor, it is essential for the management that the diagnosis be verified.

If, after a detailed history has been obtained and a careful examination has been carried out, doubt still remains about the duration of pregnancy, additional procedures may be required, such as sonography with measurement of the biparietal diameter or amniocentesis with determination of creatinine concentration, lecithin/sphingomyelin (L/S) ratio or foam test, and cytology.

While abruptio placentae is an absolute contraindication for prevention of premature birth, placenta previa is not. It is therefore essential to determine the cause of any third trimester bleeding before treatment with labor-inhibiting drugs is considered.

Premature rupture of the membranes often presents a dilemma, because of the risk of intrauterine infection. Amnionitis increases the dangers of prematurity but, on the other hand, the delay of birth by a week can mean the difference between neonatal death and survival. Each case must be treated individually, and if labor-inhibiting agents are employed, the patient must be watched very closely for signs of infection. Although the risk of infection appears to be less at home than in the hospital, treatment should at least be initiated after admission to a hospital.

PHARMACOLOGICAL ARREST OF PRETERM LABOR

Although our understanding of the mechanism of labor is incomplete, the past 2 decades have greatly increased our knowledge of the physiology and pharmacology of the uterine muscle. The myometrium appears to have a mechanism which keeps the uterus at rest until the onset of labor, although it has the capacity to contract at any time during gestation. The exact nature of this mechanism is not known, but it appears to prevent the conduction of impulses from cell to cell which is necessary for the synchronous activation of various parts of the myometrium. Animal studies indicate that steroids are involved in this mechanism. Although the myometrium could conceivably contract if this defense mechanism were removed, the uterus in vivo also seems to require an activating stimulus to contract. Several humoral agents can stimulate uterine contractions, including oxytocin, prostaglandins, and various biogenic amines such as histamine, serotonin, bradykinin, and catecholamines. While there is no evidence for a role of the amines, both oxytocin and prostaglandins are thought to be essential.

Figure 26.1 illustrates the essential factors in the myometrium and the fetoplacental and maternal hormones which in-

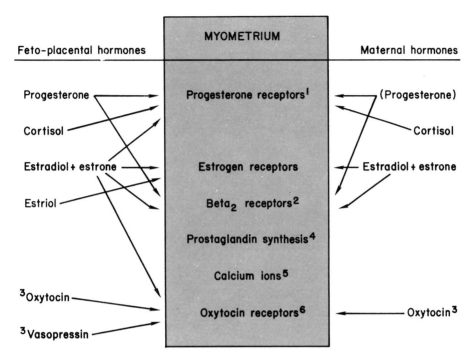

Figure 26.1. Schematic illustration of the factors known or assumed to play a role in the mechanism of labor. The central box contains the factors in the myometrium itself. These factors are activated or modulated by hormones which originate either from the fetoplacental unit or from the mother. The superscript numbers refer to the sites of action of various tocolytic agents which are discussed in the text.

fluence myometrial function. The superscript numbers refer to the possible points of attack for pharmacological control of premature contractions.

1. It has been assumed that progesterone is necessary for keeping the myometrium at rest, as certainly is the case in many animal species. This has led to the use of progestins to prevent premature birth. Although there are specific progesterone receptors in the myometrium and progesterone binds very rapidly, it takes 12–24 hours for the effect on myometrial motility to develop. It is too late, therefore, to try to reinforce the progesterone level once the uterus has begun to contract. Use of a synthetic progestin for prophylactic treatment of cases with a high risk of premature onset of labor has shown promising results but caused some concern about possible teratogenic effects on the fetus.

2. Like other smooth muscle systems, the myometrium contains α- and β-receptors. Stimulation of the β-receptors causes relaxation; although the physiological role of these sympathetic receptors is poorly understood, the presence of β-receptors has provided one of the best approaches to pharmacological control of uterine contractions. The β-receptors are divided into β_1-receptors, found in the heart, and β_2-receptors found in other smooth muscles, including the myometrium. During the past decade, a number of β-agonists have been developed which predominatly stimulate β_2-receptors; these agents have been widely used as bronchodilators for the treatment of asthma. In Europe and other parts of the world, these agents have also been widely used in preterm labor. In the United States, a betamimetic compound with the generic name *ritodrine* is the first agent approved for use in preterm labor. Betamimetic agents are usually given IV

initially, followed by oral administration until maturity of the fetus.

3. There is considerable evidence to support the assumption that uterine contractions do not develop "spontaneously" but require active stimulation of the myometrium. Therefore, inhibition of secretion or formation of activating agents should inhibit uterine activity. The most powerful uterine stimulant is oxytocin, and there is incontrovertible evidence for the presence of oxytocin in the maternal and fetal blood during parturition. The secretion of oxytocin from the neurohypophysis can be inhibited by administration of ethanol; this approach has been used in threatened premature labor, particularly in the United States where the betamimetic agents were not available for the prevention of preterm birth. Ethanol is given as an IV infusion of a 10% solution of ethanol in saline or dextrose-water in a dosage calculated to give a blood alcohol level of 0.12–0.18%. The treatment consists of an initial dose given over 2 hours to obtain the therapeutic level and a maintenance dose which is one fifth of the initial hourly dose and is given for 10 hours. Ethanol passes through the placenta very rapidly, and equilibrium between mother and fetus is established in 15 minutes. After the treatment, the mother can metabolize ethanol at a faster rate than can the fetus, but equilibrium is maintained until the ethanol has been eliminated from fetus and mother.

4. Another group of uterine stimulants are the prostaglandins which are formed in the decidua, membranes and myometrium during parturition. The formation of prostaglandins can be inhibited by prostaglandin synthetase inhibitors; such agents have been shown to be able to arrest preterm labor. However, due to the fact that prostaglandins are ubiquitous and have many physiological roles, the use of such agents could have dangerous side effects. Thus, indomethacin, a potent prostaglandin synthetase inhibitor, has been shown to cause premature closure of the fetal ductus arteriosus in animals. There have been cases described of neonatal pulmonary hypertension after indomethacin

treatment of the mother, presumably with the same pathophysiology. This group of agents must therefore be studied further, before their proven effect on uterine activity can be utilized for prevention of preterm birth.

5. Calcium ions play an important role in the cellular mechanisms of muscular contraction and relaxation. Magnesium sulfate and a number of pharmacological agents interfere with the availability of calcium ions. On this basis, both magnesium sulfate and certain drugs have been used to inhibit uterine contractions in premature labor.

6. It has recently been shown that the myometrium in rabbits and rats contains receptors for oxytocin, and studies indicate that this also applies to the human. For some 20 years, several groups have tried to develop oxytocin analogues which are devoid of oxytocic properties but which bind to the same receptors. By saturation of the receptors with the analogue, the binding of oxytocin which is necessary for its action would be prevented. One such analogue has shown considerable promise in preliminary clinical trials.

CLINICAL MANAGEMENT OF PRETERM LABOR

The preterm fetus is not as well equipped as the term fetus to withstand the stresses of labor. When arrest of preterm labor fails or is contraindicated, it is essential to conduct labor and delivery in such a way that the risk of damage of the fetus is reduced to a minimum. Delivery should take place in a hospital which is equipped to cope with all obstetric emergencies and which has the facilities for and a staff with expertise in the intensive care of the newborn.

Labor should be monitored electronically to permit immediate intervention in cases of fetal distress. Prolonged labor should be avoided; the second stage should be shortened by a generous episiotomy and by outlet forceps where applicable. Breech presentations are much more frequent before term than at term, and in recent years it has been clearly documented that the least traumatic delivery of a preterm fetus in breech presentation is by cesarean section.

Although resuscitation of the small newborn is crucial, it is recommended to delay the clamping of the cord for 60 seconds while the baby is held upside down below the level of the placenta. This permits the newborn to receive a certain amount of blood from the placenta, partly by gravity and partly by contraction of the uterus. While in principle the obstetrician is responsible for the immediate care of the newborn, it is useful to have a neonatologist present to conduct the resuscitation. Often the anesthesiologist can be helpful when intubation is required. As soon as respiration has been established, the small newborn is transferred out of the delivery room, to the neonatal intensive care unit.

In multiple gestations which are particularly prone to preterm labor, enough manpower should be available to ensure immediate resuscitation of the newborn infants, especially when they are delivered simultaneously by cesarean section.

If tubal ligation has been planned, either in connection with a cesarean section or in the puerperium, it is prudent to delay this procedure until the viability of the preterm infant has been established beyond doubt.

PREMATURE RUPTURE OF MEMBRANES

Rupture of the membranes before the onset of labor is called *premature rupture of membranes*. If it happens at 37 weeks or later, it rarely presents serious problems; labor will often begin within hours, and if not, labor can usually be induced with relative ease, using intravenous oxytocin infusion. If the membranes rupture before 37 weeks, it often causes serious problems, compounding the risks associated with preterm birth. The worst problems occur when the gestation age is between 26 and 29 weeks. While the premature fetus at this stage usually is better off in the uterus than in the nursery when the membranes are intact, this is not necessar-

ily so after rupture of the membranes, because of the risk of ascending infection which causes amnionitis and pulmonary infection of the newborn. When a patient is admitted with signs of ruptured membranes before 37 weeks, vaginal examination should be avoided, except when there is a suspicion of a prolapse of the cord or a transverse lie, to reduce the risk of ascending infection. If there is no labor, the patient may be observed for signs of imminent infection, in the hope that the fetus may gain some additional time in the uterus. In most cases, the time gained by this conservative approach is limited; on the other hand, every day gained may be critical for survival of the baby. Prophylactic use of antibiotics is a much debated issue; it is not always effective and it can mask problems in the newborn.

In summary, premature rupture of the membranes after 37 weeks are best treated by induction of labor, if spontaneous labor does not occur in 8–12 hours. Premature rupture of the membranes before 37 weeks is treated with hands-off observation as long as there are no complications and with immediate intervention if signs of infection or other complications occur. The preterm fetus has less tolerance against the stress of labor; if infected in utero, the preterm fetus is even more vulnerable.

ANTENATAL PREVENTION OF THE RESPIRATORY DISTRESS SYNDROME OF THE NEWBORN

The respiratory distress syndrome (RDS) or hyaline membrane disease (HMD) is the most common cause of postnatal complications and death among premature infants. The syndrome is due to insufficient surfactant activity in the infant's lungs. Without sufficient surfactant, more than normal pressure is required to keep the alveoli open, causing the premature infant to develop respiratory distress. The synthesis of the phospholipids providing the surfactant activity is closely related to the gestational age. It begins around 24–26 weeks, and at 36 weeks of gestation the fetal lungs have usually reached functional maturation. The best way to prevent RDS is to prevent premature birth and this provides a strong argument for pharmacological arrest of premature labor. Even a short delay can be highly beneficial, if during the interval the mother is treated with corticosteroids, as first described by Liggins and Howie in 1972. In the infants up to 32 weeks' gestation age, the incidence of RDS is lower if the mothers are treated with corticosteroids than in infants of untreated mothers. In the more mature infants, there is little difference. This management is not universally accepted, but it has many advocates. The final answer should be provided by the current collaborative trials in the United Kingdom and the United States. Most obstetricians use betamethasone or dexamethasone, but a similar effect can be achieved by a single intramuscular injection of 100 mg hydrocortisone. When rapid effect is mandatory, intravenous administration of glucocorticoids may be preferable. The mechanism of action of the steroids is not fully understood, but they do increase the synthesis of surfactant lipids as shown in fetal lambs and rabbits. In the human, the L/S ratio and the foam stability in amniotic fluid samples reflect the surfactant activity; the L/S ratio is increased after glucocorticoid treatment.

Suggested Reading

1. Brown, E.R., Torday, J.S., and Taeusch, H.W., Jr. Pharmacologic control of fetal lung development clinics. *Perinatology 5:*242, 1978.
2. Caritis, S.N., Edelstone, D.I., and Mueller-Heubach, E. Pharmacologic inhibition of preterm labor. *Am. J. Obstet. Gynecol. 133:*557, 1979.
3. Creasy, R.K. Preterm parturition. *Semin. Perinatol. 5:*191, 1981.
4. Fedrick, J., and Anderson, A.B.M. Factors associated with spontaneous pre-term birth. *Br. J. Obstet. Gynaecol. 83:*342, 1976.
5. Fuchs, F. Prevention of prematurity. *Am. J. Obstet. Gynecol. 126:*809, 1976.
6. Johnson, J.W.C. (ed.) Obstetric aspects of preterm delivery. *Clin. Obstet. Gynecol. 23:*15–179, 1980.
7. Liggins, G.C., and Howie, R.N. Controlled trial of antepartum glucocorticoid treatment for prevention of the respiratory distress syndrome in premature infants. *Pediatrics 50:*515, 1972.

CHAPTER 27

Postmaturity

RONALD M. CAPLAN, M.D.

If a pregnancy progresses to 42 weeks or beyond from the first day of the last menstrual period, it is regarded as postmature. This is an important clinical entity, as there are definite risks associated with the postmature state. As well, the postmature infant has recognizable features.

The placenta usually undergoes an "aging" process toward term (see Chapter 5: "Development and Endocrine Physiology of the Placenta"). Beyond term, the ongoing infarction and calcification of areas of the placenta impede the level of transfer of nutrients and oxygen to the fetus. This can result in unexpected fetal demise, especially if other factors or disease states exist that contribute to inadequate placental perfusion.

The postmature infant classically displays a loose, wrinkled skin with inadequate subcutaneous fat. It tends to be thin and pale in appearance. Desquamation is in evidence, especially on the soles of the feet, which otherwise show the characteristic creases of the full-term infant. Fingernails and toenails tend to be long. It is important to differentiate true postmaturity from a miscalculation in the estimated date of confinement. Such a miscalculation is still the most common reason for apparent discrepancies between the size of the developing fetus and the estimated age of gestation. An accurate history, as well as the early institution of antenatal care, can obviate many such errors. Ancillary tests, such as ultrasonography, can help to establish fetal age.

When true postmaturity is encountered, it is necessary to carefully follow the course of the pregnancy and the status of the fetus. Diminished fetal movement can be an ominous symptom. Frequent estriol determinations and nonstress tests can be utilized. Amnioscopy may be used to diagnose the presence of meconium. Ultrasonography can be used to detect a diminished volume of amniotic fluid, which suggests declining placental function. If fetal compromise is suggested, induction of labor with careful intrapartum monitoring should be undertaken.

Bibliography

1. Crowley, P. Non quantitative estimation of amniotic fluid volume in suspected prolonged pregnancy. *J. Perinatol. Med.* 8:249, 1980.
2. Hauth, J.C., Goodman, M.T., et al. Post term pregnancy. *Obstet. Gynecol.* 56:467, 1980.
3. Homburg, R., Ludomirski, A., and Insler, V. Detection of fetal risk in postmaturity. *Br. J. Obstet. Gynecol.* 86:759, 1979.

CHAPTER 28

Virus Infections of the Fetus

DONALD E. HENSON, M.D.

PHILIP GRIMLEY, M.D.

Viral infections during pregnancy can involve the fetus. Fetal involvement is most likely to occur at the time of primary virus infection in the mother during viremia, although there are some exceptions. The result can be fetal death, prematurity, congenital malformation, functional impairment such as deafness, or no apparent sequelae. Death can result from infection at any time during gestation, whereas congenital malformations from infection arise during the first 2 months during the formative stages. Fetal death usually occurs from overwhelming infection, although it can probably result from other causes, such as fever or toxins elaborated by infected cells in the mother or placenta. The most common infections that cause congenital infections are listed in Figure 28.1.

In infants who survive in utero infection, viruses cause a spectrum of disease manifestations rather than a single defined syndrome unique for each virus. This spectrum results from the many variables in the virus-host relationship. These include the time of infection in the gestational calendar, presence of maternal antibody, duration and severity of infection, virulence of the virus, and possible immune response in the fetus. Manifestations of in utero infections may be subclinical or delayed into postnatal life. If infection occurs near term, the infant may either be born with signs of infection or develop the disease in the neonatal period.

Viruses can invade the fetus during a clinical or subclinical infection in the mother. In most cases, however, the fetus is not infected and the gravida delivers a normal infant. On rare occasions the fetus does become infected and the expected outcome of pregnancy may be altered.

Rapidly growing fetal tissues are more susceptible to viruses than are adult tissues. This increased susceptibility is most evident during early embryogenesis and often persists after birth. As a consequence, viruses can produce disease and tissue damage in the fetus different from that produced in the adult.

Many different viruses can cause intrauterine fetal infections (Fig. 28.1). It is accepted that fetal infection occurs after virus invades the placenta during hematogenous dissemination. However, it is also suspected that in utero infections can result from an ascending infection in the cervix. Infection can also occur during delivery, as in the case of herpes simplex.

THE HERPESVIRUSES

There are two types of herpesviruses, I and II, which differ in antigenic structure. Type I usually infects the face and oral region, while type II infects the genital tract of women and the skin of the penis of males. Infection with both types is characterized by recurring vesicular eruptions, which are commonly called fever blisters or cold sores when they occur on the face. Type II, which is venereally transmitted, produces recurring cervicitis and vaginitis in the female. Recurrent genital infection

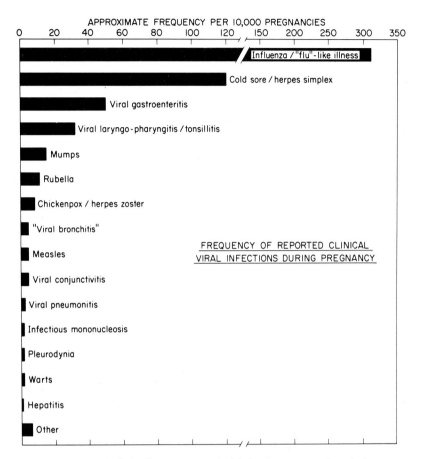

Figure 28.1. Frequency of clinically apparent viral infections occurring during pregnancy. (Reprinted with permission from Sever, J.L., and White, L.R.: Intrauterine viral infection. *Annu. Rev. Med. 19:*471, 1968.)

is the result of both reactivation of a latent infection and exposure to a new infectious source.

Neonatal infection with herpesvirus type II is not common. Infection is usually acquired during delivery when the mother has active herpetic cervicitis or vulvovaginitis. As the infant passes along the birth canal, it becomes infected from the traumatized herpetic lesions. During the active stages, these lesions are highly infectious and virus can readily be recovered from the vesicular fluid.

Neonatal infection usually becomes evident after the fourth but usually before the 21st day. Signs and symptoms include fever (or, in some cases, subnormal temperature), respiratory distress, cyanosis, tachycardia, jaundice, skin eruptions, vomiting and diarrhea. There also may be petechial hemorrhages, thrombocytopenia and gastrointestinal bleeding.

The clinical course is progressive and often fatal, although recovery has been reported. Diagnosis may be difficult if skin lesions do not appear and if genital herpes is not suspected in the mother.

Autopsy studies typically show areas of focal necrosis in the liver and adrenals, although any organ can be involved. Histologically, intranuclear viral inclusions are found around necrotic areas.

As a preventive measure, it is important to exclude active genital infection at term, especially in a woman with recurring herpes cervicitis or vulvovaginitis. In the presence of overt infection, a prophylatic cesarean section should be performed before rupture of the membranes and the infant should be isolated immediately. There is no treatment for neonatal herpes infection. Genital infections are more common in lower socioeconomic groups. Women with a history of genital herpes infection should be carefully followed during pregnancy.

CYTOMEGALOVIRUS (CMV)

CMV is the most important virus causing in utero infection, accounting for about 1 to 2% of all infant deaths. CMV is probably the most common cause of brain damage in infancy. Approximately 10% of microcephalic mentally retarded children show serologic evidence of CMV infection. There are two sources for fetal infection—primary infection in the mother or reactivation of a latent infection. Most of the maternal infections are not clinically apparent. In some cases, mothers who give birth to infected infants reported nonspecific upper respiratory tract infections during pregnancy or mild febrile illnesses that may resemble infectious mononucleosis. Fetal infection can result from reactivation of a latent infection in the mother, and virus can be transmitted to the fetus years after the initial infection even in the presence of maternal antibody.

In utero infection can lead to abortion, prematurity, permanent disability in those who survive or mild disease. Classically, infants born with cytomegalic inclusion disease are premature or of low birth weight for gestational age. They may show microcephaly or hydrocephaly, chorioretinitis, blindness, hepatosplenomegaly, jaundice and petechiae which are often present at birth. Roentgenograms of the skull may show paraventricular cerebral calcification. The clinical signs usually appear sooner and are more severe in infants under 2500 gm. Premature infants symptomatic at birth have the worst mortality and morbidity rates. Infants who survive may be left with neurologic sequelae that include blindness, mental retardation and

diplegia. Less severe effects include hearing deficits and subnormal intelligence. It seems that congenital infection must occur before 4 months' gestation to cause significant fetal damage.

Many infants are infected but show no evidence of disease. The incidence of CMV infection during pregnancy is more common than was originally suspected. About 6% of women develop significant levels of CMV complement-fixing antibody during pregnancy and 5% develop cytomegaloviruria.

Women can shed virus from one or more sites, including the pharynx, genital tract, urinary tract and breasts. Infants can become infected if exposed in the postpartum period. However, these infants have no sequelae. At present, there is no vaccine for CMV.

RUBELLA

Fetal infection with rubella is probably less frequent than with cytomegalovirus, but the associated developmental malformations are the most dramatic, with cataracts and heart defects in addition to microcephaly. Historically, the association of these organ malformations with maternal rubella stimulated modern interest in the teratogenic potential of virus infections. It is now well recognized that rubella-associated disease encompasses a broader spectrum of congenital manifestations than those which are grossly obvious. This spectrum includes abortion, stillbirth, prematurity or decreased birth weight, and growth retardation. Effects of rubella are most severe when the mother is infected during the first trimester, but rubella infection transmitted in late stages of pregnancy may produce chronic infection with delayed effects such as cryptorchidism, sterility and deficiencies of cell-mediated immunity.

In adults, rubella produces relatively mild coryza, fever and dermatitis and is spread from respiratory secretions by fomites. Patients are contagious during the exanthematous phase and virus may be shed from the oropharynx from 10 days before to 15 days after onset. Transplacental viremic spread to the fetus has been estimated to occur in 14–50% of infected mothers. The infant is most susceptible during the first trimester of pregnancy when the classical teratogenic effects are produced.

This susceptibility may be related to enhanced virus cytotropism for fetal cells or a predilection for rapidly growing tissues. Acute effects of rubella infection in the fetus include extensive dermatitis, necrotizing encephalitis and giant cell alveolitis. Clinical manifestations in the newborn include pneumonitis, diarrhea, failure to thrive and platelet deficiencies. More subtle effects are produced by rubella infection in the later stages of gestation and by chronic infection persisting into the newborn period. For example, fetal infection during the fourth month carries a 10% risk for a single congenital defect. Postpartum lactational transmission also has been reported. The long-term consequences of infection include visual problems secondary to cataracts, psychomotor retardation secondary to encephalitis, hearing impairments secondary to acoustic infections and related deficiencies in the development of communications skills or language. Diabetes mellitus is a less common delayed sequela.

Diagnosis of rubella infection depends upon detection of neutralizing antibodies which inhibit hemagglutination. Seroconversion during pregnancy augments fetal infection in up to 50% of cases, and prophylactic abortion can then be considered. Since up to two thirds of maternal infections may be asymptomatic, mandatory screening programs have been instituted in some jurisdictions. Current public health emphasis is appropriately directed toward immunoprophylaxis by exposing nonpregnant women to an attenuated live virus vaccine capable of conferring long-term immunity. Immunized individuals do not transmit rubella infection. Reinfection may occur, but virus usually remains confined to the respiratory tract. Viremia is rare, so that fetal infection in an immunized mother reexposed to rubella is extremely infrequent. Conception must be delayed for at least 3 months after vaccination, since the fetus is susceptible to live attenuated vaccine strains.

HEPATITIS VIRUS

Viral hepatitis can be caused by a number of agents including members of the herpes virus family (Epstein-Barr virus, cytomegalovirus), yellow fever virus in the togavirus group, and hepatitis A virus which is closely related to the enteroviruses such as poliovirus. In infants, hepatitis produced by members of the herpes family is generally associated with disseminated infection and is usually discovered postmortem. The hepatitis A virus infection is typically self-limited and there is no evidence for a chronic or carrier state. The most common manner of transmission is through person-to-person contact, almost always by the fecal-oral route. Contamination of food or drinking water is a common element in transmission, and high rates of hepatitis A infection are seen in economically developing countries. Antibody appears at early ages and most infections appear to be subclinical and anicteric.

Fetal or neonatal infections with hepatitis B virus are of the greatest concern due to the higher incidence of icteric disease, with the potential for chronic hepatitis or even cirrhosis. In low socioeconomic populations of the economically developing nations, vertical transmission of hepatitis B is common and probably represents a major avenue for perpetuation of this disease as compared with the more common iatrogenic or venereal transmission in developed nations such as the United States. In the Maoris of New Zealand, for example, two thirds of all cases of hepatitis B occur in children less than 15 years of age. In northern European populations, the ratio is reversed.

The hepatitis B virus is comprised of two major elements: an infectious core with the viral DNA genes measuring 28 nm in diameter, known as the Dane particle, and a surrounding surface coat of proteins which also may be found independently of the core and represent the hepatitis B surface antigen commonly detected in serum by immunoassays (HBsAg). The core material may polymerize into rodlike structures which can be very numerous in the serum of patients with active hepatitis B infection and are resolved by electron microscopy. The Dane particle is the infectious agent and corresponds to the core antigens detected by immunoassay (HBcAg). An e antigen is also associated with the core.

Vertical transmission of infectious Dane particles can occur at three stages: 1) prenatally through the placenta, 2) perinatally during passage of the infant through the birth canal, and 3) postnatally during close maternal contact with the newborn or infant. Perinatal transmission during childbirth may be due to contact of the newborn with maternal blood or abraded surfaces. Only serum and saliva have actually been determined to contain infectious hepatitis B virus in experimental transmission studies; however, hepatitis B surface antigen has also been found in feces, urine and breast milk. Clearly, saliva itself could provide an important route of transmission from mother to newborn. Assays of cord blood for hepatitis B virus in infants born to mothers with documented infection have shown that the transplacental route accounts for a relatively small proportion of the total cases (less than 10%).

Mothers who are asymptomatic carriers of hepatitis B may infect their infants on successive occasions. Prevention of neonatal infection can be difficult since many mothers are asymptomatic. Maternal screening for hepatitis B virus by radioimmunoassay is necessary. Passive immunization of the newborn with hyperimmune hepatitis B immunoglobulin can be effective in reducing infant morbidity and mortality. In any case, more than 80% of infected infants will survive 1 year. Although most newborns recover, hepatitis B may be fulminant and fatal. This is often accompanied by syncytial giant cell transformation of hepatocytes histologically.

The late sequelae of hepatitis B infection include chronic persistent hepatitis and even cirrhosis which may predispose to development of hepatocellular carcinoma.

Since transmission of hepatitis B from mother to infant is often delayed and the incubation period is generally long (6–8 weeks), infants of women found to develop hepatitis B during the last trimester of pregnancy or during the first 2 months postpartum must be tested regularly for up to 6 months of age to exclude development of infection. Clinically, it is important to distinguish viral hepatitis from congenital bile duct atresia. Unnecessary surgery in a child with hepatitis B merely serves to increase the risk of fatality. In view of the magnitude of the hepatitis B problem, it is fortunate that increased rates of abortion, stillbirth and developmental abnormalities have not been reported.

As iatrogenic and neonatal transmission of hepatitis B virus infection come under greater scrutiny and control in the industrialized nations, recognition of other causes of viral hepatitis increases. Most posttransfusion hepatitis in the United States is now attributed to non-A, non-B hepatitis, the etiologic agent or agents of which have not yet been characterized. Whether fecal-oral transmission which is common for hepatitis A or venereal and neonatal transmission which are common for hepatitis B are also important for any of the non-A, non-B agents remains to be determined.

DIAGNOSIS

The diagnosis of congenital viral infections is important for epidemic considerations, for family counseling, and for the differentiation of viral-induced malformations from idiopathic and familial malformations. Diagnosis can be made by viral isolation, measurement of fetal IgM production which is elevated during infectious processes, and histology. The specific agent can often be identified from the elevated IgM through special tests.

Bibliography

1. Monif, G.R.G. *Viral Infections of the Human Fetus.* Macmillan Corp., New York, 1969.
2. Henson, D., and Sever, J.L. Congenital virus infections. In *Advances in Obstetrics and Gynecology,* edited by Caplan, R.M., and Sweeney, W.J. Williams & Wilkins, Baltimore, 1978, pp. 135–147.
3. Krech, U.H., Jung, M., and Jung, F. *Cytomegalovirus Infections of Man.* S. Karger, Basel, 1971.
4. Mims, C.A. Pathogenesis of viral infections of the fetus. *Prog. Med. Virol. 10:*194, 1968.
5. Overall, J.C., Jr., and Glasgow, L.A. Virus infections of the fetus and newborn infant. *J. Pediatr. 77:*315, 1970.

CHAPTER 29

Pathophysiology of Placental Development

ELMER E. KRAMER, M.D.
M. YUSOFF DAWOOD, M.D.

PATHOLOGY OF THE PLACENTA

Abortion

About 15–20% of pregnant patients abort. Abortion is the termination of pregnancy before the 20th–24th week. The upper limit of the duration of pregnancy applied to abortion varies from source to source. In general, abortions may be divided into *early*, before 10 weeks' gestation, and *late*, 10–20 weeks' gestation. Generally, in early abortion the abortus is rarely normal, that is, there is a germplasm defect and/or some deficiency in implantation. In the late abortion (10–20 weeks), the abortus is generally normal and usually the factors that control the maintenance of pregnancy are incriminated. These are usually maternal rather than fetal factors.

Abortion may be classified into *spontaneous* and *induced* abortions (Fig. 29.1). The spontaneous abortions are further divided into *threatened*, *incomplete* and *complete* and then subdivided in the incomplete category into *septic* and *missed* abortions.

Threatened abortion is one in which there are infrequent uterine cramps and slight spotting; then the bleeding subsides and the patient continues with the pregnancy. *Incomplete abortion* has occurred when part of the products of conception have passed out and a portion of the placenta is retained, thus requiring completion by curettage. *Induced abortions* are generally of the elective type or therapeutic type.

Abnormalities in Placental Implantation

BLIGHTED OVUM

Normally, the embryonic pole goes in first so that it can obtain an attachment to the placental site. Occasionally there is malimplantation and it is very likely that a *blighted ovum* or a stunted embryo would result. The pregnancy would develop, there would be fluid in the gestational sac and subsequently, at 8–12 weeks, the membranes would rupture and the pregnancy would be terminated. At completion, there would be no fetus identifiable or detectable. A blighted ovum occurs in about 5% of pregnancies, so that approximately one third of spontaneous abortions are blighted ova or stunted embryos.

PLACENTA ACCRETA, INCRETA AND PERCRETA

If Nitabuch's layer does not develop completely, the villi grow down into the deeper layers of the endometrium and finally to the myometrium. This is known as the *placenta accreta*. If the villi grow into the uterine muscle, it is called *placenta increta* (Fig. 29.2). If the villi grow through the uterine muscle to the serosa, then it is known as *placenta percreta*.

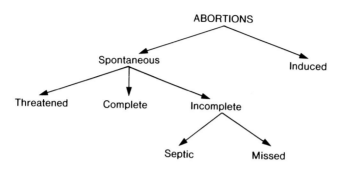

Figure 29.1. Classification of abortions.

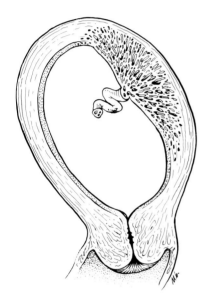

Placenta increta

Figure 29.2. Placenta increta.

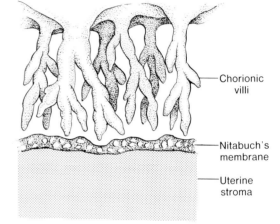

Figure 29.3. Nitabuch's membrane.

These abnormalities may occur only partially if Nitabuch's layer does not develop completely (Fig. 29.3).

PLACENTA MEMBRANACEA

The villi occupying the decidua capsularis site normally undergo degeneration and atrophy. However, if this is a deep implantation, the villi can persist and at 4–4.5 months they may start to grow again. The decidua capsularis meets the decidua vera so that placental tissue is present 360° around the pregnancy. This situation is called a *placenta membranacea* which completely surrounds the pregnancy (Fig. 29.4).

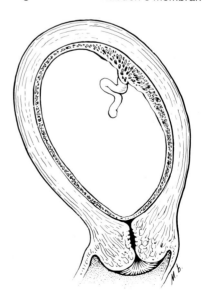

Placenta membranacea

Figure 29.4. Placenta membranacea.

VELAMENTOUS INSERTION OF THE CORD

The pregnancy is not displaced completely in its implantation site as shown in Figure 29.5A, but the embryonic pole is near the placental site and the vessels can pass through the membranes, giving rise to a *velamentous* insertion of the cord. This is seen in about 1% of single pregnancies, about 7% of twin pregnancies and 50% of triplet pregnancies.

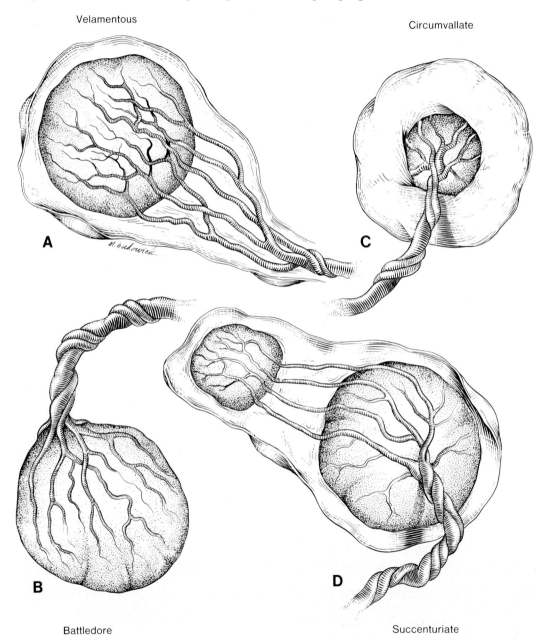

Figure 29.5. *A.* Velamentous insertion of the cord. *B.* Battledore placenta. *C.* Circumvallate placenta. *D.* Succenturiate lobe of the placenta.

Hence, several problems may develop early in pregnancy which are not faced until late in pregnancy. These are the placenta accreta, increta, percreta, membranacea and velamentous insertion of the cord. Their presence and complications are not manifested until after the infant is born and immediately during the third stage of labor.

Abnormalities in Size and Shape of Placenta

BATTLEDORE AND CIRCUMVALLATE PLACENTA

The placenta can be of any size and shape—oval, round, square, rectangular, figure of 8—and occasionally the cord is attached to the periphery of the placenta—*battledore placenta* (Fig. 29.5B). Occasionally, the *circumvallate placenta* develops, in which the membranes double up to form a whitish ring (Fig. 29.5C). The etiology of this condition is unknown. Some feel that it is due to decidual necrosis.

SUCCENTURIATE LOBES

Accessory or succenturiate lobes of the placenta are occasionally present (Fig. 29.5D). This is one of the reasons the placenta should be examined on both sides immediately after delivery. In examining the membranes the vessels are checked for; if they are torn, then it indicates the likely presence of an accessory lobe which may be retained in utero, and exploration of the uterus becomes necessary. The development of an accessory lobe is thought to be due to either a lack of decidual receptivity or a lack of trophoblastic aggressivity, so that placental tissue or villi did not form in the space between the main portion of the placenta and the accessory lobe. That is, a patchy development of the placenta occurs.

BIPARTITE PLACENTA

Occasionally, the placenta will be in two equal parts so that we refer to it as a *bipartite placenta*, in three equal parts it is called *tripartite placenta* and so forth. These are situations which are not uncommon but are mainly of academic interest.

SENILE CHANGES OF THE PLACENTA

The placenta has a life span of 9 months but it does not wait until that time to undergo senile changes. In certain complications such as toxemia of pregnancy and reduced blood flow through the placenta, senile changes of the placenta may start to take place as early as 6 months. There is hyalinization and calcification to some degree in most placentas. The placenta has a tremendous reserve and if the complication does not reduce placental function by about 30% or more, the pregnancy continues normally. If the placental function is reduced by 30% or more, then the fetus may succumb in utero, so that this is of some concern when the patient goes overdue. Before stating that the patient is overdue, it is necessary that the date of her last menstrual period and the expected date of confinement should be accurate. According to Naegle's rule, 2 weeks are allowed one way or the other before a patient is considered early or overdue. Once she is 2 weeks past the expected date of confinement, then there is concern about postmaturity and senile changes that may occur in the placenta.

Changes in Position of Implantation

PLACENTA PREVIA

The placenta is partially or totally implanted on the lower uterine segment. This occurs in about 1–1.5% of pregnancies. The placenta can be totally across the internal os, *total or complete placenta previa* (Fig. 29.6), or it can be off to the side, *incomplete placenta previa*. This can also be called a partial or a marginal placenta previa. The etiology of placenta previa is felt to be multiparity. It is believed that after several pregnancies, the endometrium has been damaged for a subsequent implantation and if the placenta site is studied, endarteritis and scarring are seen. Hence over the years, another site is chosen and finally the placenta comes to lie low in the uterus, giving rise to a placenta previa. This is one of the causes of third trimester bleeding and is painless. (See Chapter 30: "Third Trimester Bleeding.")

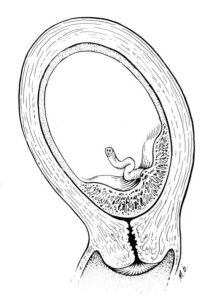

Placenta previa

Figure 29.6.   Complete placenta previa.

ECTOPIC PREGNANCY

A pregnancy that implants in a site other than the uterine cavity is an ectopic pregnancy. It can be in the tube, the cervix, the ovary or in the abdominal cavity (Fig. 29.7). Ninety-five percent are in the tube, often the ampullary portion. Commonly, the condition may be due to previous salpingitis, leading to defective timing in the transport of the fertilized egg, so that at the time of implantation the egg is still in the tube.

The patient in the first trimester may complain of vaginal spotting or frank bleeding and low abdominal pain on the side corresponding to the ectopic gestation.

Examination may reveal blood in the vagina. The uterus may be smaller than expected for the length of gestation. A fusiform small tender mass may be palpable in the affected adnexal region.

Radioreceptor assay or radioimmunoas-

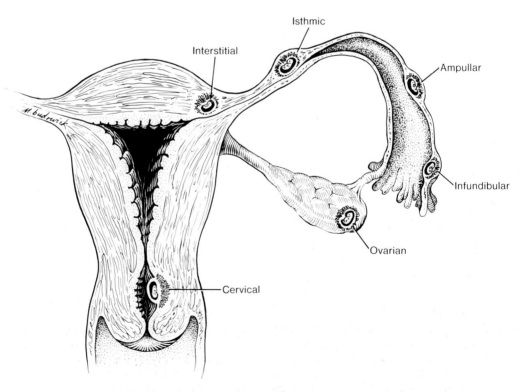

Figure 29.7.   Some possible sites for ectopic pregnancy.

say for hCG may yield a level lower than expected for the age of gestation. Ultrasonographic findings are helpful. (See Chapter 15: "Ultrasonography.") Diagnosis may be confirmed by laparoscopic examination of the pelvic organs.

If allowed to persist, the growing pregnancy will eventually rupture the tube, leading to intraperitoneal hemorrhage and shock. Culdocentesis will then reveal the presence of intraperitoneal blood.

The treatment is surgical. If an early unruptured tubal pregnancy is discovered, it is often possible to open the tube, remove the pregnancy, and close the tube microsurgically. Once rupture has occurred, it is usually necessary to remove the affected portion of the tube.

DISORDERS OF THE AMNION

Hydramnios

The amnion is a single layer of cells that surrounds the amniotic cavity which contains the amniotic fluid. The fluid is normally about 1000 ml at term. If the volume of fluid is more than 2000 ml, then it is called *hydramnios*. The causes of hydramnios include:

1. *Maternal reasons*
   a. Twins
   b. Diabetes mellitus
   c. Rh isoimmunization
2. *Fetal reasons*
   a. Anencephaly
   b. Spina bifida
   c. Esophageal atresia

Fifty percent of polyhydramnios cases are due to these causes, but the other 50% have no known cause and are idiopathic. The patient complains that she feels bigger than she should be and that she has edema of the extremities and shortness of breath, particularly after exertion. Examination will reveal that the uterine fundus is relatively high for the duration of gestation. There is a feeling of a great deal of fluid between the fetus and the palpating hands of the examiner, and the sound of the fetal heart may seem distant and be difficult to hear.

It is not known how the amniotic fluid enters the amniotic cavity but it is completely exchanged every 3 hours; therefore if there is a slight shift in this mechanism and an extra 10 ml is put in while 10 ml less is put out every 3 hours, then there will be an increase in amniotic fluid within a few days.

Twins

All twin placentas should be checked in an effort to ascertain if it is a single or a double ovum twin pregnancy. *Single ovum* or *identical* twins occur in 33% of twin pregnancies. *Double ovum* or *fraternal* twins occur in 66% of twin pregnancies. The double ovum is the inherited type, whereas the single ovum is due to chance splitting of the ovum. In the double ovum, there are two placentas and there are 4 layers of amniotic membranes, i.e., *dichorionic-diamniotic placentas* (Fig. 29.8). In the single ovum twin, there is usually one placenta and a *monochorionic-diamniotic sac*, i.e., there are 2 layers of amniotic membranes (Fig. 29.9). If there is late division or splitting in the single ovum twin then there are no intervening membranes

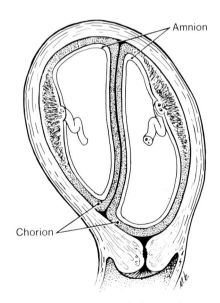

Dichorion-diamniotic membrane

Figure 29.8. Dichorionic-diamniotic placenta.

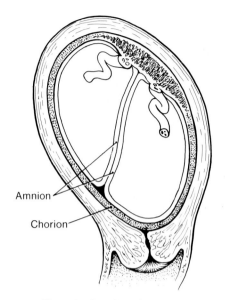

Monochorion-diamniotic membrane

Figure 29.9.   Monochorionic-diamniotic sac.

between the twins, giving rise to a *mono-chorionic-monoamniotic placenta*. Fortunately, this is the rarest type of single ovum twin pregnancy; they have the most serious complications, which include cord complications with intrauterine death of one of the fetuses, collision of twins when both fetuses attempt to engage, and locking of the twins.

Occasionally the chance splitting of the ovum occurs so early that each twin develops its own membranes and amniotic cavity so that it is similar to the double ovum twins. This occurs in 10%, so that 10% of the dichorionic-diamniotic placentas are due to single ovum twins. The only positive way of telling whether they are single ovum or double ovum twins is to wait until the twins are about 8–10 years of age and then check them out for weight, height, appearance, physical characteristics, the various blood groups and blood factors, fingerprinting (which will show identical number of whorls), loops and triradii and finally skin grafts which will take if the twins are identical. The need for determining the type of twins is 1) the possible need for transplant, single ovum twins will accept grafts from the other

twin, and 2) single ovum twins may have the same diseases; identical twins who are female are known to have developed the same type of cancer in the same quadrant of the same breast; identical twins have both had the same type of leukemia.

Single ovum twins frequently have minor vascular connections in the placenta. If the connections are significant a transfusion syndrome occurs in which the donor becomes anemic whereas the recipient becomes hypertensive and usually develops hydramnios. Recognition of this situation may be lifesaving.

Infections

Some patients may have premature rupture of the membranes before the onset of labor. Some of them may develop *intrauterine infection*. With slight contractions, the organism ascends via the membranes from the opening below to the placental site and an amnionitis develops which is then followed by chorioamnionitis. (See chapter on "Preterm Labor.") The distance from the amnion to one of the chorionic vessels is a fraction of a millimeter. This is how the infant develops septicemia.

DISORDERS OF THE CHORION

Thrombosis: (Also known as Infarcts)

TWO MAJOR TYPES

Obstruction of maternal blood flow through the placenta (maternal thrombosis) involving the spiral artery occurs in toxemia and other hypertensive complications. Obstruction of fetal blood flow through the placenta involving the chorionic artery is known as fetal thrombosis. The etiology is unknown. Both are of academic importance unless one third or more of the placental mass is involved. This eventually leads to fetal hypoxia and even fetal death.

Maternal thromboses are usually triangular or wedge shaped, with the apex toward the basal plate. In the early stage they are dark red, but after organization and scarring they are firm and whitish. In the beginning the villous capillaries are congested but eventually necrobiosis leads to the formation of "shadow" or "ghost" villi. Thrombosis of a fetal artery produces a wedged shaped area with the apex toward the chorionic plate. The area is pale and the villous vessels are obliterated. Eventually, after organization the area looks similar to an organized maternal thrombosis.

Trophoblastic Disease

HYDATIDIFORM MOLE

This is a disease of the chorion. Hydatidiform mole is a hydropic degeneration of the placenta. In 94% of cases there is no fetus present. Hence, some believe that the fetus is absent from the beginning. The circulation never becomes established in the villi; they become hydropic and appear as a bunch of grapelike vesicles. Often the diagnosis is made by the patient when she spontaneously passes grapelike vesicles via the vagina. In other instances, the patient may present with a history of threatened abortion and a uterus that feels doughy to palpation and usually larger than it should be for the period of amenorrhea. Several ancillary tests or aids may help in the diagnosis of the disorder and include: 1) sonography, which reveals a "snow-storm" appearance with absence of a fetus and the gestational sac, and 2) amniography, in which a radiopaque dye is injected into the uterine cavity and x-rays are taken which reveal a honeycomb or soap-bubble appearance.

In syncytial endometritis and myometritis, the cells are single and infiltrate between the muscle bundles and do not cause any hemorrhage or destruction of tissue. By contrast, choriocarcinoma being a tumor will invade the blood vessels and cause hemorrhage around it.

Once the vesicles are passed out, the clinician can make the diagnosis by microscopic examination, which will show large hydropic villi with marked trophoblastic proliferation which are the histologic hallmark of hydatidiform mole. From the trophoblastic proliferation, an assessment of whether it is a suspicious or malignant mole is attempted. The diagnosis of a malignant or invasive mole is, however, not possible unless the uterus is also available for examination or unless the patient has metastases to the lungs on chest x-ray. Hydatidiform mole occurs in about 1 in 2000 pregnancies in Western countries but is as frequent as 1 in 75 in some Far Eastern countries.

CHORIOCARCINOMA

Choriocarcinoma occurs infrequently. There is an antecedent hydatidiform mole pregnancy in 50% of the patients, an abortion precedes in 25% of the patients and in 25% of them the preceding pregnancy was normal. About 5–15% of hydatidiform moles develop malignant sequelae or choriocarcinoma depending on the region of the world, with the higher rate occurring in Far Eastern countries. Since 50% of the choriocarcinomas seen in Western countries arise from hydatidiform moles and 70–80% of choriocarcinomas in Far Eastern countries arise from hydatidiform moles, it is extremely important that patients with hydatidiform molar pregnancies be followed closely so as to detect choriocarcinoma early and thus obtain good response with chemotherapy. More than 2 decades ago, choriocarcinoma was a dreaded disease with a high mortality rate but it is the first gynecological malignancy to have been successfully treated with chemotherapy and now gives the best remission and survival rates with chemotherapy for any type of gynecological malignancy. It is therefore important to recognize and diagnose choriocarcinoma early so that chemotherapy can be started before hepatic and cerebral metastases occur.

The most frequent primary site of choriocarcinoma is the uterus. The tumor is very vascular and there are hemorrhagic areas in it. Metastatic spread is blood borne. Secondaries occur in the lung, the brain and the vagina in that order of frequency. Other sites of metastases include the liver, intestines, pancreas, fallopian tubes, ovaries and almost any part of the body. In choriocarcinoma, there is a solid sheet of anaplastic cells. This should be carefully distinguished from the syncytial endometritis and myometritis which is seen under every placental site. Syncytial endometritis is due to invasion of the endometrium by the normal trophoblasts.

THE DECIDUA

Premature Separation of Placenta

This occurs usually in toxemic and hypertensive patients in the third trimester. A small hemorrhage begins in the decidua and gradually pushes off the placenta, and the patient experiences pain. There are two types of premature separation of the placenta, namely, the type in which the margin of the placenta is pushed off and there is visible bleeding; this is sometimes referred to as the *revealed* type, and the type in which the bleeding occurs behind the placenta and pushes it off in an umbrella-like fashion, this is sometimes referred to as the *concealed* type. This type constitutes 10% of the cases of premature separation of the placenta. It is usually a serious situation and occurs most frequently in a multiparous patient. The patient is usually not alerted to it since she thinks that her labor is beginning. When the uterus becomes rigid and the fetal heart is lost, the diagnosis is obvious. Apart from hemorrhage, hypofibrinogenemia and disseminated intravascular coagulation are major complications and therefore serum fibrinogen should be determined whenever premature separation of the placenta is diagnosed. (See Chapter 30: "Third Trimester Bleeding.")

COMPLICATIONS OF THE CORD

Two Vessel Cord

Besides the false and true knots, the most unusual finding is the two vessel cord which occurs in 1% of pregnancies. There are two vessels instead of the usual three.

If a two vessel cord is found, the pediatrician should be alerted and generally will do a full workup of the baby, including a chest x-ray and an intravenous pyelogram to determine if there are any abnormalities.

Spiral Cord

The etiology of this condition is unclear; perhaps the infant was very active in utero.

DISEASES OF THE PLACENTA

Rh Isoimmunization

The normal placenta at term is one fifth to one sixth the fetal weight. With a markedly hydropic infant the placenta can weigh as much as one half of the fetal weight. On the maternal side, the placenta is dirty gray instead of beefy red as in the normal term placenta. It is friable and cotyledons may therefore be missing since they remain adherent to the uterus. This is one of the reasons the maternal side of the placenta is checked for missing cotyledons.

Syphilitic Placenta

The placenta is similar to the Rh isoimmunized placenta. It is markedly enlarged and is dirty gray on the maternal side. Because of the law requiring blood screening for syphilis and because the blood group and Rh type are routinely performed in the antepartum clinic, these disorders are discovered early in pregnancy and effective treatment is given.

Suggested Reading

1. Novak, E.R., and Woodruff, J.D. (eds.) *Novak's Gynecologic and Obstetric Pathology with Clinical and Endocrine Relations*, ed. 8. Saunders, Philadelphia, 1978.
2. Gruenwald, P. (ed.) *The Placenta and Its Maternal Supply Line.* University Park Press, Baltimore, 1975.

CHAPTER **30**

Third Trimester Bleeding

FREDERICK SILVERMAN, M.D.

Third trimester antepartum bleeding (TTAB) complicates pregnancies 3% of the time. The majority of episodes are mild, and properly managed do not jeopardize either mother or child. However, occasionally severe antepartum bleeding may lead to fetal intrauterine death and maternal exsanguination, with all the possible sequelae such as disseminated intravascular coagulation, renal shutdown, hysterectomy, or, rarely, death.

CAUSES

The major causes by virtue of frequency of occurrence or severity of the mishap are:

1. Premature separation of the normally implanted placenta
2. Placenta previa
3. Antepartum rupture of the uterus

The most likely source of pathologic bleeding in late pregnancy is the site of placental attachment. Antepartum rupture of the uterus usually occurs at the site of an old operative scar in the corpus (1–2% of the time), in cases of prior hysterotomy, extensive myomectomy, classical cesarean section or uterine unification operations. Spontaneous rupture of the intact gravid uterus is quite rare, as is trauma, as an etiologic factor. Rupture through a lower uterine segment cesarean section scar, most of which are transverse in location, is most likely to occur in labor (0.1–0.2%).

The clinical picture with antepartum rupture of the uterus frequently is quite dramatic, with pain, hemorrhagic shock and absent fetal heart tones. Diagnosis hinges on clinical and ultrasonographic evaluation. The fetus may be outside the ruptured contracted uterus in the abdominal cavity, and severe intraabdominal hemorrhage may occur. Laparotomy with repair of the uterus or hysterectomy along with appropriate replacement of blood and fluids comprises therapy. "Silent rupture" of the old low segment cesarean scar discovered postpartum in the patient delivered subsequently from below warrants laparotomy for repair.

Frequent, but much less important, causes of late antepartum bleeding include the "bloody show" of impending labor, vaginitis, postcoital bleeding and cervical polyps traumatized by digital examination.

Rare causes include prolapse of the cervix out of the introitus, invasive carcinoma of the cervix, and vasa previa, the latter secondary to a defect of the umbilical cord wherein a fetal vein is torn and fetal blood appears at the introitus.

MAJOR ENTITIES

Premature separation of the normally implanted placenta (PSP) is twice as common in incidence as is placenta previa, in which part or all of the placenta is in the lower uterine segment (LUS). Premature separation of the placenta occurs in 1:50 to 1:155 third trimester pregnancies. Most episodes of premature separation of the placenta do not lead to serious or fatal compromise of fetus or mother. Indeed, those cases of minor late pregnancy antepartum bleeding in which no apparent cause can be assigned are probably due to separation of the placental edge with slight tears. About 10–30% of PSP can be classified as severe, that is, more than half of the placenta has separated and the fetus is dead, with the mother in danger of exsanguination. Severe PSP is also known as *abruptio placentae*, although some authorities may extend the use of this term to all degrees of PSP. The incidence of severe PSP appears to be decreasing as women of high parity become rarer. Severe PSP correlates with maternal chronic hypertensive vascular disease but not with hypertension peculiar to the latter part of pregnancy, that is, toxemia of pregnancy. The exact cause of PSP is unknown in most instances. Trauma or nutritional deficiencies do not play an etiologic role. Sudden uterine decompression as with the loss of fluid in large amounts with polyhydramnios, or as in the case of twin gestation, after delivery of the first baby with sudden uterine contraction, separation of the placenta and resultant compromise of the fetus left in situ, occurs uncommonly. PSP may recur in subsequent pregnancies at a far higher rate (1:12) than if there were no prior history with a previous pregnancy.

Usually there is a good correlation (80%) between the amount of blood seen escaping per vaginam and the degree of hemorrhage occurring in the uterus. Occasionally, however, much of the blood entering the uterine cavity as a result of PSP is retained in the uterus, either concealed behind the placenta or in the amniotic sac. The latter event is often associated with the more severe degrees of PSP: the patient in hypovolemic borderline or frank shock, the fetus severely compromised or dead.

The pathophysiology involves the appearance of a blood clot in the decidual base, separating a variable amount of placenta from its base. As the hematoma enlarges, it separates a larger area of placenta and (unless grossly concealed) makes its way down between the inner uterine wall and the membranes, out the cervix and vagina and is visible externally.

The clinical manifestations of severe PSP are striking. The patient is brought to the labor and delivery floor in hypovolemic, hemorrhagic shock. The uterus exhibits an almost boardlike rigidity, in "tetanic contraction", wherein periods of relaxation are virtually impossible to detect. The fetal heart is almost always absent to the electronic monitor. Notable uterine tenderness and pain are evident, especially if an anterior wall placental attachment is present. If the placenta is primarily posterior the most severe pain may be in the lower back. Generally, labor is present or rapidly ensues, with emptying of the uterus occurring with dispatch, yielding a freshly stillborn fetus, the placenta separated, and almost immediately expelled in short order. In a minority of cases of severe PSP (25%), hemorrhage is of such proportion that coagulation abnormalities appear, as evidenced by gross failure of good clotting phenomena and by abnormalities in qualitative assays such as the "quick fibrinogen test" or rapid quantitative tests for fibrin degradation products. Whole blood transfusion, proper fluid and electrolyte replacement, careful monitoring of the input via CVP line or Swan-Ganz catheter and of output via indwelling urinary bladder catheter, as well as appropriate hematologic consultation and therapy almost always prevent the feared complications of renal failure, Sheehan's syndrome (partial pituitary failure) and death.

Severe PSP may be accompanied by blood making its way into the uterine wall and appearing under the serosa to give the uterus a mottled blue color due to the poor oxygen content of the blood. This is known as the Couvelaire uterus. Blood flow to the placental site is 500–800 cc/min. Laparotomy is done in those instances in which cesarean section is utilized to save a compromised but live fetus when delivery is not imminent, for maternal indications although the fetus may be dead intrapartum, with uterine atony unresponsive to other forms of therapy such as oxytocics and massage or packing, or where bleeding continues although the uterus is empty and no apparent clotting abnormalities are evident. Hypogastric artery ligation may obviate the need for hysterectomy.

Fortunately, most cases of PSP are mild to moderate in severity. Bleeding usually ceases with the fetus stable as noted by the electronic monitor, and the hematocrit, clotting tests and vital signs remaining within normal levels. Aseptic vaginal examination in the operating room ("double set-up examination"), with the option of doing an immediate cesarean section if so indicated by the presence of palpable placenta in the lower uterine segment, can be carried out. If placenta previa is not found, labor can often be instituted by rupturing the membranes. Progress is generally rapid to vaginal delivery. Cesarean section is rarely the mode of delivery in PSP, in contrast to those pregnancies complicated by one degree or another of placental previa where cesarean section is almost always the technique of delivery.

Ultrasonic localization of the placental site as well as continuous fetal electronic monitoring have facilitated accurate diagnosis and intelligent management. Perinatal mortality, however, may range as high as 50% if the series is heavily weighted by cases of severe PSP.

PLACENTA PREVIA

Placenta previa exists when part or all of the placenta is in the lower uterine segment, close to, partly covering, or completely covering the internal uterine os. The placenta normally is situated in the upper uterine segment. This is the main site of cervix-dilating expulsive force in labor as well as contraction-retraction phenomena postpartum, preventing hemorrhage from the placental site. The lower uterine segment (a functional designation) has relatively more fibrous tissue and less muscle than the upper area and is formed from the isthmus-cervix segments of the uterus. Far less well endowed with contractile abilities, the highly vascularized lower uterine segment site of placental implantation tears when subjected to trauma. Successful management of delivery and prevention of unnecessary blood loss and trauma in this condition usually necessitates cesarean section.

Placenta previa is categorized as to degree, depending upon the approximate percentage of coverage of the internal uterine os. The "low-lying placenta" is said to be present when part of the placenta is close to but not overlapping the internal cervical os. Also known as a "low implantation," this degree of placenta previa accounts for one half of all cases of previa. When part of the internal os is covered, partial placenta previa exists—about 25% of all cases. The most striking degree of previa is present when the entire internal os is covered, that is, complete placenta previa—conprising 25% of all cases of placenta previa. Generally, the greater the area of internal os covered, the earlier in the pregnancy bleeding appears. This is not an invariable rule as, occasionally, at cesarean section done for an abnormal fetal presentation (transverse, oblique or breech) the operator notes placenta previa to be present, without a history of bleeding but almost certainly playing a role in the appearance of an abnormal presentation "by competing for space" in the pelvis.

As the number of women of high parity continues to decrease, so does the observed incidence of placenta previa. The cause of previa is unknown. The incidence correlates with increasing age of the gravida, previous endometrial trauma, prior implantation sites scarred by preceding pregnancies, or with uterine surgery such as cesarean section, hysterotomy, and myomectomy. The resultant placenta in the lower uterine segment is thinner and wider in diameter than is the placenta normally implanted in the upper uterine segment.

The bleeding is thought to be triggered by normal changes in the lower uterine segment in late pregnancy, that is, an increase in uterine irritability, thinning of the lower uterine wall and beginning effacement and dilatation of the cervix. The net effect is a shearing action on the placenta-decidual bed relationship, culminating in a tearing loose of part of the placenta with resultant opening of the vascular bed and bleeding. The first bleeding episode usually ceases spontaneously without jeopardizing mother or fetus unless an untimely examination (vaginal or rectal) detaches a greater part of the placenta, with resultant copious bleeding. The untraumatized patient would, however, bleed again ultimately.

About 25% of the cases of placenta previa are first manifest while significant prematurity still exists, prior to 34 weeks of gestation. It is this minority that is subjected to "the expectant treatment" of bed rest and nonintervention unless labor or recurrent heavy bleeding forces the obstetrician to deliver the baby.

The definitive diagnosis of placenta previa is made with a double set-up examination in the operating room, where the obstetrician is immediately able to perform a cesarean section once placenta previa is diagnosed. However, for those situations in which expectant management is appropriate, in enabling a significantly premature infant to grow in utero, ultrasound localization of the placenta has been of major importance as a harmless, highly accurate technique of diagnosis. Not only is the placental locale established but also fetal presentation can be diagnosed, as well as the duration of pregnancy ascertained via fetal biparietal head measurements. Occasionally, gross anomalies of the fetus may be diagnosed by the ultrasound; this is of some note with previa, in which the incidence of anomalies is mildly increased.

Delivery of the fetus is almost always via cesarean section, usually low transverse but occasionally low vertical where the lower uterine segment is not yet well developed. This mode of delivery avoids uterine trauma, as attempts to deliver the baby through the highly vascularized lower uterine segment can result in cervical and uterine tears, with massive accompanying hemorrhage. Perinatal mortality ranges up to 20% in various series. Improved premature care in modern neonatal intensive care units has notably brightened the outlook for survival without significant deficit for the small premature infant.

References

1. Danforth, D.N. (ed.) *Obstetrics and Gynecology*, ed. 3. Harper & Row, Hagerstown, Md, 1977, pp. 378–390.
2. Niswander, K.R. *Obstetrics—Essentials of Clinical Practice.* Little, Brown, Boston, 1976, pp. 197–211.
3. Lester, E.P., et al. Disseminated intravascular coagulation in pregnancy. *J. Reprod. Med.* 19: 223–232, 1977.
4. Bear, R.A., et al. Essential hypertension and pregnancy. *Can. Med. Assoc. J.* 118:936–940, 1978.
5. Bonnar, J. Hemostatic function and coagulopathy during pregnancy. *Obstet. Gynecol. Annu.* (7) 195–217, 1978.

Section 3

Labor and Delivery

CHAPTER 31

Home vs. Hospital Birth

JOHN DWYER, M.D.

Until the 1920s the great majority of deliveries occurred in the home, but by the 1960s 98% of deliveries occurred in hospitals.

With the advent of "natural childbirth" and the greater participation of the patient and her family in "family centered maternity care," new demands were being made on the providers of maternity care—the physicians and the hospitals. When a segment of the population perceived that the providers were not responding to their demands, home deliveries began to rise. Some hospitals responded by creating a more "homey" atmosphere, i.e., a birthing room, or a more sympathetic provider of obstetrics, i.e., the certified nurse midwife.

In this chapter, we will attempt to describe these alternate forms of obstetric care and to present what statistics are available as to the results.

HOME BIRTHS

Deliveries outside hospitals tend to fall into four categories.

1. Accidental delivery—usually a rapid labor and this group is probably decreasing as multiparity decreases.
2. Religious groups who refuse formal medical care and hospitals—this group is probably not on the increase and represents relatively small numbers.
3. Indigent patients who cannot afford hospital care or through ignorance or custom do not seek such care—they tend to be delivered by a lay midwife and hopefully this group is declining.

4. Those who deliberately elect to deliver at home and may be attended by a person of varying obstetric experience such as a physician, a certified nurse midwife, a lay midwife or a family member. It is this latter group which represents a new trend.

Statistics on home deliveries are not readily available. The American College of Obstetricians and Gynecologists sent a survey to the State Health Departments in the United States. They received replies from 48 departments, representing greater than 80% of deliveries. However, only 12 states were able to link mortality in the fetus and newborn with the place of delivery and only 4 of these identified stillbirths occurring at home.

Tables 31.1, 31.2, and 31.3 show statistics obtained from this survey. They are grouped according to the criteria used by the various states, but in all groups it is clear that the fetal loss is several fold higher in those deliveries occurring out of the hospital. Supporters of this movement claim that these figures are not reliable since many births at home are not recorded. However, most officials believe that the complications in out of hospital deliveries are underreported. According to Oregon State Health officials, a large number of unregistered stillbirths that occur at home are not reported.

A study of home births from 1973 to 1976 was done for New York State (excluding New York City) by Dr. Andrew Fleck then Director of Child Health, New York State Department of Health. The "at

Table 31.1.   Perinatal Mortality Rate

	Hospital Deliveries	Out of Hospital Deliveries
Iowa	18.4/1000	63.6/1000
California	20.0	42.3
Oklahoma	20.5	57.6
Kansas (1976)	19.9	103.7
(1972–1976)	22.3	95.3

Table 31.2.   Newborn Death Rate (28 Days)

	Hospital Deliveries	Out of Hospital Deliveries
Hawaii	9.6/1000	35.4/1000
Oregon	9.7	17.0
Michigan	10.5	42.7

Table 31.3.   Infant Deaths Within First Year of Life

	Hospital Deliveries	Out of Hospital Deliveries
West Virginia	17.5/1000	58.0/1000
Wyoming	12.0	25.6
Colorado	15.8	37.2
Virginia	16.8	34.8

home rate" increased from 2.2 to 3.9/1000 live births during that period. Table 31.4 shows the neonatal mortality rate between at home and hospital deliveries. The mortality rate is clearly higher in the home deliveries. However, some disturbing statistics in this study showed that 13.1% of the home deliveries occurred in babies less than 2000 gm and 13.4% had no prenatal care. These figures are higher than those in comparable groups delivering in hospitals and suggest that at least in some cases such deliveries occur in high-risk patients, which would adversely affect the statistics.

Finally there is a report by Dr. Mehl and associates of 1146 elective home births in Northern California in which the perinatal mortality rates as well as other parameters of fetal well-being such as Apgar scores were better than those in a comparable hospital group.

More studies involving large comparable groups are needed to compare outcomes. An ongoing study in Oregon involving the medical school and out of hospital groups may provide further information in this area, but current statistics certainly imply that having a baby at home significantly increases risk factors, especially to the baby.

ALTERNATIVES TO HOME BIRTHS

Maternity Center

Because there is evidence of hazards to the mother and especially to the fetus with a home delivery and in an attempt to make the birth of a child a more pleasant experience for all, hospitals have changed many of the traditional rules and regulations.

However, another alternative to home delivery exists. The Maternity Center Association in New York City, which is a 60-year-old agency interested in improving maternity care established a Childbearing Center in 1975. The deliveries were attended by certified nurse midwives, with physicians and hospital backup when needed. The actual deliveries occur in a townhouse which lacks facilities for any substantial emergency therapy. The criteria for selection of patients are very rigid so that a low-risk population is selected. However, since a "no risk" population cannot be selected by any current criteria, a significant number of patients are referred out prior to and during the delivery. Table 31.5 shows that of the first 714 people who sought the program only 244, or 34.2%, were delivered there. Further analysis of the statistics show good Apgar scores in those who delivered there, but nine babies had to be transferred because of problems mainly related to respiratory distress. In 9 cases, significant meconium was noted; in 2 cases, mothers were transferred when no fetal heart tones were noted. As with home deliveries, when larger numbers are

Table 31.4.   Neonatal Mortality New York State, 1973–1976

	Hospital	Out of Hospital
White	9.7/1000	38.3/1000
Non white	18.9	29.4

Table 31.5. Maternity Center

	No.	%
First visit	714	—
Ineligible first visit	77	10.8
Spontaneous abortion	25	3.5
Moved or withdrew	63	8.8
Referred or transferred	177*	24.8
Delivered	244	34.2
Transferred postpartum	5	—
Remaining in program	128	17.9

* One hundred nineteen antepartum.

available some further judgment can be made as to whether this is an economically as well as obstetrically sound alternative to hospital based deliveries.

CHANGES IN HOSPITAL BASED OBSTETRICAL CARE

In the 1960s the first changes in hospital regulations involved allowing the father of the baby to be present during the process of labor and to support his wife during this period. Later these changes allowed the father to be present in the delivery room during a normal delivery. This was later extended to problem deliveries and finally in recent years has been extended to being present for a cesarean section. Not all hospitals allow the full range of activities, especially in relation to cesarean section, and many require that courses be taken before such procedures are allowed.

With the growing interest in parent-infant bonding, changes in regulations allow more immediate and prolonged contact between the newborn and its parents except when newborn emergencies prevent such contact. A more active role by the parents when the child is in the nursery is being encouraged, and many hospitals provide "rooming-in" which allows the newborn to remain in the mother's room most (if not all) of the postpartum period. Most parents who express an interest in rooming-in are interested in breast feeding and this is encouraged in most centers.

In the interest of "family centered maternity care," many hospitals provide for sibling visitation so that siblings have the opportunity to visit their mother as well as the new member of the family. In most hospitals the nursing service screens the visiting children for potential infectious disease.

There is a segment of the population who wish to deliver in a more "homey" atmosphere than the usual hospital labor and delivery rooms. This has resulted in the development of "birthing rooms." These rooms are equipped to look like a room at home but still have equipment close enough to handle obstetric problems. The room should be close enough to a delivery room so that if the need arises the patient can be quickly transferred. The birthing room has rugs, drapes, bedspreads, rocking chair, and pictures; it also has a screen in the background which hides resuscitating equipment for the newborn. Patients labor and deliver in the same bed in such rooms; some hospitals have special beds which convert to traditional delivery tables. To this segment of the population, the concept is often more important than the physical equipment. Table 31.6 describes the experience at the Roosevelt Hospital from February 1978 to October 1979. Rigid criteria are necessary such as a low-risk population, active labor, good progress and constant attendance by a nurse, nurse midwife or a physician. When complications are noted, patients need to be promptly transferred.

Another major area of change in hospital based obstetrics is the change in the

Table 31.6. Birthing Room Experience, The Roosevelt Hospital, 1978–1979

Patients	
Midwifery service	211
Clinic service	18
Private service	13
Total	242
Transferred	
Lack of progress	7*
Meconium	1
Sulcus repair	1
Postpartum hemorrhage	1
Retained placenta	1
Unspecified	1
Total	12
Baby	
Low Apgar	1
Premature	1

* Two underwent cesarean section.

person performing the delivery. In the early part of this century, lay midwives (people usually with no formal training) performed a large segment of the deliveries. General practitioners gradually replaced this group as hospital based obstetrics started to grow.

By the 1950s the number delivered by board certified obstetricians and gynecologists began to grow and the number delivered by the physician in general practice decreased. By the 1960s the certified nurse midwife began to appear in hospitals. A certified nurse midwife is a registered nurse who has 1 or 2 years additional approved training in obstetrics in an approved program and is examined and certified by the American College of Nurse Midwifery. Initially her work centered on a clinic population and involved mainly low-risk patients in this group. In 1965 the Roosevelt Hospital became the first voluntary hospital to employ nurse midwives, and in 1975 a pilot private practice program was started. In this program, patients were screened by the nurse midwife and those with high-risk problems were eliminated on the initial visit. If problems developed during the antepartum or intrapartum period, a physician was consulted and if necessary he assumed the care of the patient. A review of the first 2 years of this experience was reported. Basically it showed that it was possible to select a low-risk group, but even in this group problems ensued and therefore again established that it is not possible to select a no-risk group. An attempt was made to determine the reason the patients selected this program. They tended to be college educated and somewhat older than average. They sought the program for a multitude of reasons, including the feeling that the midwives provided more support and looked on the process as a natural event as opposed to physicians who were thought to perceive labor and delivery as a potential disease process. Many patients sacrificed their insurance coverage since the third party payer would not pay the midwives but would cover the hospital costs. As the

numbers grow larger (and the demand increases yearly), more information can be obtained as to the impact of such a program.

Certified midwives are now employed in several similar programs throughout the country. In addition, they now staff inpatient as well as outpatient facilities in indigent high-risk areas in New York City and elsewhere. Many obstetricians have now added certified nurse midwives to their practice, with a general patient acceptance and an easing of the burden of the busy obstetrician.

The future role of the nurse practitioner and the growing number of physicians now board certified in family practice is unclear at the present time. Unfortunately the lay midwife (a person with little if any formal training) continues to play a small but significant role in the care of those people who elect home delivery. There is political pressure in many areas to license them.

Most hospitals now allow the father of the baby to be present in the labor and delivery areas. Only rare problems seem to have arisen as a consequence. As with any new trend there have been demands now for other relatives and friends to be present and where to draw the line has become an issue.

The rugs, drapes, and flowers present in many birthing rooms may be a potential source of infection, but this has not been shown to be a significant problem. In addition there are less facilities in such rooms to handle emergencies, and therefore a critical delay may occur before such a patient can be transferred to a better equipped facility.

Similarly, facilities such as the maternity center are not equipped to handle significant emergencies and the delay in transfer of either mother or baby to a hospital can be hazardous. In addition the selection criteria are so rigid that only one third of those applying eventually deliver in such a facility.

Sibling visitations may introduce the hazard of bringing children with infectious disease in contact with mothers or new-borns. Screening by physicians or the nursing service tends to reduce but not eliminate such hazards.

A general complaint in this area is that this segment of the population will continue to demand more and more so that all control of obstetric care will be lost or compromised. An open attitude should be maintained to the requests of consumers, as long as there is no evidence that the medical well-being of either mother or baby will be compromised.

The ultimate goal is to provide safe optimal care to the mother and the newborn in a manner that is rewarding to them.

References

1. Dillon, T.F., Brennan, B.A., Dwyer, J.F., et al. Midwifery 1977. *Am. J. Obstet. Gynecol. 130*:917, 1978.
2. Faison, J.B., Pisani, B.J., Douglas, R.G., Cranch, G.S., and Lubic, R.W. The childbearing center: An alternative birth setting. *Obstet. Gynecol. 54*:527, 1978.
3. Fleck, A.C. Home births for upstate New York, 1973–1976 (unpublished).
4. Mehle, L.E., Peterson, G.H., Whitt, M., and Hawes, W.E. Outcomes of elective home births: A series of 1146 cases. *J. Reprod. Med. 19*:281, 1977.
5. Nelson, L.P. Results of the first 124 deliveries in the birth room at Roosevelt Hospital in New York City. *Birth Fam. J. 6*:97, 1979.
6. Pearse, W.H. Home birth (editorial). *J.A.M.A. 241*:1039, 1979.

CHAPTER **32**

Measurement of the Pelvis

ROBERT WIECHE, M.D.

Pelvimetry simply defined is the evaluation of the bony pelvis and its estimated potential capacity to accommodate a vaginal delivery. This capacity is one of the significant factors that we are concerned with in the process of labor—the others being the quality of labor, the presentation and position of the fetus, its size, as well as its physiological status.

The two means that we have available for pelvimetry are clinically by palpation and radiographic under certain circumstances when more precise information is needed.

CLASSIFICATION OF PELVES

The Caldwell-Moloy classification of pelves is the one that is commonly used. This is basically a radiologic classification that has been employed clinically by correlating palpable features of the bony pelvis with the known characteristics of the four pure types of pelves (Fig. 32.1):

1. Gynecoid (round or normal female)
2. Android (heart shaped or male)
3. Anthropoid (long, narrow, oval in the anteroposterior diameter)
4. Platypelloid (flat, oval in the transverse diameter)

The final classification in the Caldwell-Moloy terminology is done by describing the posterior and anterior halves of the inlet. The widest transverse diameter of the inlet is used to divide the pelvis into the two halves. The posterior half describes the *type* of pelvis, and the anterior half describes the *tendency*. Thus, a pure gynecoid pelvis would be called *gynecoid-gynecoid*. If the posterior half was gynecoid and the anterior half was longer and with some narrowing of the forepelvis, it would be called *gynecoid-anthropoid*, or gynecoid with anthropoid tendency (Fig. 32.2).

The general morphological features of the pure type of pelves are as follows.

Gynecoid Pelvis

The inlet is round. The transverse diameter of the inlet is equal to or slightly greater than the anteroposterior diameter. The sacrum has a good hollow and is not inclined either anteriorly or posteriorly. The sidewalls are straight, and the ischial spines are blunt and not prominent. The sacrosciatic notch is rounded and not narrow. The pubic arch is rounded and wide—a Norman type of arch.

Android Pelvis

The inlet is heart or wedge shaped, with the posterior sagittal portion of the anteroposterior diameter being shorter than the anterior portion. The posterior half of the inlet is wedge shaped, with the anterior portion being longer, narrower, and triangular. The sacrum is straight and inclined forward. The sidewalls are convergent, the sacrosciatic notch is narrow, and the subpubic arch is pointed and narrow—Gothic type. The pelvis basically funnels, with anteroposterior as well as transverse diameters progressively decreasing from the inlet of the pelvis to the outlet.

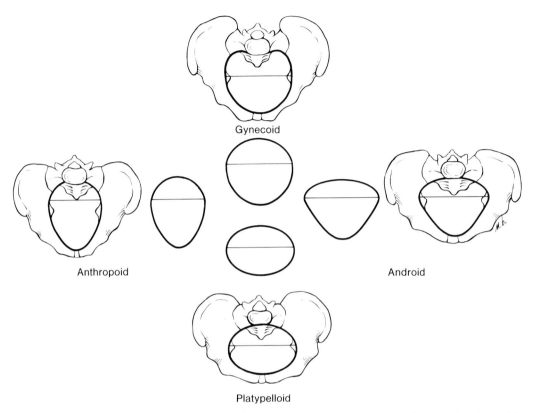

Gynecoid

Anthropoid

Android

Platypelloid

Figure 32.1   The four ''pure'' types of pelves: gynecoid, android, platypelloid, and anthropoid.

Anthropoid Pelvis

The inlet is an oval in its anteroposterior diameter, with the transverse diameter being much smaller. The anterior half of the inlet, or forepelvis, is often pointed or narrowed. The sacrum is frequently straightened and may be inclined posteriorly. The sidewalls are usually somewhat convergent and the spines may be prominent. The sacrosciatic notch is usually large. The subpubic arch is slightly narrowed and Gothic, or pointed, in shape.

Platypelloid Pelvis

The flat pelvis is simply an ovoid type, with the oval in the transverse direction; thus, the transverse diameter of the inlet is much greater than is the anteroposterior diameter. The sacrum in its upper portion is often straightened and its inclination is usually average, or posterior. The sidewalls are straight, spines are not prominent, and the sacrosciatic notch is usually rounded and of average size. (NOTE: The notch has both anteroposterior and transverse dimensions to it so that usually it is extremely limited only in the android pelvis.) The subpubic arch is well rounded and wide.

CLINICAL PELVIMETRY

The inlet or superior strait of the pelvis is not clinically palpable or measurable. However, palpable features of any pelvis aid in developing a probable picture of the inlet and its approximate size.

The CO (obstetrical conjugate) is the shortest distance between the area of the sacral promontory and the back of the pubic symphysis.

The conjugate vera is the distance be-

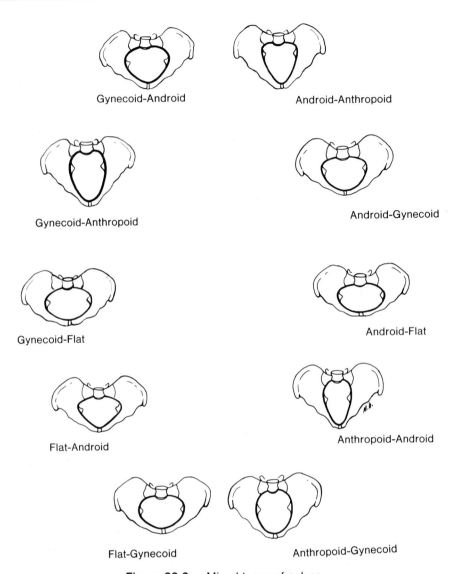

Figure 32.2.   Mixed types of pelves.

tween the sacral promontory and upper border of the pubic symphysis (Fig. 32.3).

The diagonal conjugate, or CD, is the distance between the lower border of the symphysis and the sacral promontory. Because the inclination of the pelvis can vary so greatly, there is no consistent relationship between the CO and the CD. However, if one is able to clinically palpate the sacral promontory, it is quite likely that the pelvis is small or is shortened in its anteroposterior diameters.

Transverse diameters of the inlet and the midpelvis are not measurable by clinical palpation, although the characteristics and palpability of the ischial spines give suggestive information regarding the midpelvis transverse diameter.

The TI (transverse diameter of the outlet between the ischial tuberosities) is palpable and, although instrument measurement is no longer in general use, close correlation with actual measurement may be done by clinical estimate. The subpubic

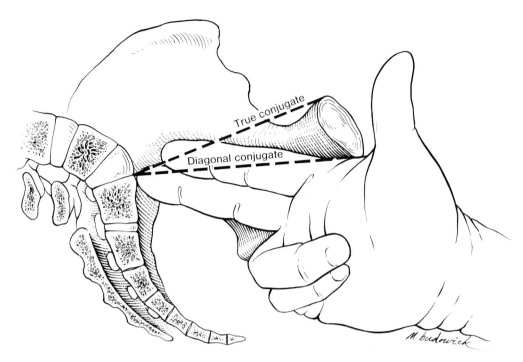

Figure 32.3.   The diagonal conjugate and the true conjugate.

arch morphology, TI estimate, characteristics of the ischial spines, and relationship of the sidewalls of the pelvis are the palpable features of a pelvis which clinically are employed to develop a picture of the transverse diameter of the inlet.

OUTLINE OF CLINICAL PALPATION

With the patient on the examining table, feet in stirrups, hips at edge of table and knees drawn up and separated widely, the examiner can palpate with the tips of his thumbs the medial aspect of the subpubic arch. At the point where it flares out, he holds the tips of his thumbs for a short time, so that a good clinical estimate of the TI can be made (Fig. 32.4).

Then the examiner stands with one foot on a stool and with elbow of the examining hand resting on his knee. The index and middle fingers are introduced into the vagina, while the ring and little fingers are flexed into the palm of the hand. This position gives stability to the examining hand and allows palpation to be carried

out smoothly and with minimum discomfort to the patient.

The sidewalls of the pelvis are palpated (Fig. 32.5) and most important is whether they are straight and parallel to one another or whether they are convergent—and, if so, slightly or markedly.

The ischial spines are palpated (Fig. 32.6), and it is noted whether they are sharp or blunt, prominent or not prominent. The transverse diameter between the spines is most important; if one suspects clinically that it is somewhat limited, this serves as an alert for future clinical management in labor.

From the tip of the ischial spine, the sacrospinous ligament is palpated to the lateral border of the sacrum. If this is less than $2\frac{1}{2}$ fingerbreadths, there is a strong clinical suggestion that the sacrosciatic notch is narrowed. Clinically, this often correlates with a limitation of the posterior portion of the inlet.

Next, the coccyx is felt, and it is noted whether it is flexible or fixed and whether or not it juts forward.

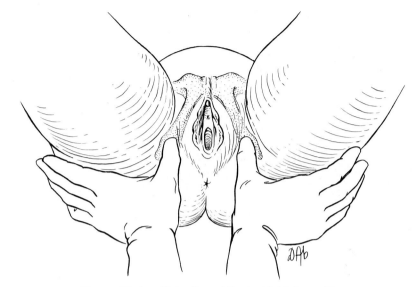

Figure 32.4.   Palpation of the ischial tuberosities.

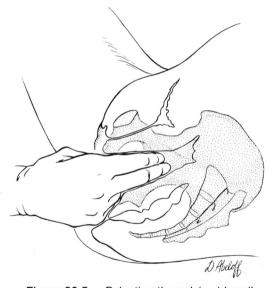

Figure 32.5.   Palpating the pelvic sidewall.

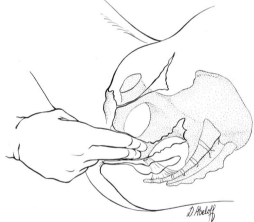

Figure 32.6.   Palpating the ischial spine.

Finally, the anterior surface of the sacrum is felt. It is noted whether the sacrum is hollow or straightened, and whether or not it is inclined anteriorly. Then one attempts to reach the sacral promontory. With the knuckles of the flexed fingers of the examining hand pushing into the perineum, and employing the fulcrum action of the elbow resting on the knee, the index and middle fingers are carried up the anterior surface of the sacrum. If the promontory is reached by the tip of the middle finger, it is held at this point, the hand elevated until the radial surface of the index finger touches the lower border of the symphysis, and this point is marked by the index finger of the other hand. The CD (diagonal conjugate) reached is then read on the fixed wall scale.

An individual's maximum reach may be

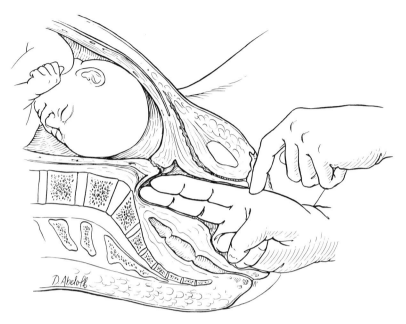

Figure 32.7.   Measuring the diagonal conjugate.

read on the wall scale by marking a point on the radial surface of the hand about one third of the distance between the knuckles of the index finger and the thumb (Fig. 32.7).

There is no absolute relationship between the CD and the true CO but certainly when the CD is reached at 12.0 cm or less, one should be clinically alerted that the pelvis may be less than average size.

Convergence of sidewalls, straightening and forward inclination of the sacrum, prominence of the spines and their jutting inward, narrowing of the base of the sacrosciatic notch, and, finally, pointing and narrowing of the subpubic arch with estimation of the TI being below 9.5 cm, all represent less than ideal features of the pelvis.

All are relative, but the above features should be well-documented and serve as alerts to reevaluate the pelvis when the pregnancy is at term.

Conversely, if the pelvis is originally felt to be clinically adequate but the presenting part remains high as term approaches, reevaluation should take place.

X-RAY PELVIMETRY

The purpose of x-ray pelvimetry is to elucidate the size and shape of the bony pelvis. In the majority of instances, clinical palpable pelvimetry will suffice and exact measurements and morphology are not necessary for proper management of labor.

Additional consideration must be given to the fact that there is ionizing radiation involved. There are those who would advocate that all radiographic pelvimetry should be eliminated. Suffice it to say that a more conservative approach would be to request it only in a limited number of selected cases in which the information obtained will play a significant role in the management of labor, especially in breech presentation when vaginal delivery is contemplated.

The isometric method of x-ray pelvimetry is used at the Lying-In division of the New York Hospital. In it, the patient is positioned on the the x-ray table so that the inlet of the pelvis is essentially parallel to the surface of the table. A notched centimeter metallic ruler is placed vertically against the symphysis. The lateral view of

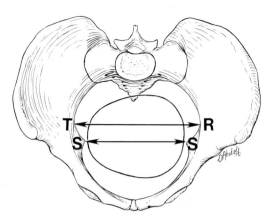

Figure 32.8.   The pelvic inlet. *S:* ischial spine at midpelvic level. *T-R:* transverse diameter of inlet. *S-S:* transverse diameter of midpelvis (interspinous diameter).

the pelvis can then be used to read the important anteroposterior diameters of the pelvis because they are distorted exactly as the metallic ruler on the film is.

The AP view of the pelvis (Fig. 32.8) shows the morphology of the inlet. In addition, the transverse diameters of the inlet and the midpelvis can be obtained.

A distorted scale has been made by tak-ing x-rays of the metallic centimeter ruler at 1 cm levels above the table. From the lateral film, one can determine at which levels the transverse of the inlet and the midpelvis diameters (interspinous) are and use the appropriate scale for their exact measurement.

Many years of experience have revealed that there are certain critical dimensions in association with high percentages of cesarean sections or difficult deliveries. Obviously, today the majority of the latter have also become abdominal deliveries.

The critical measurements by experi-ence at the New York Lying-In Hospital are as follows:

CO	11.5 cm
Transverse of inlet	11.5 cm
Interspinous	9.5 cm

As the dimensions progressively de-crease below these measurements, the in-cidence of abdominal or difficult deliveries increases.

Obviously, morphology, size of head, moldability and position are significant factors and can shift the outcome one way or the other.

CHAPTER 33

Uterine Contractility

RONALD M. CAPLAN, M.D.

The *tonus* is the lowest intraamniotic pressure that can be recorded between uterine contractions. It represents the resting pressure of the uterus between contractions and normally does not exceed 12 mm Hg.

The *intensity*, or amplitude, of each contraction is measured by the rise of pressure (mm Hg) it produces in the amniotic fluid.

The *frequency* is expressed as the number of contractions per 10 minutes.

Uterine activity is the product of the intensity and the frequency of the uterine contractions and is expressed as millimeters of mercury per 10 minutes.

PREGNANCY

During the first 30 weeks of gestation, uterine activity is minimal. The contractions themselves are very small, localized in a discrete area of the uterus. The contractions of "false" labor, the so-called Braxton-Hicks contractions, are stronger, measuring 10–15 mm Hg, and are spread to a larger area of the uterus. The frequency is low, approaching one contraction per hour in the 30th week. After the 30th week, the uterine activity gradually increases due to an increase in the *intensity* and *frequency* of the contractions. Their coordination is improved and they spread more diffusely throughout the uterus. This period of increasing uterine activity, which lasts for several weeks, is called *prelabor*. During this period, the uterine cervix is progressively ripened, presumably as a consequence of the contractions of the uterus.

ONSET OF LABOR

As the 40th week approaches, the uterine activity progressively increases. There is no clear-cut demarcation between prelabor and labor, but rather there is a gradual and progressive transition between these stages. The small, localized incoordinated contractions typical of early pregnancy tend to disappear as prelabor advances and are absent during normal labor, in which only strong and rhythmical contractions normally occur. Labor is said to be in a latent phase until progressive cervical dilatation commences: the active phase of labor.

FIRST AND SECOND STAGES OF LABOR

The uterine activity progressively increases until the fetus is delivered. The intensity of the contractions increases from 30 mm Hg at the commencement of labor to 50 mm Hg at the end. The frequency increases from 3 to 5 contractions per 10 minutes, and the tonus from 8 to 12 mm Hg. The intensity of the contractions is usually greater in primigravidas than in multiparous patients.

THIRD STAGE OF LABOR

After the fetus is delivered, the uterus continues to contract rhythmically. The frequency of these contractions diminishes progressively. The first, second, or third contraction usually expels the placenta from the upper uterus to the birth

251

canal. These contractions have similar intensity to those of the second stage.

EARLY PUERPERIUM

The uterine activity diminishes very rapidly. The frequency of the contractions usually decreases first, being reduced to one contraction per 10 minutes some hours after delivery. The intensity of the contractions diminishes more slowly. The rate of propagation of the contractile wave through the uterus is also progressively reduced.

NORMAL UTERINE CONTRACTION OF LABOR

The wave originates near the uterine end of one of the fallopian tubes where the pacemaker is located. It then spreads at a rate of 2 cm per second, invading the entire uterus within 15 seconds. The greater part of the wave is propagated downward (descending propagation).

The activity of the different parts of the uterus is so well coordinated that the acme of the contraction is attained almost simultaneously in all parts. The farther the wave moves away from the pacemaker, the shorter is the duration of the contraction phase. The intensity of the contraction also diminishes from top to bottom due to the reduction in the thickness of the myometrium and in the concentration of the contractile protein, actomyosin.

The normal contractile wave has a triple descending gradient: 1) propagation, 2) duration and 3) intensity. These three gradients are essential for the contraction to dilate the cervix. The contraction of the upper parts of the uterus, adjacent to the pacemaker, starts before and is stronger and of longer duration than that of the lower parts, which yield to and are distended by the contraction.

As all parts of the uterus reach the acme of the contraction almost simultaneously, the sum of these effects causes a great increase in the amniotic pressure. The existence of good coordination between the different parts of the uterus is evident when the amniotic pressure wave assumes a regular form with a single peak. The synchronous relaxation of all parts allows the amniotic pressure to fall to 10 mm Hg, the level of normal tonus. Incoordination of the different parts of the uterus results in amniotic pressure waves having irregular form, diminished intensity, greater frequency, and increased tonus.

Contractions are perceptible by abdominal palpation only after their intensity exceeds 10 mm Hg, a value influenced by the thickness and tonus of the abdominal wall and by the experience of the observer. The clinically apparent duration of the contraction, possibly 70 seconds, is much *shorter* than its actual duration measured by recording the intrauterine pressure. When the intensity of the contraction reaches 40 mm Hg, the uterine wall is so hard that it resists depression. There is usually no pain until the intensity exceeds 15 mm Hg, as this is the minimum pressure required to distend the lower segment and the cervix during the first stage and the birth canal during the second stage. The pain threshold varies from patient to patient and is raised by analgesic drugs and "natural childbirth" training.

In prelabor and labor, during each contraction the upper segment shortens and exerts a longitudinal traction on the cervix, causing progressive ripening, effacement and dilatation. The traction is transmitted by the lower segment, which also contracts but with less force than the upper segment. During labor, after each contraction the upper segment remains shorter and thicker, while the cervix becomes more effaced and dilated. The pressure exerted by the presenting part or the amniotic sac also contributes to the effects of the contractions on the lower parts of the uterus.

As it pulls above the presenting part, the lower segment of the uterus undergoes circumferential dilatation and consequent thinning. Longitudinal shortening of the lower segment occurs during the second stage.

DESCENT OF THE FETUS

Because the lower part of the uterus is attached to the pelvis by the uterosacral and cardinal ligaments, the shortening of the contracting uterus pushes the fetus downward. The contractions of the round ligaments, which are simultaneous to those of the upper segment, tend to pull down the uterine fundus, thus contributing to the fetal descent.

In the second stage, the bearing-down efforts produce strong (50–70 mm Hg) rapid and short-lasting (20 seconds) elevations of the intrauterine pressure which are superimposed on the slower, smoother and more prolonged rises of pressure caused by the uterine contractions.

ABNORMAL CONTRACTILITY

Uterine contractions may be hyperactive, that is, abnormally increased in intensity or frequency. These changes may be accompanied by hypertonicity. In the extreme the tonus is over 30 mm Hg, resulting in what clinically is one long hard contraction: the so-called *tetanic contraction.* Cephalopelvic disproportion, hypertensive disorders of pregnancy, and excess dosage of oxytocic drugs are some possible causes of uterine hyperactivity. Hyperactivity may result in precipitate (abnormally rapid) delivery and fetal asphyxia. Conversely, contractions may be *hypoactive,* that is, decreased in intensity or frequency, leading to prolonged labor. The uterine tonus is usually low.

The normal triple descending gradient of propagation, duration, and intensity may be inverted so that contractions are stronger and last longer in the lower part of the uterus. Abnormal contractile waves may be present, localized in various regions of the uterus: this situation is known as *uterine incoordination.*

ABNORMAL LABOR PATTERNS

Labor is defined as abnormal if it progresses too slowly, too quickly, or actually fails to progress.

The preparatory or latent phase of labor (Fig. 33.1) comprises that period from the onset of regular uterine contractions to the onset of progressive cervical dilatation. Friedman defines a *prolonged latent phase* as one which lasts more than 20 hours in a primigravida or more than 14 hours in the multiparous patient.

In the dilatational phase of labor, Friedman recognizes two abnormalities. *Protracted active-phase dilatation* is diagnosed in the nulliparous patient whose cervix is dilating 1.2 cm/hour or less and in the multipara who is dilating 1.5 cm/hour or less. The other essential component of progressive labor is the descent of the fetal presenting part through the birth canal. *Protracted descent* is recognized in the primigravida if descent is 1 cm/hour or less and in the multipara if descent is 2 cm/hour or less.

A deceleration phase, with a decreased rate of cervical dilatation, normally follows active-phase dilatation just prior to the appearance of the full dilatation of the cervix that defines the onset of the second stage of labor. The *deceleration phase* is considered by Friedman to be *prolonged* in the primigravida if it lasts 3 hours or more. One hour or more in the deceleration phase is considered prolonged in the multiparous patient. A cessation of active phase progression for 2 hours or more is called a *secondary arrest of dilatation.* If descent of the fetus has ceased for 1 hour or more, an *arrest of descent* is deemed to have occurred.

Once the cervix is fully dilated, the second stage of labor begins. Maternal "pushing" efforts add to the expulsive force of the uterine contractions. In effect, the mother inspires and, by holding her breath and contracting the diaphragmatic muscles, performs a Valsalva maneuver, thus increasing the intra-abdominal pressure ("bearing-down"). These combined forces should result in gradual, continued descent of the fetus through the maternal pelvis and to birth.

A *failure of descent* is defined by Friedman as the lack of expected descent during the deceleration phase and the second stage of labor.

A labor that progresses abnormally quickly is said to be precipitate. *Precipitate dilatation* is present in the primigravida whose cervix is dilating 5 cm/hour or more

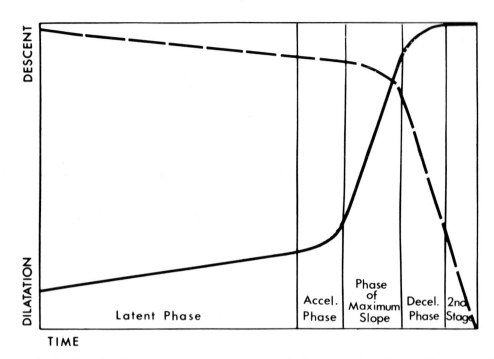

Figure 33.1. Cervical dilatation and descent patterns in the labor of nulliparas. The time period from the onset of the acceleration phase to the end of the deceleration phase is known as the active phase. (From E.A. Friedman, in *Advances in Obstetrics and Gynecology*, edited by R.M. Caplan, and W.J. Sweeney. Williams & Wilkins, Baltimore, 1978, p. 247.)

and in the multipara whose cervix is dilating 10 cm/hour or more.

Descent of the fetus through the birth canal at 5 cm/hour or more in the primigravida or 10 cm/hour or more in the multiparous patient is classified as *precipitate descent*.

INDUCTION OF LABOR

Induction of labor refers to the institution of progressive uterine contractions by artificial means. Stimulation of labor involves the enhancement of uterine contractions by artificial means.

Induction of labor should be carried out only for medical indications (Table 33.1). These include evidence of diminished fetal well-being, such as falling estriol levels, nonreactive nonstress tests (see Chapter 18: "Stress Testing and Nonstress Testing") and rising optical density difference levels in Rh isoimmunized patients (see Chapter 24: "Rh Isoimmunization"). Evi-

Table 33.1.   Indications for Induction of Labor

Fetal compromise
    Intrauterine growth retardation (placental
      insufficiency)
    Falling estriols
    Nonreactive nonstress tests
    Rh isoimmunization
    Postmaturity
Intrauterine fetal death
Maternal disorders
    Hypertensive disorders of pregnancy (toxemia)
    Diabetes
    Cardiac disease
    Rupture of membranes—prolonged

dence of diminished fetal well-being is likely to be seen in mothers with diabetes, Rh isoimmunization, hypertensive disorders and postmaturity. Maternal well-being may be a factor as well, for example in patients with toxemia. The so-called elderly primigravida, over 35 years of age, is one type of patient who might have a fetus with intrauterine growth retardation

(IUGR) secondary to placental insufficiency.

Evidence of fetal maturity should ideally be obtained prior to an attempt at induction of labor (see Chapter 19: "Determination of Fetal Age and Fetal Maturity" and Chapter 15: "Ultrasonography").

Whenever possible, induction is deferred until the cervix has begun to efface (shorten) and dilate (open). Ideally, the fetal head should be engaged in the maternal pelvis. Malpresentation is a contraindication to induction, as is cephalopelvic disproportion of significant degree. If these conditions are fulfilled, induction may be quite simple.

An enema is given to evacuate the rectum, thus leaving more potential space in the pelvis for the fetus and stimulating the maternal bowel, which empirically seems to enhance uterine contractions. Monitoring of both the fetal heart rate and the uterine contractions should be employed. This must be done externally until rupture of the membranes either occurs spontaneously or is undertaken artificially. Once the membranes are ruptured, an internal fetal scalp electrode and internal amniotic pressure catheter may be placed (see Chapter 36: "Fetal Monitoring in Labor").

Pitocin (oxytocin) is given intravenously by infusion pump, starting at 1 mU/minute and gradually increased until adequate uterine contractility is achieved in the physiologic range, leading to progressive effacement and dilatation of the cervix.

Usually, with average intensity of contractions at 50 mm Hg and 4 to 5 contractions per 10 minutes, the first stage may progress satisfactorily.

After the baby is delivered, the pitocin infusion is maintained to ensure contraction of the uterus, thus closing the intrauterine vessels and keeping maternal blood loss to a minimum.

Prostaglandins may be utilized to induce labor. However, at the present time, this approach tends to be reserved for midtrimester abortion, and pitocin stimulation remains the method of choice for induction of labor.

Bibliography

1. Caldeyro-Barcia, R. Entrait due Deuxieme Congres International de Gynecologie et d'Obstetrique de Montreal en 1958–Tme I, p. 65.
2. Friedman, E.A. *Labor: Clinical Evaluation and Management*, ed. 2. Appleton-Century-Crofts, New York, 1978.
3. Friedman, E.A. Patterns of labor. In *Advances in Obstetrics and Gynecology*, edited by Caplan, R.M., and Sweeney, W.J. Williams & Wilkins, Baltimore, 1978, pp. 246–252.
4. Jeffcoate, T.N.A. Dystocia due to or associated with abnormal uterine action. In *British Obstetric and Gynecologic Practice*, edited by Holland. Heinemann, London, 1955.
5. Jeffcoate, T.N.A. Physiology and mechanism of labour. In *British Obstetric and Gynecologic Practice*, edited by Holland. Heinemann, London, 1955.
6. Reynolds, S.R.M. *Physiology of the Uterus*, ed. 2. Hoeber, New York, 1949.
7. Seitchik, J. Quantitating uterine contractility in clinical context. *Obstet. Gynecol.* 57:453, 1981.

CHAPTER 34

Mechanism of Labor

RONALD M. CAPLAN, M.D.

A pregnant woman evolves into labor, and labor itself is a fluid, dynamic process. It is important to remember this truth when confronted with the concepts of the "start" of labor, "false" and "true" labor, "Braxton-Hicks" as opposed to "labor" contractions, and the fragmented concepts of "engagement," "descent," and "rotation." All these entities are complementary to each other and occur in an evolving pattern.

VERTEX PRESENTATION

One must study the size and configuration of the normal human female pelvis to realize that the distance traversed by the fetus in labor, from inlet to outlet, is relatively short. Therefore, a centimeter is a significant distance and can be critical in evaluating the prognosis of the labor.

The key movements of the fetus in a vertex presentation during labor are:

1. Engagement
2. Descent
3. Flexion
4. Internal rotation
5. Extension
6. External rotation
7. Expulsion

Engagement (Fig. 34.1) is defined as the passage of the widest diameter of the presenting fetal part into the inlet of the maternal pelvis. In the case of the well-flexed fetal head, it is the entry of the *biparietal diameter* (Fig. 34.2) of the head into the plane of the inlet that defines engagement. This biparietal diameter at term measures 9.5 cm. In the case of the well-flexed head, when the biparietal diameter is in the inlet the occiput is at the level of the ischial spines. The relation of this leading part to the level of the ischial spines is referred to as the *station*. In this case, the station is "spines zero" (Sp-0). Clinically, by Leopold's maneuvers the examiner may determine that the fetal head is well-fixed and may be engaged, and by sterile vaginal examination the clinician may confirm that the occiput has reached the level of the ischial spines. The examiner infers from this data that the biparietal diameter is at the pelvic inlet and, therefore, that engagement has occurred. However, the mere fact that the lead point of the presenting part is at the level of the ischial spines does *not* define engagement (Fig. 34.3), as with increasing extension of the fetal head there is a longer distance between this leading part and the widest diameter of the fetal head being presented to the pelvis. This is an important clinical point, as the examiner will prognosticate differently on the eventual course of the labor depending on whether or not it is believed that engagement has occurred. Engagement may occur in the primigravida (patient having a first pregnancy) as early as 36 weeks' gestation or it may not occur until labor is well established.

With uterine contractions, the fetus gradually descends through the birth canal. Descent occurs with engagement and all subsequent mechanisms, until the fetus is expelled. As the fetus descends, due to the soft tissue resistance encountered by the presenting part in the birth

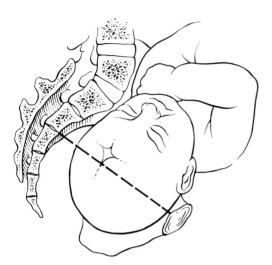

Figure 34.1. Engagement. The widest diameter of the fetal head is into the pelvic inlet. The occiput is at the level of the ischial spines (not shown).

canal, by a lever principle the head gradually flexes so that the fetal chin is in contact with the fetal chest. In a well-flexed head, the effective diameter being presented to the maternal pelvis is the *suboccipitobregmatic diameter* (Fig. 34.2), which is 9.5 cm and is the smallest effective diameter that the fetus can present to the pelvis. Internal rotation refers to that rotation which occurs while the fetal head is within the birth canal. In the vertex presentation, at the start of labor the head may be in a variety of positions in relation to the maternal pelvis. Most commonly, it will start out with the sagittal suture in a position transverse to the maternal pelvis (Fig. 34.4), with the occiput either to the left or to the right (left occiput transverse = LOT; right occiput transverse = ROT) or with the occiput at a 45° angle from the maternal symphysis pubis (left occiput anterior = LOA; right occiput anterior = ROA). Less commonly the initial position of the occiput is posterior, with the occiput 45 degrees from the maternal sacrum; thus the head will have to undergo 135 degrees of rotation so that the occiput will impinge under the maternal symphysis pubis (left occiput posterior = LOP; right occiput posterior = ROP).

With increasing uterine contractions and descent, the head will rotate due to the configuration of the birth canal to bring the occiput directly under the maternal symphysis pubis, at which time the fetal sagittal suture will be exactly in the anteroposterior diameter of the maternal pelvis.

With the occiput impinged under the symphysis, continuing uterine contractions cause extension of the head to occur and the maternal vulva bulges. As the head *crowns*, the chin gradually sweeps over the perineal body and is born in this way by extension. External rotation is that rotation which occurs with the baby's head outside the maternal pelvis. The first component of this is *restitution* to the oblique: the baby's head returns to its original position if it was at a 45° angle (LOA, ROA). The external rotation then continues until the sagittal suture is transverse, thus completing an external rotation of 90 degrees.

At this point, the anterior shoulder impinges under the symphysis, and the posterior shoulder is born first, by lateral flexion, as it sweeps over the maternal perineum. The anterior shoulder is then born as the fetal spine straightens, and the rest of the body follows easily.

VAGINAL EXAMINATION DURING LABOR

The progress of labor is ultimately gauged by noting progressive *effacement* and *dilatation* of the cervix, as well as the position, engagement, descent, flexion and rotation of the presenting part. This is accomplished by careful monitoring of uterine contractions and of the fetal heart rate as a sign of the response of the fetus to the labor, by abdominal palpation (Leopold's maneuvers) and by sterile vaginal examination. The cervix is palpated and if it is very thin, it is clinically said to be fully effaced. At this point the entire cervical canal between the external cervical os and the internal os has been taken up into the lower uterine segment—the definition of full effacement. The degree of effacement is a rough measurement, starting with no

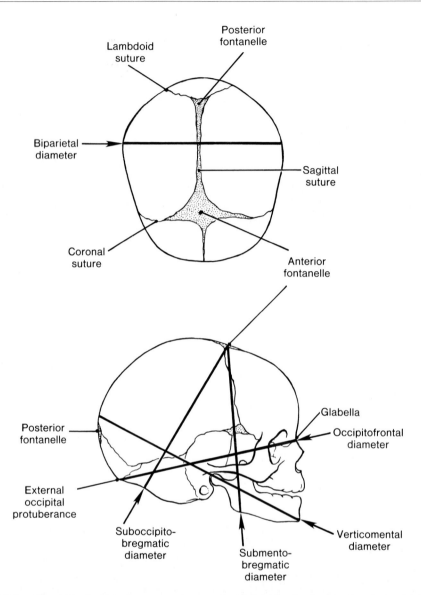

Figure 34.2. Fetal skull, showing some important diameters in the mechanism of labor. The biparietal diameter is the widest transverse diameter; the suboccipitobregmatic diameter is the shortest anteroposterior diameter. The submentobregmatic diameter is operative in face presentations, and the verticomental diameter is operative in brow presentations. In the case of "deflexion"—the military attitude—the occipitofrontal diameter is operative.

effacement (the long cervix of the nonpregnant woman or woman in early pregnancy). Effacement of the cervix gradually starts, usually in the latter weeks of pregnancy, and may or may not be complete prior to the onset of labor.

Dilatation of the cervix refers to the opening of the cervical os. This is measured in centimeters, and full dilatation is deemed to have occurred when the diameter of the open cervical os has reached 10 cm. At this point, on vaginal examination,

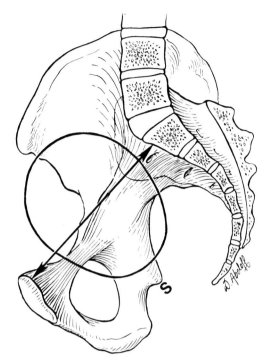

Figure 34.3. Fetal head at approximately 2 cm above the ischial spines (Sp−2). Note that engagement has not yet taken place. The widest (biparietal) diameter of the head is above the level of the pelvic inlet. S = ischial spine.

no cervix can be felt, but only the presenting part of the fetus. On vaginal examination, the vertex presentation is confirmed by feeling the symmetrical, hard, spherical head through the opening of the cervical os. It can be ascertained whether the "membranes" (amniotic sac) are intact by feeling a ballooning compressible bulge between the fetal head and the examining fingers. Of course, a prior assessment of this should have been made on history (the patient will have noted a gush or leakage of fluid from the vagina) and on inspection of the vagina for the presence of fluid, as well as testing of the pH of the vaginal fluid (amniotic fluid is alkaline). If there is a leakage of amniotic fluid, its appearance should be noted: the presence of fetal feces (meconium) may be a grave prognostic sign. The presence of blood should be noted prior to instituting a pelvic examination. Although a small amount mixed

with mucus may only represent "show" (blood and mucus present in the cervix—"the mucus plug"), it may also be a sign of pathology that precludes vaginal examination without strict precautions (see Chapter 30: "Third Trimester Bleeding").

The position of the fetal head is determined by palpating the sagittal suture, determining its direction, and then allowing the two examining fingers to glide along this suture to the fontanelles. The anterior fontanelle on palpation is four-sided, due to the junction of the coronal suture with the sagittal suture, while the posterior fontanelle is three-sided (triangular), as the sagittal suture does not progress beyond its meeting with the occipital suture.

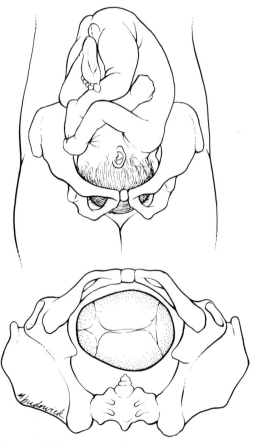

Figure 34.4. Left occiput transverse position. The widest transverse diameter of the fetal head is the biparietal diameter.

If the posterior fontanelle is located anteriorly in the maternal pelvis and to the mother's left side, with the sagittal suture at 45 degrees to the anteroposterior diameter of the maternal pelvis, then the position is left occiput anterior (LOA). Rotation is gauged on successive examinations by noting gradual movement of the posterior fontanelle under the maternal symphysis. Maximal information is gained by examining the patient during a uterine contraction. At this point it can be determined if the fetal head is applied closely to the cervix: the cervix will dilate more, and the head may be actually felt to rotate somewhat and then to fall back to its previous position at the end of the contraction. The examination is often made more difficult by the presence of *asynclitism*. This is an obliquity of the head (lateral flexion) either anteriorly or posteriorly. If the anterior parietal bone presents with the sagittal suture more toward the maternal sacrum, this is anterior asynclitism. If the posterior parietal bone presents, this is posterior asynclitism. Other factors which may complicate this examination are the presence of *caput succedaneum* and *molding*. The former condition is simply scalp edema in the presenting part of the head not covered by cervix (that is, in the cervical os). Molding refers to the overlapping of the fetal skull bones so that commonly the occipital bone margin lies under the parietal bones. These conditions are more prevalent in cases of protracted labor and are more marked when a degree of *cephalopelvic disproportion* exists (maternal pelvis small in relation to the fetal head). In a well-flexed head, the posterior fontanelle should be easily palpable and the anterior fontanelle palpated with difficulty, or not at all. If the anterior fontanelle is readily apparent and the posterior fontanelle is palpated only with difficulty, then a degree of extension (deflexion) exists: the so-called *military attitude*.

The determination of whether or not the fetal head has engaged has already been described. First, it is necessary to ascertain the degree of flexion, both by abdominal palpation and by vaginal examination (preceding paragraph). With the well-flexed head, it may be inferred that engagement has occurred if the occiput is at the level of the ischial spines, provided that it is the occipital bone that is being palpated, keeping in mind that caput succedaneum and molding may distort this perception.

By convention, progress in descent is delineated by noting the distance of the occiput from the spines: if the occiput, for example, is 2 cm above the spines (no engagement has occurred), this is noted as Sp−2 (Fig. 34.3). If, on the other hand, the occiput is 1 cm below the levels of the spines, this is noted as Sp+1.

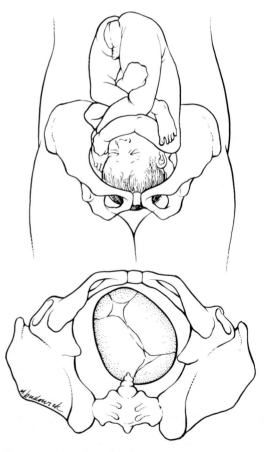

Figure 34.5. Longitudinal lie cephalic presentation, left occiput posterior position.

OCCIPUT TRANSVERSE AND POSTERIOR POSITIONS

In the occiput transverse (LOT, ROT) position, which is the most common starting position in labor, the mechanism is exactly as described, except that internal rotation of 90 degrees must occur to bring the fetal occiput under the maternal symphysis pubis (Fig. 34.4).

In the occiput posterior (LOP, ROP) position, a 135 degree internal rotation must take place (Fig. 34.5). Therefore, labor is often of longer duration. In infrequent cases, the occiput does not turn 135 degrees anteriorly but instead turns 45 degrees posteriorly, thus bringing the occiput into the hollow of the sacrum and the fetal chin under the symphysis. In this case, the chin impinges and the occiput is born first, bulging and sweeping over the perineum, and the head then is born by extension. External rotation then brings the anterior shoulder of the baby under the symphysis, and the remainder of the delivery proceeds normally.

Bibliography

1. Dennen, E.H. *Forceps Deliveries.* F.A. Davis, Philadelphia, 1955.
2. Oxorn, H., and Foote, W.R. *Human Labor and Birth*, ed. 3. Appleton—Century—Crofts, New York, 1975.
3. Taylor, E.S. *Beck's Obstetrical Practice*, ed. 8. Williams & Wilkins, Baltimore, 1966.

CHAPTER 35

Abnormal Lies, Presentations, and Positions

RONALD M. CAPLAN, M.D.

BREECH

The breech presentation has implications that are dangerous for the fetus. The head is the largest part of the fetus prior to and at term, and the presenting of another portion of the fetus to the pelvis in labor, especially in a primigravida, suggests the possibility of some degree of cephalopelvic disproportion. As the head, which is largest, comes last in a breech delivery, it is often impossible to be completely sure that the delivery can be easily completed until the body is out. Prematurity is often associated with breech presentation, and the relatively long and potentially asphyxiating breech delivery process has especially grave implications in these cases.

Delivery of the breech is a fluid, continuous process but may be considered in three stages: the birth of the buttocks, then the shoulders, followed by the head.

The key movements of the fetus in a breech presentation during labor are:

A. Buttocks
   1. Engagement
   2. Descent
   3. Flexion
   4. Internal rotation
   5. Lateral flexion

B. Shoulders
   6. Internal rotation
   7. Lateral flexion

C. Head
   8. Internal rotation
   9. Flexion.

During labor, the breech gradually and continuously descends. The breech has engaged when the bitrochanteric diameter is at the level of the pelvic inlet. Lateral flexion of the spine occurs so that the anterior hip leads. For a right or left sacrum anterior position, 45 degrees of rotation then occurs to bring the anterior hip under the pubic symphysis, so that the resulting position is right sacrotransverse (RST) or left sacrotransverse (LST).

With the anterior hip impinged under the symphysis, lateral flexion in the opposite direction to that previously described now occurs, so that the posterior hip is born first. As the spine straightens, the anterior hip is born.

The fetus then rotates 45 degrees back to the original oblique position, and with continuing descent the shoulders engage. As the anterior shoulder impinges under the symphysis, 45 degrees rotation back to RST or LST occurs. The posterior shoulder is born by lateral flexion, followed by the anterior shoulder.

As the head engages, rotation occurs so that the occiput impinges under the sacrum. The head is born by continuing flexion over the perineum, with the chin being born first.

Assisted Breech Delivery

The breech is allowed to deliver spontaneously to the inferior angles of the scapulae, keeping the external parts of the fetus wrapped in a warm towel, making sure the umbilical cord is not taut, and following the descending vertex down with the attendant's hand on the maternal abdomen to maintain flexion of the fetal head.

If the arms do not deliver spontaneously, they are delivered one at a time by sweeping the attendant's fingers in a splinting fashion across the fetal back and gently down along the humerus as rotation of the body occurs.

A Mauriceau-Smellie-Veit maneuver may then be carried out to create traction on the fetal shoulder area, while flexion of the head is maintained with the attendant's left hand (Fig. 35.1). An assistant continues to "follow" the fetal head with an examining hand on the maternal abdomen.

Breech Extraction

Active interference is commenced by the attendant prior to the appearance of the inferior angles of the fetal scapulae. Because of the enhanced possibility of damage and asphyxia to the fetus, it is not commonly utilized.

FACE PRESENTATION

In many cases, this position infers a significant degree of cephalopelvic disproportion, and cesarean section becomes the mode of delivery.

After extension, the mentum (chin) must internally rotate anteriorly under the symphysis and the head is born by increasing flexion, sweeping over the perineum.

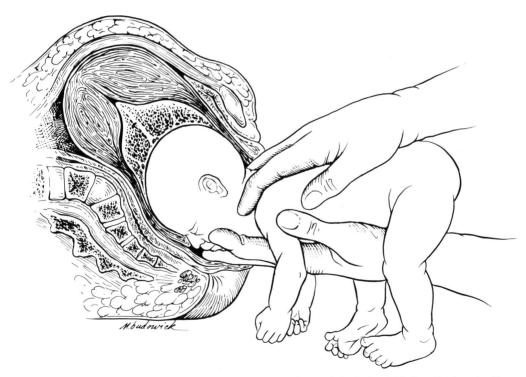

Figure 35.1.   The Mauriceau-Smellie-Veit maneuver. An assistant should follow the head with an examining hand on the maternal abdomen, to maintain flexion of the fetal head and to create fundal pressure to aid in delivery.

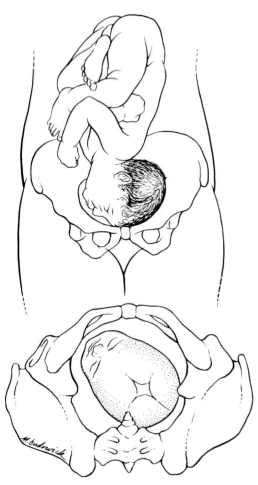

BROW PRESENTATION

Unless this presentation easily and spontaneously converts to either a vertex or a face presentation, cesarean section is the rule, as the presenting vertex-mental diameter measures 13.5 cm.

The frontum (forehead) presents. Vaginal delivery, although rarely advisable, is technically possible if the frontum rotates anteriorly, so that the occiput is posterior (Fig. 35.2).

TRANSVERSE AND OBLIQUE LIES

These abnormal lies are undeliverable vaginally if they do not convert to longitudinal lies. Therefore, cesarean section must be carried out.

Bibliography

1. Sweeney, W.J., Hawks, G.G., and Caplan, R.M. Breech presentation. In *Gynecology and Obstetrics*, edited by Gerbie, A.B., and Sciarra, J.J. Harper & Row, Hagerstown, MD, 1980, vol. 2, chap. 77.

Figure 35.2. Brow presentation. On vaginal examination, the anterior fontanelle and brow are palpable; the posterior fontanelle is not.

CHAPTER 36

Fetal Monitoring in Labor

ALAN BERKELEY, M.D.

In 1958 Edward Hon reported on a practical method for continuous electronic fetal heart rate monitoring (EFM). He suggested that dynamic monitoring of the fetal heart rate (FHR) could give more information about changes in the intrauterine environment than could single, isolated periods of listening. Since the introduction of monitoring, there have been many improvements in the hardware and an increase in our understanding of the meaning of the various patterns. Further refinements such as fetal pH determinations obtained from fetal scalp sampling have increased the ability to interpret monitoring data.

Each fetal monitor (Fig. 36.1) is a two-channel oscilloscope, one for fetal heart rate display and the other for uterine activity recording. The leads that plug into the monitors may be either external (from the maternal abdomen) or internal (from intrauterine leads placed after membranes are ruptured artificially or spontaneously).

EXTERNAL (INDIRECT) MONITORING

There are three types of abdominal transducers for FHR detection: Doppler ultrasound, phonocardiograph and fetal EKG. The ultrasound is the one most commonly used during labor and delivery (Fig. 36.2). Ultrasound waves that are reflected off moving surfaces undergo changes in frequency (Doppler effect) that can be converted to an electronic signal and then amplified. The transducer emits and receives ultrasound waves that change fre-

quency during their reflection from the cardiac valves; the motion of the heart valves becomes the basis for the calculation of the FHR. Since the motion of fetal valves appears during systole and diastole as movement toward and away from the transducer with each cardiac cycle, one could expect the monitor to count two beats for each one that actually exists because of the two changes in electronic frequency generated by the waves with each cycle. Therefore, there is a refractory period built into the monitors so that only "half" the beats are counted. One must remember that if the FHR slows below this refractory period, the monitor may falsely record double the true rate because both heart motions are not "seen." In addition, if the ultrasound beam is directed at a strong maternal pulse, it may preferentially record this rate rather than the fetal rate. One must always be careful to check that it is not the maternal pulse that is being recorded.

The second method of FHR detection involves phonocardiography. The closure of the fetal heart valves creates sounds that can be detected by a phonocardiographic transducer after electrical amplification. This abdominal microphone is quite accurate in its perception of the fetal heart sounds but unfortunately is also equally adept at picking up other ambient sounds such as maternal pulse or bowel sounds and fetal movement. For this reason it is not a useful method for a patient in active labor but may be appropriately used in antenatal testing where other noises can be controlled.

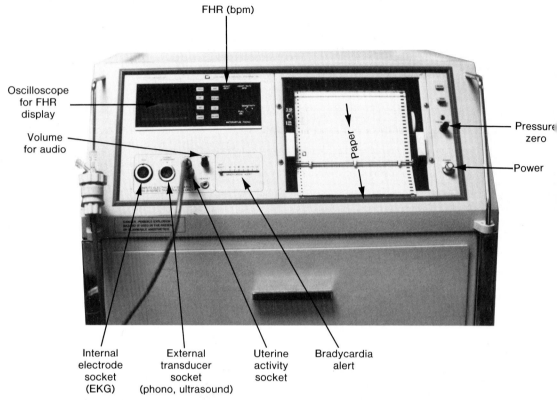

Figure 36.1.   Electronic fetal monitor (Corometrics Model 112).

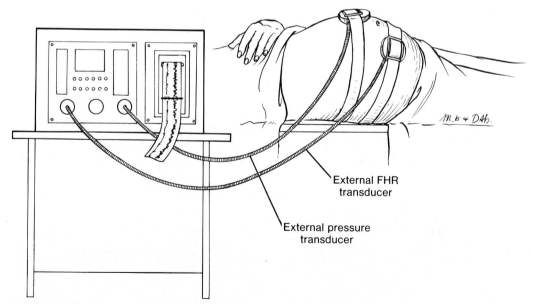

Figure 36.2.   Mother being externally monitored with both fetal heart rate and pressure transducers.

A third method of external auscultation is to obtain a fetal EKG tracing directly from the maternal abdomen. Since the fetal signal is of low amplitude, there can be difficulty in distinctly separating the fetal from the maternal EKG as well as from extraneous noise. Although potentially very accurate, this method has little application to patients in active labor.

An abdominal tocodynamometer is used in conjunction with the external FHR transducer. This tocodynamometer has either a diaphragm or plunger that senses uterine motion below the maternal abdominal wall; the sensor translates this motion into electrical energy and records the changes on an oscilloscope. This external transducer records only the presence and approximate duration of a contraction; it in no way measures the actual strength of a contraction. In the vast majority of cases, where there is no question of FHR abnormality and no other problems with the progress of labor, this external system is adequate for satisfactory monitoring. However, when a more accurate measure of activity is required, an internal system must be used.

The most important facets of external monitoring are proper placement of the leads and the recognition that maternal or fetal movement can alter previously good placements. With vertex presentations the FHR is usually heard best below the umbilicus, while in breech presentation it may be higher on the maternal abdomen. The external pressure transducer usually records best in the fundal area but, particularly in obese patients, it may be difficult to obtain a readable tracing. One must constantly guard against the impulse to restrain the laboring patient in a flat or supine position, leading to the supine hypotension syndrome and its complications. In this syndrome, the pregnant uterus compresses the inferior vena cava when the mother is supine; this leads to decreased venous return, decreased cardiac output, hypotension and decreased uterine blood flow, with resulting fetal compromise.

The only physical risk of external monitoring is supine hypotension. Much more serious can be the complications that some observers believe result from either the unnecessary or the misdirected application of external monitoring. As with any methodology, inappropriate use or misinterpretation of the derived information can lead to inappropriate actions. With appropriate physician and nursing education and with increased clinical experience, EFM can safely be applied to a wide variety of patient situations.

INTERNAL (DIRECT) MONITORING

Direct methods of FHR detection and contraction analysis are more accurate than indirect methods. In order to insert internal leads, membranes must be ruptured and the fetal position accurately identified. Errors in recognition of position can result in application of the scalp electrodes to vital fetal structures. For this reason the value of the information gained from direct methods should be weighed against potential risks. One must also not consider the internal scalp electrode and the uterine pressure catheter an inseparable pair. Each has its own indications and complications; their use should be individualized.

The fetal electrode is a spiral wire that can be applied to the fetal scalp and directly record the fetal EKG. The R-R interval is used as the basis for determining rate; the reciprocal of this R-R measurement is the FHR. The monitor records each R-R interval in milliseconds instantaneously so that an accurate recording of beat-to-beat change in FHR (variability) can be obtained by this method. Normally, the amplitude of the R wave is much larger than any other "noise" that can be detected by the electrode. Unless there is some abnormality of the fetal complex that causes the scalp electrode to fire on other than the R wave or on more than one component of the complex, the internal tracing will be very accurate and free from artifact. In the event of intrauterine fetal death, the transmission of the maternal R complex to the electrode is possible, with the subsequent recording of the maternal rate on the monitor tracing.

The complications of applying the electrode to the fetus include rare but occasionally serious fetal scalp infections, fetal hemorrhage and the problems with misapplication.

The indications for the use of the scalp electrode include all those situations in which adequate information cannot be obtained from the external leads. These include:

1. Evidence of fetal stress or distress on external leads
2. Decreased beat-to-beat variability
3. Meconium-stained fluid
4. External tracing of such poor quality that presence or absence of fetal stress or distress cannot be determined

Since in many cases membranes are intact, the decision to apply internal leads often involves a concomitant decision to artificially rupture membranes. One must, therefore, balance the expected increase in accuracy in information about fetal status against the risks of amniotomy, namely cord prolapse, infection and the possible deleterious effect on the fetus of removing its amniotic fluid cushion.

The most accurate method of measuring uterine activity is by use of a fluid-filled polyethylene catheter inserted between the fetal head and the uterine wall. The intrauterine end of the catheter has many small openings; once the catheter is filled with sterile water, the pressure inside the closed fluid-filled space of the uterus is transmitted directly through the catheter to the diaphragm of a strain gauge. The motion of the diaphragm is converted to an electrical potential that can be displayed on the monitor tracing in millimeters of mercury.

Indications for the insertion of an internal pressure catheter include:

1. FHR abnormalities that require an internal catheter for correct interpretation of their timing
2. Abnormalities in the pattern of labor
3. The administration of oxytocin

Complications of insertion have been reported. Trauma to the fetus is extremely rare. More common are uterine injuries such as perforation. Placental abruption can be produced if the catheter is inadvertently introduced between the placenta and the uterine wall. There has been controversy about whether the internal leads, particularly the catheter, cause an increase in intrauterine infection. The multiplicity of confounding variables such as duration of ruptured membranes, number of examinations and ultimate mode of delivery make any definitive statement difficult. In Haverkamp's prospective trial comparing electronically monitored (internal) with nonelectronically monitored patients, no difference was found in either maternal or fetal infection rates. Ledger, however, suggested that the infection rate may be higher in the monitored group, particularly in those patients who ultimately undergo cesarean delivery. For these reasons, the decision to insert a pressure catheter should be taken seriously and not be routine with every patient.

The technique of insertion of the catheter is extremely important. In most institutions, the perineum is sterilely prepared and draped. If the patient has had an ultrasound examination and the placental location is known, an attempt can be made to avoid this area of the uterine cavity. A firm plastic introducer is placed about 1 cm inside the posterior aspect of the cervical os (which needs to be only minimally dilated) and then the softer, more malleable catheter is introduced through it. Approximately 18 inches of catheter are inserted. Most catheters have a mark 18 inches from the tip to prevent introduction of excessive catheter length. If any resistance is met, the catheter should not be forced, but rather the location of insertion should be changed from the usual posterior half of the cervix to a more anterior portion of the cervix. The catheter should be flushed before insertion. The catheter is then attached to the strain gauge via a three-way stopcock with the strain gauge placed at the level of the catheter tip (Fig. 36.3). Discrepancies between the height of the gauge and the patient will lead to either

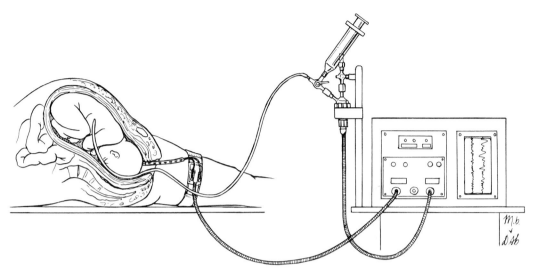

Figure 36.3. Mother being internally monitored with both scalp electrode and intrauterine pressure catheter.

falsely high or low values on the pressure readings. Once the circuit is complete, the stopcock should be opened to air so that atmospheric pressure can be used as a reference point for zero intrauterine pressure. Then direct communication between the catheter tip and the strain gauge is established. In most patients there is a baseline tone of 5–15 mm Hg, with contractions registering 25–100 mm Hg. If the patient is experiencing contractions that are not being appreciated by the monitor, one must systematically check the various components to make sure each is working; occasionally the line is kinked and simply withdrawing it a few centimeters will correct the problem. Rarely, the entire catheter needs to be removed and replaced. The scalp electrode is placed after the catheter so as not to displace an already attached scalp electrode.

FETAL HEART RATE PATTERNS

Most monitor paper in the United States is divided into two sections. The horizontal axis on both sections measures time, with each 3 cm representing 1 minute (some machines have a 1 cm/minute option). The lower (or right-sided as one faces the monitor) grid has a vertical scale from 0 to 100

mm Hg that is valid only for the internal lead. The upper (left-sided) grid is for recording FHR from 30 to 240, with divisions every 30 beats. Above 240 beats per minute, the R-R interval becomes so short that the built-in logic will often halve the rate because two beats occur before the programmed refractory period ends.

The major difficulty in interpreting these tracings involves the FHR; many studies have shown that a normal tracing is a very good predictor of fetal well-being. The key to successful management in labor is the recognition of the meaning of deviations from normal. A normal FHR (Fig. 36.4) varies between 120 and 160 beats per minute (bpm), has a short-term beat-to-beat variability of 3–5 bpm and has a long-term cyclicity of 3–5 cycles per minute. In addition, a healthy fetus often increases its heart rate in response to its movements; this information is the basis of antenatal nonstress testing. Deviations from normal include:

1. Early deceleration (head compression pattern, type I)
2. Late deceleration (uteroplacental insufficiency pattern, type II)
3. Variable deceleration (cord pattern, type III)

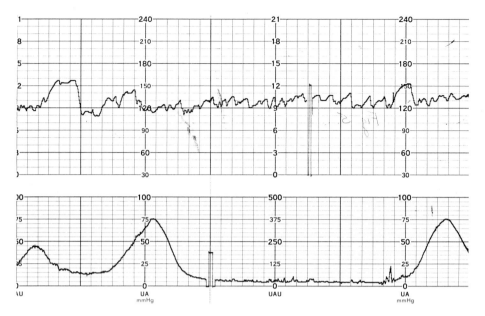

Figure 36.4.   Normal tracing. Baseline FHR = 130 bpm, with short-term beat-to-beat variability of 3–5 bpm and good cyclicity. There are accelerations with movement and contractions. Uterine activity is excellent, with contractions of 75 mm Hg and low baseline tone.

4. Baseline tachycardia
5. Baseline bradycardia
6. Loss of variability
7. Prolonged bradycardia
8. Fetal arrhythmia
9. Artifactual changes in variability

The FHR is the result of the interplay of the sympathetic and parasympathetic systems in the fetus, with normal short-term beat-to-beat variability dependent on this continuous interaction. This can be demonstrated by giving atropine to the mother to effect fetal vagal blockade. There will be a fairly rapid increase in baseline FHR, with a loss of short-term variability. In addition, accelerations will appear with each contraction, suggesting a sympathetic betamimetic effect that had been inhibited by the vagus. If one now gives propanolol, a beta blocker, these accelerations will disappear and there will be a decrease in the FHR. There is also evidence that the FHR is under central control, as various types of brain injuries and anomalies can lead to a decrease in beat-to-beat variability.

Early Decelerations (Fig. 36.5)

As originally described by Hon, these head compression patterns or type I decelerations were felt to be the direct result of increased intracranial pressure, with concomitant decreased cerebral blood flow leading to vagal stimulation. This symmetrical deceleration usually coincides with the onset and cessation of a uterine contraction; on the monitor strip, the contraction and deceleration often "mirror" each other. Most studies of fetal acid-base status suggest that this type of change is not associated with hypoxia or acidosis and requires no therapy. They are most prominent during active labor and during the second stage of labor.

Late Decelerations (Fig. 36.6)

Maternal-fetal oxygen exchange occurs in the intervillous blood space. With each uterine contraction there is a decrease in uterine blood flow and, secondarily, oxygen exchange. If this decrease is enough to cause fetal hypoxemia with or without

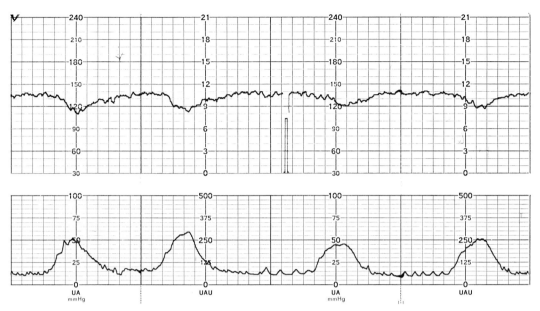

Figure 36.5.   Head compression pattern (type I deceleration) of patient in active labor. Note that decelerations are uniform in shape and "mirror" the contractions. Their onset is with the start of a contraction and they finish with the end of the contraction. There is a slight decrease in variability in this tracing secondary to the recent administration of a narcotic analgesic.

acidemia, a late deceleration based on uteroplacental insufficiency will occur. This acute insult with each contraction should be differentiated from chronic insufficiency states such as intrauterine growth retardation associated with hypertension. The deceleration is traditionally late in onset in relation to the start of the contraction and returns to baseline after the end of the contraction; the return to baseline tends to be gradual. The basis for this deceleration is probably initially a reflex fetal baroreceptor and chemoreceptor response, leading to parasympathetic stimulation and later direct myocardial depression in the presence of acidemia. One cannot tell simply by looking at the tracing which mechanism is predominant (that is, whether or not acidemia is present). However, late decelerations are an indication of fetal stress, and it is up to the obstetrician to determine if distress is present.

Variable Decelerations (Fig. 36.7)

This pattern, so named because of its variable onset and disappearance in rela-tion to uterine contractions, is felt to be a result of umbilical cord compression during uterine contractions. Again, there may be multiple mechanisms at work, and the degree of abnormality may be modified by the amount of amniotic fluid present. The degree of abnormality also depends upon whether the occlusion compromises blood flow in the umbilical vein or artery or both. With umbilical vein compression there is decreased return to the fetal circulation, with hypovolemia, stimulation of baroreceptor and a reflex FHR acceleration. When the artery is occluded there is fetal hypertension, leading to parasympathetic vagal slowing of the FHR. In addition, the decreased blood flow through the cord may lead to fetal hypoxemia and myocardial depression. The retention of CO_2 also contributes to fetal acidosis. Therefore, the more severe form of variable decelerations may be associated with fetal distress and thus requires further investigation. Variable decelerations have arbitrarily been classified as mild, moderate or severe. Mild decelerations last less than 30 seconds ir-

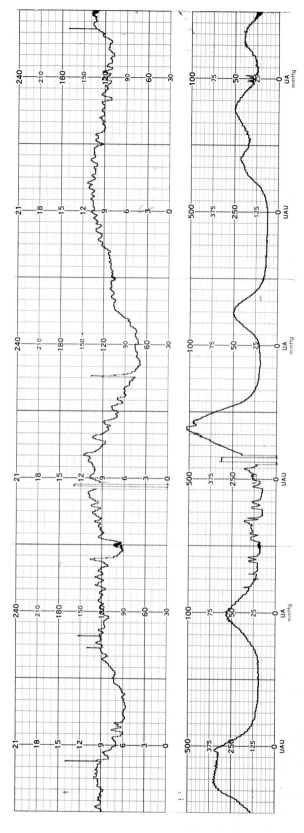

Figure 36.6. Uteroplacental insufficiency pattern or late deceleration (type II deceleration) during active labor. Onset is after the peak of the contraction and the return to baseline is gradual and occurs after the contraction is finished. Note that with a particularly strong 100 mm Hg contraction, the deceleration is severe. This type of tracing would be an indication for either scalp sampling or delivery, if possible.

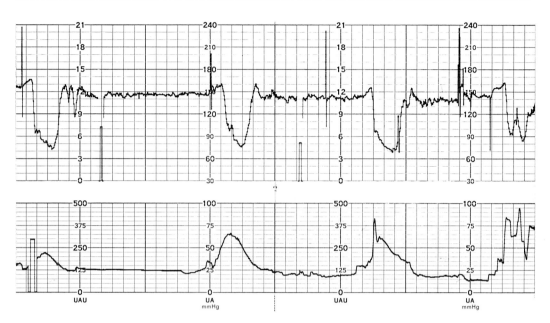

Figure 36.7. Cord compression pattern or variable deceleration (type III) in early labor. Note rapid drop in rate after initial short increase. The return to baseline is rapid. Each deceleration lasts 30–35 seconds and would be classified as "mild" variable deceleration. One might expect that as labor progresses, these patterns would become worse, particularly if there were a nuchal cord or occult cord prolapse.

respective of rate. Severe last 60 or more seconds and fall to 60 bpm or less. In between these two extremes fall the moderate changes.

Baseline Tachycardia

While minimal elevations of the FHR can be variants of normal, rates above 170 certainly need to be investigated. Although parasympatholytic and betamimetic agents (like atropine and ritodrine) have this effect, usually one has to rule out maternal infection or illness (chorioamnionitis or hyperthyroidism). Only rarely does this change represent fetal disease (heart failure, anemia or tachyarrhythmia). The tachycardia may also be one of the signs of fetal hypoxia, before decelerations appear.

Baseline Bradycardia

This condition is not as common as tachycardia. Moderate bradycardia of 100–120 usually represents a variant of normal when it occurs without decelerations or loss of variability. Rates below 100 are abnormal and should be investigated. With the loss of variability, they may represent severe fetal compromise and require immediate intervention. Rarely, bradycardia may indicate fetal heart block which can be shown by fetal EKG.

Loss of Variability (Fig. 36.8)

It is now accepted that the presence of beat-to-beat variability is one of the most reassuring patterns of fetal well-being. The presence of variability is considered to be a sign of an intact central and autonomic nervous system and adequate fetal reserve. There has been controversy about the relative importance of variability and decelerations, with some authors of the opinion that loss of variability is a more ominous sign than all but the worst decelerations. Conversely, an increase in variability may be the earliest sign of distress as the reflex increase in vagal tone predominates in the short term until the more severe effects of hypoxemia become apparent. Loss of var-

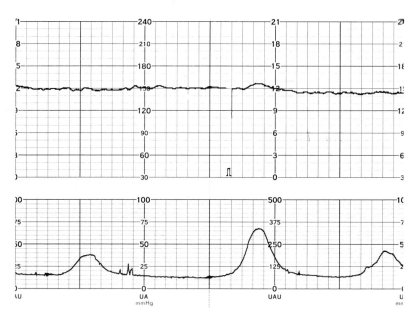

Figure 36.8. Decreased short- and long-term variability. Baseline FHR = 150 bpm. Note flatness with beat-to-beat change of only 1–2 bpm and scant to absent cyclicity. There is acceleration of 10 bpm with some of the contractions.

iability, in and of itself, is not an indication for any immediate action; however, it is a major warning signal and in some situations (such as the presence of meconium-stained fluid) may be an indication for fetal scalp sampling.

Prolonged Decelerations

These are sustained decelerations of longer than 2 minutes duration, with a rate of less then 100 bpm and usually with a loss of variability. The two most common causes on most delivery services are hypertonus during oxytocin stimulation and supine hypotension with or without epidural anesthesia (Fig. 36.9). This deceleration can also be seen with placental abruption and the administration of a paracervical block. The treatment of this disorder is the correction or elimination of the underlying cause. The appearance of an unexplained prolonged bradycardia during an antenatal stress test may also have ominous implications.

Fetal Arrhythmias

The monitor is capable of recording some abnormalities of rhythm. Because of the logic program built into the monitors, many of the external systems will have difficulty picking up all but the most obvious of changes. Complete heart block with rates of less than 80 must be distinguished from a severe bradycardia or the transmission of a maternal pulse with a fetal death (Fig. 36.10). This can be done by simultaneous auscultation with a head stethoscope and palpation of the maternal pulse. Fetal paroxysmal atrial tachycardia (PAT) can also be appreciated at least until the rate exceeds 250 bpm when the machine may halve the true rate. Less serious changes like atrial premature contractions (APCs) and ventricular premature contractions (VPCs) may be diagnosed with certainty only by direct fetal EKG analysis.

Artificial Changes in Variability

Each of the three types of external transducers has a problem correctly evaluating the beat-to-beat variability. As perceived by an ultrasound transducer, the "variability" of cardiac motion often creates a false impression of FHR short-term variability where little or none exists. Attempts have been made to "edit" this false beat-

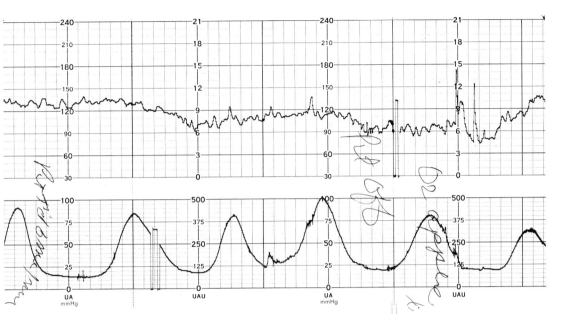

Figure 36.9. Sustained 6-minute bradycardia with hyperstimulation during oxytocin augmentation of labor. Strong 75–100 mm Hg contractions occur every 90 seconds, with less than 1 minute return to baseline tone between contractions. Once the bradycardia is recognized, the oxytocin is discontinued, O₂ applied and the patient turned to her left side. The tracing then returns to normal.

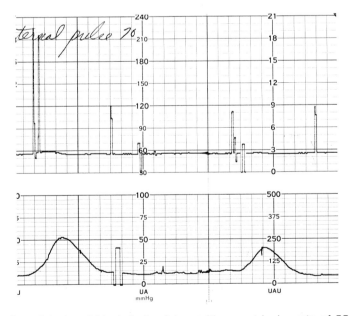

Figure 36.10. Complete heart block in the fetus, with a ventricular rate of 55. Note complete lack of variability. This diagnosis was confirmed by fetal EKG. Note that maternal rate is 70. This fetus was delivered vaginally and did well.

to-beat variability by various methods of computer averaging of each beat with several preceding beats. However, the only conclusion one can draw from an external ultrasound tracing is that an absence of variability is probably true while its presence may or may not be. Because of the accuracy of phonocardiographic perception of fetal sounds, there is rarely evidence of FHR variability when none exists. The abdominal EKG has a different problem caused by coincidence in the occurrence of fetal and maternal beats; accurate counting of the fetal rate is dependent on subtracting the maternal rate. When the two coincide, the computer logic built into the monitor creates a new R-R interval equal to the prior one, thus giving the impression of less variability than may actually exist.

MONITORING IN LABOR

Since its introduction approximately 20 years ago, EFM has gained wide acceptance among a large segment of obstetricians. However, a vocal and thoughtful minority of observers have raised many questions about the safety and efficacy of monitoring. There is no uniform agreement about who should be monitored, ranging from the belief that optimally everyone should be monitored to those who believe monitoring is totally an electronic infringement on what should be a natural event. However, at this time certain fairly definite conclusions can be made:

1. In large series in multiple centers and with differing patient populations, there is a consistent decrease in intrapartum fetal death from about 1.5/1000 to 0.5/1000.
2. While there are certain patients who are at extremely high-risk for complications in labor on any given delivery service, a significant proportion of untoward events will occur in patients designated as low-risk.
3. While there is probably a benefit to monitoring high-risk labors, there is still disagreement as to whether or not the low-risk parturient requires monitoring. In the often-quoted studies by Haverkamp, three groups of patients were studied: an internally monitored group, an internally monitored group where scalp sampling was used to furth. evaluate abnormal patterns and a third group observed closely by trained labor nurses. The maternal and neonatal outcomes were the same for all groups; the cesarean rates were higher in the electronically monitored group (intermediate when sampling was used). Two other prospective studies suggest a benefit to the monitored patient. Clearly, more study is required.
4. In almost all hospitals after monitoring is introduced, there is a dramatic increase in the cesarean section rate for the first few years, followed by a gradual decline as doctors become more familiar with the various patterns and equipment. Opponents of monitoring have called many of these cesareans unnecessary.
5. Monitors are only a tool; they in no way replace physician judgment; in fact, they may even demand a more advanced level of obstetrical judgment. One can never replace the need for bedside evaluation of both maternal and fetal status and appropriate interpretation of all information.

Taking all this information into account, a solid argument could be made for monitoring all patients in labor. At the minimum, the following would be a partial list of indications for patients who definitely should be monitored.

1. Patients with abnormal fetoscopic auscultatory findings
2. Abnormal fetal presentations
3. Abnormal labor patterns
4. Meconium-stained amniotic fluid
5. Patients with poor prior obstetric outcome
6. Patients with high-risk medical conditions such as diabetes, hyperten-

sion, hemoglobinopathies, asthma, bleeding disorders, and heart disease

7. Patients with abnormal antenatal test results

8. Patients with obstetric complications such as preeclampsia, placental abruption, placenta praevia, premature labor, premature rupture of membranes, prematurity and postmaturity

FETAL SCALP SAMPLING

It should be increasingly obvious that even with a thorough understanding of all the mechanisms of abnormal monitor patterns, there is still great difficulty in differentiating fetal stress from distress. In the continuum of fetal metabolic changes, it is clear that some tracing abnormalities involve neither hypoxemia nor acidemia while others involve both. In an attempt to distinguish these various possibilities, the technique of fetal capillary scalp sampling was developed. The indications for scalp sampling include those cases in which vaginal delivery is not imminent and the monitor tracing has evidence of fetal distress, most often severe variable or late decelerations with loss of variability. The requirements for performing this test are ruptured membranes and a cervix dilated enough (about 3–4 cm) to admit the cone-shaped introducer.

When performing this test (Fig. 36.11), one should not lose sight of the stress it represents to the mother. She is laboring, often in pain and apprehensive about herself and her child. She will need to be in either the lithotomy or the lateral Sims position (where there is less risk of supine hypotension). After the cone and light source have been introduced (and only after one is sure the lab is ready to perform blood gas determination) the scalp is cleansed, dried with silicon gel to promote beading of the blood sample, punctured with a standard 2-mm blade and blood is collected in a heparinized capillary tube.

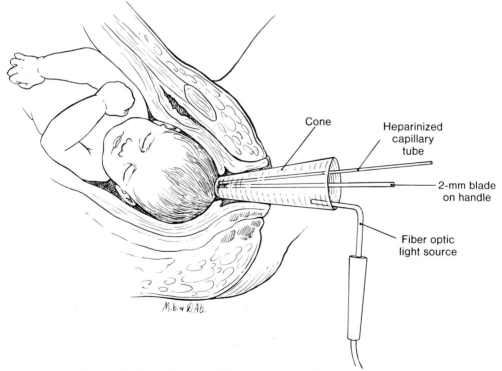

Cone

Heparinized capillary tube

2-mm blade on handle

Fiber optic light source

Figure 36.11.   Diagram of fetal scalp sampling with cone in vagina.

Pressure must be applied afterward to be sure there is no bleeding, as small blood volumes represent significant blood loss to the fetus, particularly if it is compromised. Even after the instruments have been removed from the vagina, one must be alert to unusual bleeding.

The physiologic basis for scalp sampling is that with hypoxemia the fetus, like the adult, utilizes anaerobic metabolism, with the production of lactic acid and the consumption of the buffer base. Unique to the fetus is a "respiratory" component with umbilical cord compression leading to CO_2 retention, although in this instance there is usually no consumption of buffer base. Normal fetal pH is usually 7.25–7.35, about 0.1 less than normal maternal pH. Levels below 7.20 are considered definitely abnormal, with 7.20–7.25 the borderline zone. If one does the sample during a contraction when CO_2 is being retained, one could obtain an acidotic value, but if base excess is determined it would be near normal— warning that the problem is respiratory rather than metabolic acidosis. Comparison must also be made with maternal pH to make sure that the values from the fetus do not represent metabolic changes in the mother rather than intrinsic fetal problems. What is most important of all is to realize that metabolic changes are not single-point events but rather part of a continuum of change; therefore, serial samples are needed to evaluate trends or continuing abnormalities.

There has been fairly accurate correlation between EFM, scalp pH and neonatal outcome. Occasionally, local tissue edema can cause falsely low pH values, sometimes respiratory and metabolic changes are confused, and often the time from obtaining the sample until delivery is so long that the conditions that pertained at the time of the sample no longer apply. In general, those fetuses with lower scalp pH are more likely to have low apgar scores at 1 and 5 minutes than are fetuses with normal pH. It is the fetuses with severe variable or late decelerations with loss of variability that are most likely to have low pH.

For the future, work is now being done with continuous scalp pH or oxygen electrodes. The benefit of a continuous reading of fetal metabolic status is apparent. Two major problems need to be overcome before this will become a practical approach. First, there is a practical problem of refining a continuous pH electrode that can safely be applied to the fetal scalp during labor. Most of the present prototypes have glass components and can break in the fetal scalp. Assuming that this problem will ultimately be worked out, there is still some question whether scalp pH represents central pH, particularly in the presence of marked caput succedaneum. It has been argued that the scalp samples may give falsely low pH values, particularly as labor advances. One could hope that in the near future some type of more aesthetic and practical method of evaluating fetal metabolic status will be developed. With experience, the obstetrician can be fairly accurate in the interpretation of monitor patterns, but there are always situations in which more definitive data would be of extreme value.

MANAGEMENT OF ABNORMAL FHR PATTERNS

Once the decision to monitor has been made, one must have a plan in mind for the management of abnormalities if they should arise. The preceding discussion has pointed out the basis for many of the patterns that are commonly seen; the following is a plan of action for the evaluation of fetal distress that will be generally applicable for most patients.

1. If the signs of distress are externally derived, one should apply an internal scalp electrode if the membranes are ruptured; if membranes are intact, one must decide if the abnormality justifies artifical rupture of membranes. If one is faced with severe variable decelerations or late decelerations with loss of variability and a cervix that is closed with a high presenting part, abdominal delivery may be indicated. If there is any question

about the timing of decelerations or the accuracy of the pressure tracing, an internal catheter should be inserted.

2. Underlying maternal disease that can compromise fetal status, such as uncontrolled hypertension or diabetes, requires treatment.

3. The mother should be turned on her side (preferably left side) if she has been supine; if she is hypotensive, IV hydration is also required.

4. If the patterns are compatible with hypoxemia in the fetus, oxygen in high concentration should be administered by mask to the mother.

5. One should carefully evaluate possible iatrogenic causes of distress. If augmentation of labor with oxytocin is being carried out, the oxytocin should be discontinued until the distress is resolved.

6. If there has been a recent epidural anesthetic, one should be alert to relative hypovolemia and hypotension. Correction of these changes with hydration, change in position and possible drug therapy are indicated.

7. If narcotic analgesics have been used, consideration should be given to their deleterious effect on FHR variability.

8. Vaginal examination should be performed to check cervical dilatation and to rule out cord prolapse. If frank or occult cord prolapse is diagnosed, the patient should be placed in Trendelenburg position and cesarean section done.

9. If abnormal patterns persist despite all these maneuvers, one must assess the feasibility of obtaining a scalp sample. If scalp sampling is either impossible or not available and delivery is not imminent, one should consider immediate abdominal delivery if there are severe variable or late decelerations. If sampling is performed, a pH above 7.25 will be very reassuring; however, if the abnormal patterns persist, repeat samples every 30–45 minutes may be necessary to reconfirm the normalcy of the fetal

environment. Values below 7.20 (after checking maternal pH) are an indication for immediate delivery by the most appropriate route. Intermediate values require repetition of the sample until either resolution of the problem or delivery.

The goal of this management plan should be the delivery of a nonacidotic infant. No purpose is served in chemically documenting the progression from a stressed fetus to a frankly distressed one. One should intervene before severe acidosis is present. In addition, if severe acidosis is documented but an underlying etiology for the acidosis is also present, it may be appropriate to delay or even avoid an emergency delivery until "intrauterine resuscitation" has been attempted and evaluated. This resuscitation may include many or all of the maneuvers listed above. There are also now reports of the use of betamimetic agents in these situations in an attempt to increase uterine blood flow by decreasing uterine activity.

Although the intrauterine pressure catheter is usually used to help evaluate abnormalities in the progress of labor, occasionally its placement is required to aid in accurately delineating the relationship of the decelerations to the contractions; often, abnormal progress is associated with fetal stress or distress and the indication for insertion of the catheter will be doubly strong.

Placement of the catheter can be of benefit in other ways. It is often difficult to adequately assess uterine activity; a patient's obesity or high or low pain tolerance can make this assessment even more difficult. The early placement of the catheter will eliminate unnecessary delays in stimulating labor with oxytocin as well as identify those situations in which the addition of oxytocin might be of little benefit. On occasion, the pressure tracing will indicate either baseline tone (above 25 mm Hg) or hyperstimulation secondary to oxytocin, and reduction or discontinuation of the oxytocin will result in a more normal labor pattern.

The advent of monitoring has given us the opportunity to constantly assess fetal status. The controversies about its possible abuse in certain situations should not obscure its definitive value in preventing intrapartum death and chronic distress not appreciated by auscultation alone. As physicians become more familiar with all aspects of monitoring, the benefits from its widespread use should become even more apparent.

Bibliography

1. Banta, H.D., and Thacker, S.B. Costs and benefits of electronic fetal monitoring: A review of the literature. Department of H.E.W. publication (PHS) 79–3245.
2. Freeman, R.K., and Garite, T.J. *Fetal Heart Rate Monitoring*. Williams & Wilkins, Baltimore, 1981.
3. Gassner, C.B., and Ledger, W.J. The relationship of hospital-acquired maternal infection to invasive intrapartum monitoring techniques. *Am. J. Obstet. Gynecol. 126*:33, 1976.
4. Haverkamp, A.D., et al. A controlled trial of the differential effects of intrapartum fetal monitoring. *Am. J. Obstet. Gynecol. 134*:399, 1979.
5. Hon, E.H. The electronic evaluation of the fetal heart rate. *Am. J. Obstet. Gynecol. 75*:1215, 1958.
6. Kelso, I.M., et al. An assessment of continuous fetal heart rate monitoring in labor: A randomized trial. *Am. J. Obstet. Gynecol. 131*:526, 1978.
7. Klavan, M., Laver, A., and Boscola, M. *Clinical Concepts of Fetal Heart Rate Monitoring*. Hewlett-Packard Company, 1977.
8. Quilligan, E.J. Identifying true fetal distress. *Contemp. Obstet. Gynecol. 13*:89, 1979.
9. Renou, P., et al. Controlled trial of fetal intensive care. *Am. J. Obstet. Gynecol. 126*:470, 1976.
10. Tejani, N., et al. Correlation of fetal heart rate—uterine contraction patterns with fetal scalp blood pH. *Obstet. Gynecol. 46*:392, 1975.
11. Williams, R.L., and Hawes, W. Cesarean section, fetal monitoring and perinatal mortality in California. *Am. J. Public Health 69*:864, 1979.

CHAPTER 37

Analgesia and Anesthesia

EDWINA SIA-KHO, M.D.

Obstetrical analgesia and anesthesia differ from surgical anesthesia in a number of ways. There are two lives to consider and monitor.

Labor requires prolonged analgesia. Since all drugs pass the placental barrier freely, dosages should be the least that will provide maximum analgesia without affecting the fetal welfare.

The danger of vomiting and aspiration is increased in the obstetrical patient. Patients come to the hospital at any time. They are apprehensive and uncomfortable and often unable to cooperate. The anesthesiologist sees them for the first time when they come in already in labor.

The modern trend of obstetric analgesia and anesthesia is to have an alert baby and a pain free, happy mother who is conscious and participating in the birth of her baby. A properly managed labor and delivery is a rewarding experience for the mother.

The relief of pain in labor depends on many factors. Medications play an important role, but psychological factors are equally important. There has been increased emphasis in recent years on preparation for childbirth, not only of the mother but also of the father, who can assist and support his wife in labor. Several methods have been used to try to avoid medications during labor and delivery: hypnosis, psychoprophylaxis, the method of Lamaze, acupuncture and natural childbirth. The breathing exercises, so popular in the childbirth preparation class, use positive conditioning by teaching the woman to focus her eyes on a specific location during contraction and maintain a proper breathing rhythm as coached by her husband. She also learns the voluntary control of her abdominal pelvic muscles.

These exercises have helped most women pass through the early stages of labor; in the later stages as the cervix is increasingly dilated and there is more distention, pain, and pressure, the patients often become fatigued or lose control and they require some form of analgesia. Even when they do not need any medication during labor, many women require local infiltration of the perineum, pudendal block, nitrous oxide supplement, or regional anesthesia for delivery.

Not all mothers and babies benefit from natural childbirth. The breathing exercises can produce hyperventilation in overzealous patients. Severe hyperventilation produces nausea, vomiting, light-headedness or dizziness. It can lead to respiratory alkalosis associated with a decreased cerebral blood flow and decreased uterine blood flow. A decreased cerebral blood flow can produce carpopedal spasm and tetany in the mother; a decreased uterine blood flow causes hypoxia and metabolic acidosis in the fetus.

Epidural analgesia can reverse all these effects. Shnider et al. showed that maternal stress in labor increases the plasma norepinephrine level. Uterine blood flow is reduced and there is inefficient contraction of the uterus. When pain is decreased by epidural analgesia, the patient's uterine contractions become coordinated and active. Therefore, analgesia can avoid unnecessarily traumatic experiences during childbirth and also can be used in the management of uncoordinated labor.

In dealing with the anesthetic management of obstetrical patients, there are two syndromes of importance: the Mendelson syndrome, or acid aspiration syndrome, and the supine hypotensive syndrome, or aortocaval compression syndrome.

MENDELSON'S SYNDROME

In 1946 Mendelson described the aspiration of stomach contents into the lungs during general anesthesia for obstetrics without a protected airway. This syndrome is characterized by cyanosis, bronchospasm, tachycardia, rales, expiratory wheezing and hypotension, which may prove fatal if not treated instantaneously.

The low pH of gastric juice (about 1.5) produces tracheobronchial tree changes, resulting in an increase in pulmonary vascular resistance, with outpouring of plasma-like fluids from the respiratory epithelium into the lungs, leading to hypoxia. The PO_2 falls to 40–50 torr. The pathology shows marked peribronchiolar exudative reaction, with interstitial hemorrhage and edema.

While aspiration of gastric juice is dangerous, aspiration of gastric contents can be fatal. The patient can die on the delivery table from obstruction of the airway. (Patients have been known to regurgitate undigested food eaten days before labor began.)

The tendency to aspiration pneumonitis is enhanced by the anatomical and physiological changes of pregnancy. The increased level of progesterone in pregnancy relaxes the cardioesophageal junction. Gastric motility is decreased and there is an increase in acid and chloride in the stomach. The gravid uterus pushes the intestinal cavity up toward the diaphragm, retarding the evacuation of gastric contents. It also produces an incompetent cardioesophageal sphincter, unable to resist regurgitation. In addition to these physiological factors, narcotics and sedatives administered during labor also delay gastric emptying time, and fear, anxiety and the stress of labor inhibit gastric emptying time. The lithotomy position, often used during vaginal delivery, increases intragastric pressure. The supine hypotensive syndrome or hypotension from any cause also produces nausea and vomiting. General anesthetics abolish the laryngeal reflexes and there is danger of silent regurgitation of food.

Recent advances in obstetrical anesthesia include a routine antacid regimen for patients in labor and before cesarean section. Antacid brings the gastric pH to more than the critical level of 2.5. At least 30 minutes must be allowed for the antacid to dilute the gastric juice. Antacids also relax the pylorus and increase gastric motility, thus speeding gastric emptying time. If aspiration occurs and pneumonitis ensues, it is a milder form if antacids were given preoperatively. Patients usually remain clinically well.

Modern anesthetic practice for obstetrics favors regional or local anesthesia, but if general anesthesia must be used, an endotracheal tube is mandatory.

Maternal aspiration pneumonitis is still the number one cause of maternal mortality and morbidity due to anesthesia. The statistics have improved in recent years because of recognition of the Mendelson syndrome and methods for its prevention, but aspiration and its consequences still occur, often following a difficult intubation.

AORTOCAVAL COMPRESSION

Pregnant women near term manifest hypotension when lying supine on their back. The first symptom is nausea or vomiting, or the woman appears pale and sweating. This hypotension is caused by compression of the inferior vena cava by the gravid uterus, impeding venous return to the heart and causing a fall in cardiac output. The condition is often called the supine hypotensive syndrome.

In 1968 Bieniarz et al. demonstrated that aside from the vena caval occlusion there is also uterine compression of the aorta which begins at the level of L1 and reaches its maximum at the level of L4 and L5 at the area of lumbar lordosis. Since then, the syndrome also became known as aortocaval compression. In addition to the nausea, women manifest tachycardia (or bradycardia if a high regional block has been used), dizziness, vertigo, irritability and central nervous system ischemia. All these symptoms are due to one cause—hypotension.

The accepted systolic blood pressure for maintenance of adequate placental uterine perfusion is 100 torr. Any drop in pressure below this may produce these symptoms. Usually, a compensatory increase in peripheral resistance and an increase in the ovarian uterine arterial anastomosis around the site of compression will maintain the maternal blood pressure. This compensatory mechanism gives a false sense of security because occlusion of the aorta and vena cava is "concealed." The fetus is at risk, because there is still a compression of the aorta which causes uterine hypoperfusion. If maternal hypotension and uterine hypoperfusion persist, the result is asphyxia and fetal acidosis.

All these symptoms are reversible by a simple maneuver. Turn the woman to the left side to relieve the compression of the aorta and vena cava. Symptoms disappear once the patient is turned. All obstetrical patients should lie on their left side or at least at a 20–30 degree left lateral tilt during labor and delivery, especially in the presence of exaggerating factors such as anesthesia and surgery.

General anesthesia causes widespread vasodilatation. Epidural, caudal and spinal anesthesia, with resultant sympathetic block, produce vasodilatation of the lower limbs due to the loss of autonomic vasoconstrictor reflexes normally present in the lower half of the body. Positioning of the patient for surgery or manipulation of the uterus may cause greater compression, sudden bleeding and loss of vasomotor tone. The patient may be unable to compensate for this increased hypotension.

The dangers of neglected aortocaval occlusion are placental abruption, acute circulatory collapse and profound shock. Prevention is simply turning the patient to the left. Additional measures are rapid infusion of intravenous fluids, oxygen, and elevation of the patient's legs to permit autotransfusion. A vasopressor such as ephedrine, 10–15 mg, can be given intravenously as a last resort.

SYSTEMIC MEDICATIONS

Systemic medications are used during the early first stage of labor. Narcotics are the main drugs used, while sedatives or tranquilizers are added to potentiate the action of the narcotics. Tranquilizers and sedatives do not have analgesic effects; they are used only to allay anxiety. If they are used alone they produce only sedation and not pain relief, and during a contraction the patient may become disoriented and uncontrollable. Narcotics cause respiratory depression in the mother and newborn, while sedatives and tranquilizers cause sedation in the mother and newborn. Both types of drugs can produce changes in the neurobehavioral response of newborns.

The commonly used drugs are narcotics (Demerol, etc.) and sedative-tranquilizers (Valium, barbiturates).

Demerol (Meperidine Hydrochloride, Pethidine)

Of all the narcotics, Demerol is the most commonly used drug. It causes fewer side effects and has a shorter duration of action when compared with morphine.

Although Demerol is widely used, it is not effective in relieving labor pain completely. About 70–80% of patients feel less pain during contractions. The remainder have partial relief and they are drowsy between contractions due to the sedative effect of Demerol.

The most common side effects of Demerol are nausea and vomiting, due to the drug's stimulation of the chemoreceptor zones. Milder effects are dizziness, giddiness, flushing, sweating, vertigo and dry mouth. Although intravenous administration of Demerol is considered a more reliable route, nausea and vomiting are seen more frequently after intravenous administration.

Maternal hypotension (and especially postural hypotension) is another common side effect of Demerol, probably as a result of peripheral vasodilatation and decreased peripheral resistance. If the hypotension persists, it can diminish oxygen transport and uterine perfusion, putting the fetus in jeopardy.

The main drawback of Demerol is that it causes maternal respiratory depression which in turn causes fetal respiratory depression, as Demerol passes the fetal blood-brain barrier. After an intramuscular injection of Demerol, the peak narcotic effect is seen in 2–3 hours. It can affect the baby soon after it is given intravenously; intramuscularly the effect on the baby is delayed by 1 hour. If Demerol is given less than 1 hour or more than 4–6 hours before the estimated time of delivery, there is less narcotic effect in the newborn.

There are reports that a baby takes 3–6 days to excrete the drug. Its elimination half life in neonates is 23 hours; in an adult it is only 3–5 hours. The effect on the fetus is related to the dose given and the time interval between the mother receiving the Demerol and the time of delivery. In the fetus, the drug is found to produce respiratory acidosis due to hypoventilation, and a generally lower Apgar score and depressed neurobehavioral functions, such as decreased alertness, sucking, Moro response, or rooting behavior. Demerol should be particularly avoided in premature births because of the frequency of undeveloped lungs in premature infants.

Demerol should be given cautiously to cardiac patients because of the tachycardia it produces after intravenous injection. Increased metabolic demands during pregnancy and stress of labor can cause tachycardia, and if Demerol is given intravenously to obstetrical patients who have mitral stenosis it can cause a severe tachycardia or atrial fibrillation that may decrease cardiac output and produce pulmonary edema.

Demerol delays labor if it is given too early, because it diminishes uterine activity and tone, especially if repeated doses are given. After 100 mg of Demerol, labor can be retarded or stopped. Demerol has mild spasmogenic action in the stomach and it delays gastric emptying time. If a patient requires general anesthesia, the risk of gastric aspiration is increased when the patient is rendered unconscious.

Because of its many disadvantages, Demerol should be used only in the acceleration phase of labor. In this way, the drug will not prolong labor and the dose can be limited to the least amount needed to achieve analgesia, without causing respiratory depression. The dose depends on the pain threshold of the individual, her age, her emotional status, her weight, and the route of administration.

The onset of analgesia is in 30 seconds when Demerol is given intravenously. It reaches its peak effect in 10–15 minutes. Pain relief lasts 2–3 hours. When it is given intramuscularly, its peak effect is in 40–50 minutes. Pain relief lasts 3 hours. When Demerol is combined with barbiturates, pain relief lasts from 3 to 4 hours.

Intravenous administration gives a more rapid effect, but 50 mg of Demerol in a single intravenous bolus can cause euphoria followed by mild depression of the cortex. Therefore, a single intravenous bolus should not exceed 25–35 mg. It can be given in a dose of 1 mg/kg body weight (25–35 mg IV, the rest IM) at 3–4 cm dilation in the primigravida or at 2–3 cm in the multipara. An optimum intramuscular dose varies from 50 to 100 mg. Demerol can be repeated after 3–4 hours; preferably it should not be repeated in less than 4 hours. However, it should not be given late in the first stage or during the second stage of labor, for fear of causing neonatal asphyxia. The maximum dose should not exceed 200 mg.

Narcan (Naloxone Hydrochloride)

Narcan is a narcotic antagonist, a synthetic congener of oxymorphone. It is the preferred narcotic antagonist because it has no agonist activity. It has no cardiorespiratory or central nervous system depressant effect. It acts by displacing the narcotic from the receptor sites in the central nervous system. When Narcan is administered intravenously, the reversal effect is seen within 2 minutes, and only slightly longer when the drug is administered intramuscularly or subcutaneously. It should be given in small increments and repeated until adequate ventilation and alertness are obtained. The usual initial adult dose is 0.4 mg (1 ml). The usual initial infant dose is 0.01 mg/kg body weight. In the delivery room, infants who do not respond to resuscitation, or who take initial breaths and then gradually decrease their respiratory efforts, should receive Narcan. It is given intravenously through the umbilical vein. It can also be given intramuscularly or subcutaneously. Narcan should be used cautiously in newborns of mothers who are known narcotic addicts, since it can produce acute withdrawal symptoms. In adults, abrupt reversal of narcotic depression with an excessive dose of Narcan can cause adverse reactions such as nausea, vomiting, sweating, tachycardia, increased blood pressure and tremulousness. Patients who respond satisfactorily to Narcan reversal should be under constant observation for respiratory depression in particular, since Narcan has a shorter duration of action than do narcotics. It can be repeated if the respiratory depressant effect of the narcotic lasts longer than the Narcan.

Valium

Valium (diazepam) is a benzodiazepine derivative used for its tranquilizing effect and anticonvulsant action. It has a mild sedative effect, but no analgesic action. It also has amnesic effects and it is a mild centrally acting muscle relaxant. It is used during the first stage of labor, in combination with narcotics, to potentiate the narcotic effect. It is safer than a sedative drug for cardiac patients because it does not cause a fall in blood pressure. The dose of Valium varies from 5 mg to 10 mg intramuscularly. It can be repeated once, not exceeding a total of 20 mg. Since it passes the placenta readily, excessive doses can cause hypoactivity and flaccidity of the skeletal and smooth muscles of the newborn, causing poor sucking reflexes, bowel

and bladder hypotonia, and hypothermia for 24–48 hours after birth. These depressed neonatal reflexes persist for the first 3 or 4 days of life and the neonatal blood level of Valium can be elevated for as long as 1 week. Another problem associated with Valium is the stabilizer contained in its injectable form, called sodium benzoate, which is a bilirubin-albumin uncoupler. It displaces the bilirubin from its albumin-binding site and this can cause physiological jaundice. For all these reasons, Valium must be given in small doses. Intravenously, a dose of 2.5 mg is injected slowly; Valium is known to cause apnea if injected rapidly. Its use in cesarean section, after delivery, is becoming popular because of the amnesic effect. Light general anesthesia in cesarean section is given before the baby is delivered and patients may have some awareness of the surgery. Valium provides a retrograde amnesic effect.

Valium may also be given intravenously to apprehensive patients prior to administration of regional anesthesia. The usual dose is 2.5 mg.

Valium is the drug of choice as an anticonvulsant both as a prophylactic agent and as a therapeutic agent to combat local anesthetic toxicity. It raises the CNS threshold toxicity effect from local anesthetic.

Barbiturates

Short-acting barbiturates can be used for sedation during the early latent phase of labor when delivery is not anticipated for at least 12 hours. Barbiturates cross the placenta rapidly (within minutes) and are known to cause depression of the neonate and prolonged neurobehavioral changes. They are now losing their popularity in obstetrics. These drugs were used for their anticonvulsant action in severe preeclampsia and to combat local anesthetic toxicity, but Valium is now preferred for this purpose.

Perhaps the only indication for barbiturates nowadays is in a single dose for induction of general anesthesia for cesarean section. The drug should be given during a uterine contraction when the umbilical cord is compressed. In this way there is minimal transfer to the fetus. A dose of less than 4 mg/kg will not expose the fetal brain to a great concentration of the barbiturate because most barbiturates enter the fetal liver first, are diluted in the liver, and then are diluted further by blood coming from the lower extremities and viscera. By the time the drug reaches the fetal brain, it is not potent enough to cause depression if the induction dose is kept to a minimum.

Ketamine is a phencyclidine derivative that produces "dissociative anesthesia" with analgesia and superficial sleep. It can be used in conjunction with Nembutal in cesarean sections.

INHALATION ANALGESIA AND ANESTHESIA

Inhalation analgesia is the administration of subanesthetic doses of an inhalation agent for pain relief during labor and delivery without rendering the patient unconscious. It is given through a mask, with constant supervision of the patient. The patient is awake with her protective laryngeal reflexes intact at all times. Since inhalation agents are delivered in very low concentration, they do not produce significant depression of the fetus regardless of the duration of labor.

Inhalation analgesia is indicated when the patient refuses systemic medication and regional anesthesia or when both are contraindicated. It is used as a supplement during delivery to ease the uncomfortable pulling and pressure sensation under epidural anesthesia.

The common inhalation agents used during labor are nitrous oxide and Penthrane (methoxyflurane). Trilene (trichlorethylene) is used in the United Kingdom but not in the United States. Nitrous oxide is a compressed gas. It is a nonirritating, sweet smelling, nonflammable, weak anesthetic. It is used mixed with oxygen.

There are two ways to give nitrous oxide for patients in labor. The most effective way is continuous administration in a concentration of 30–40% nitrous oxide in 60–70% oxygen. Another method is intermittent administration with 70% nitrous oxide and 30% oxygen. Timing is important in this technique because it takes 45–50 seconds for the patient to get the analgesic effect. She must start to breathe the nitrous oxide before the start of a uterine contraction. Between contractions she should be breathing pure oxygen.

Nitrous oxide must be delivered in a high flow. If it is given alone, without local or regional anesthesia, it is not suitable for forceps delivery or for repair of episiotomy. It must be supplemented by local infiltration or pudendal block or regional block to provide a painless delivery. Since complete analgesia is rarely accomplished without deepening the concentration and hyperventilation, the patient can easily enter the stage of delirium, excitement, nausea and vomiting, risking aspiration pneumonitis. Therefore, the patient's sensorium must be checked by constant conversation. If she becomes drowsy or excited, the inspiratory concentration must be decreased. If the concentration of nitrous oxide is not more than 50% and there is constant supervision by the anesthesiologist, the patient will not enter the second stage of anesthesia or the excitement stage.

Nitrous oxide can also be used with Penthrane in a mixture of 60% nitrous, 40% oxygen, and 0.25–0.3% Penthrane. This combination may produce a better analgesic effect if the patient is still uncomfortable with nitrous oxide alone. Again, the patient's consciousness must be checked constantly during administration.

Penthrane (methoxyflurane) is 2,2-dichlorofluroethyl methyl ether. It is a nonflammable agent. A concentration of 0.25–0.3% provides a subanesthetic level for the first plane of surgical anesthesia. It must be given under supervision. The physiological respiratory changes in pregnancy reduce anesthetic requirements. This is due to a reduction of functional residual capacity and an increase in alveolar ventilation. If a patient inadvertently receives a higher concentration of Penthrane, resulting in disorientation and vomiting, there is an increased possibility of aspiration pneumonitis.

Penthrane is known to have nephrotoxic effects in high concentrations if it is administered for a prolonged period of time. It should be avoided in toxemic patients and in patients with a history of renal impairment.

Inhalation anesthesia is the administration of inhalation agents that render the patient unconscious with an anesthetic concentration that is higher than that used for inhalation analgesia. In this higher anesthetic concentration, all the inhalation agents cross the placenta and they can produce a dose- and time-related depression in the fetus and neonate. These agents can also cause a related depression of the uterine tone and contraction and this may result in postpartum hemorrhage. For these reasons it is not advisable to put a patient to sleep during vaginal delivery unless there is a reason to depress uterine activity. Two inhalation agents, halothane and ethrane, are used for this purpose because of rapid onset of effect and predictability.

Halothane is a fluorinated hydrocarbon. When used in a concentration of 0.75–2%, it produces rapid relaxation of uterine muscle. Halothane should be used only by an experienced anesthesiologist and a cooperative obstetrician; excessive relaxation of the uterus will result in hemorrhage. Halothane is best avoided in patients with a history of jaundice and hepatic disease.

Enflurane (Ethrane) is a short-chain fluorinated ether. It is a nonflammable inhalation agent. It is used in obstetrics in a concentration of 1–3% for relaxation of the uterus.

Some anesthesiologists advocate the use of halothane and enflurane during cesarean sections when a higher oxygen concentration is necessary to better oxygenate the fetus. Most cesarean sections are done with 60–70% nitrous oxide; if increased oxygen is necessary, the nitrous oxide must be decreased to 40–50% and supplemented with 0.5% halothane or 0.75% Ethrane or 0.2% Penthrane, with care not to hyperventilate the patient. Such concentrations are claimed not to produce uterine atony because they are immediately discontinued after delivery of the baby.

REGIONAL ANALGESIA

Regional analgesia includes epidural, caudal and spinal analgesia. It is the most effective means of pain relief during labor and it can be used for operative obstetrical intervention. The mothers are awake and participate in the birth of their infants. Women who have had regional analgesia for childbirth generally consider it a most rewarding experience.

The mother is completely devoid of pain and the fetus is less likely to develop depression. With the woman awake, there is no danger of aspiration and its disastrous consequences. Of course, there are potential dangers in regional analgesia as there are in other forms of analgesia and anesthesia, but if properly conducted it can be the safest and best choice of analgesia for both the mother and fetus.

EPIDURAL ANALGESIA

The epidural space is a potential space formed by the two layers of dura mater fused superiorly at the level of the foramen magnum and inferiorly limited by the sacrococcygeal ligament that closes the sacral hiatus. It contains adipose tissue, lymphatics, areolar tissue, venous plexuses, blood vessels and nerves. It is also called extradural, peridural, or interdural space. There are 31 pairs of spinal nerves with their dural prolongations that pass through this space and exit at the intervertebral foramina. It is these spinal nerves that come in contact with local anesthetics injected into the epidural space. The onset of nerve block starts at the smallest fibers and the nonmyelinated fibers. The autonomic nerves are blocked first, followed by the sensory and then the motor nerves.

The landmark used to perform epidural analgesia is the same as in spinal analgesia. An imaginary horizontal line is drawn between the two upper iliac crests. This line corresponds to the L4 interspace. The L4 interspace is frequently chosen because the spinal cord ends at the level of L2 vertebrae in 60% of patients; in another 30% it ends at L1, and in still another 10% it ends at L3.

The following layers are encountered: skin, subcutaneous tissue, supraspinous ligaments, interspinous ligaments, and ligamentum flavum. There is a gradual increase in resistance as the epidural needle passes the above ligaments until it reaches the ligamentum flavum and a loss of resistance is encountered upon entering the epidural space. This is the so-called loss of resistance technique.

PAIN PATHWAY OF THE PARTURIENTS

In the first stage of labor, pain is caused by contraction of the body of the uterus and cervix and dilatation of the lower uterine segment. It travels along the sensory pathways (visceral afferents) that accompany the sympathetic nerves that enter the spinal cord at the thoracic levels of T10, T11, T12 and lumbar level of L1. During the latter part of the first stage, when the fetal head descends, and also during the second stage of labor (delivery of the fetus), pain is caused by continuing contractions and dilatation and also by the distension of the lower birth canal, vulva and perineum. This pain travels along sensory pathways (somatic afferents) which are components of pudendal nerves that enter the spinal cord at sacral levels 2, 3, and 4. The third stage of labor (delivery of the placenta) has the same pain pathway as the first stage of labor. Therefore, a level of analgesia from T10 to S5 is essential for the entire delivery.

The center of the spinal dermatome, T10, is at the level of the umbilicus; T12 is at the level of the symphysis pubis; L1 is at the level of the upper pubis and affects the inguinal region, midsacral area and inside upper thighs. S1 affects the soles of the feet. S2–S4 (pudendal nerves) affect the vulva and anal areas, and S5 is at the coccyx.

Pain relief for the first stage of labor can be achieved with the so-called segmental epidural block. That is a block at the level of T10, T11, T12 and L1. Segmental epidural analgesia preserves the muscle tone of the pelvic floor to facilitate the rotation and flexion of the fetal head, thus decreasing the incidence of persistent posterior position or transverse position of the fetal head. It is useful in multiple births or breech presentation. The mother can have pain relief from T10 to L1 but there is no block of the pelvic floor. The fetus can rotate and the mother has expulsive power. In addition, only a small dose of anesthetic agent is required to produce segmental epidural analgesia, thus lowering the incidence of hypotension and toxic drug levels. A larger refill dose is needed when the patient is in the late first stage or approaching the second stage (delivery).

The level of epidural analgesia must be extended cephalad to at least T6 to T8 for cesarean section, but unless a level of T4 is obtained the patient will feel sensations of burning, pressure, and pulling. The spinal dermatome of T4 corresponds with the nipple line; T6 corresponds with the xyphoid area, and T8 with the costal margins.

Epidural analgesia is used when the parturient is in active labor; the fetal presenting part is engaged; cervical dilatation is 3–4 cm in the multipara and 5–6 cm in the primigravida; and uterine contractions are regular, with good intensity, at less than 3 minutes intervals and lasting 35–50 seconds or longer. However, epidural analgesia can be used in incoordinate uterine activity. The stresses of labor enhance the release of catecholamines (epinephrine and norepinephrine) which interferes with uterine contractions and results in resistance to the progress of labor. Since epidural segmental block relieves the anxiety and pain of labor, it may restore incoordinate uterine contractions to normal.

Epidural analgesia offers advantages over spinal analgesia. 1) A continuous catheter is left in place to control the level of analgesia. 2) Absence of headache in the postpartum period enables the mother to move around and care for her baby. 3) The onset of sympathetic blockade is gradual; hypotension is easier to prevent or control. There is less motor block than with spinal analgesia; the mother can push out the fetus. 4) Analgesia can be continued after delivery for postpartum tubal ligation.

Parturients have the option of regional analgesia for pain relief in uncomplicated pregnancy, and it has become popular in recent years in cesarean sections when women want to see their baby immediately after birth.

For patients with respiratory or cardiac disorders, epidural analgesia can reduce cardiopulmonary effort. It is beneficial as well in controlling blood pressure in hypertensive preeclamptic patients and in those who have renal disease. It is useful in relieving the pain due to oxytocin infusion. It facilitates operative vaginal delivery to shorten the second stage of labor.

SPINAL ANALGESIA

Spinal, or subarachnoid, analgesia is the injection of local anesthetic into the spinal space containing cerebrospinal fluid. The so-called saddle block is used for normal spontaneous delivery; the block is limited to the sacral dermatomes for perineal analgesia. If forceps delivery is anticipated or cesarean section is to be done, the block should be extended to a higher level. If forceps delivery is anticipated, the block should extend to the T10 level. If cesarean section is to be done, a larger dose of anesthetic agent is required to reach the T4 or T5 level. A higher dose with a higher level may cause a rapid onset of hypotension. Hypotension is also seen more frequently than with epidural analgesia because the sympathetic block is immediate.

Advantages of spinal analgesia: Only a very small dose of local anesthetic is used. The onset of analgesia is rapid. The block provides good muscle relaxation for an operative procedure. A spinal is an easy block to perform.

Disadvantages of spinal analgesia, aside from rapid hypotension: The level of an-

algesia is unpredictable. The intense motor block takes away the expulsive power or bearing down reflex which may be necessary to push out the fetus. If headache occurs in the postpartum period the mother is unable to care for her baby, but the use of a 25- to 26-gauge spinal needle will reduce the incidence of headache.

CAUDAL ANALGESIA

Caudal analgesia provides immediate perineal analgesia when it is required. It should be done when the woman is near the end of the first stage of labor. Cervical dilatation should be at least 7 cm in the primigravida and 6 cm in the multipara. If the block is done at an early stage, before the head has descended, the loss of muscle tone in the pelvic diaphragm will result in failure of rotation of the fetal head during descent. Caudal analgesia is a form of epidural analgesia with the site of injection at the lower end of the epidural space, called the caudal space. The landmark is the sacral hiatus that is covered by the sacrococcygeal membrane.

Caudal analgesia has some disadvantages compared with epidural analgesia. There is a greater risk of toxic effect of local anesthetics because a caudal block requires a larger dose. There is a greater possibility of spread of infection into the caudal canal due to the proximity of the perineum to the site of injection. There is a risk of inadvertent fetal scalp puncture caused by the faulty position of the caudal needle at the junction of the sacrum and coccyx; the needle can pierce the rectum and enter the descended fetal head. More anomalies are found in the caudal anatomy than in the lumbar spinal vertebrae. Technically, the procedure is more difficult than is the lumbar epidural approach. There is a possibility of inadvertent dural puncture. The lower extent of the dural sac ends at the level of the second sacral foramina, at the level of the posterior superior spines. If the caudal needle is advanced beyond the second sacral foramina, dural tap can occur.

CONTRAINDICATIONS OF EPIDURAL, SPINAL AND CAUDAL ANALGESIA

A patient who refuses regional analgesia should not receive regional analgesia.

Absence of an intravenous route, lack of resuscitative equipment, and unskilled personnel are contraindications.

If a patient knows she has an allergy to a local anesthetic drug, she can receive a different agent. Cross allergies can happen within the same class of local anesthetics but not between esters and amides.

Absolute contraindications are: systemic or local infection, such as pilonidal abscess or skin disease such as rash, psoriasis, etc. at the site of needle insertions; uncontrolled hemorrhage or hypovolemic shock from acute blood loss, seen in placenta previa and abruptio placenta. Any sudden massive bleeding can result in hypovolemia and the hypovolemia can aggravate the hypotension that is already present with regional analgesia.

Anticoagulant therapy or coagulopathies can cause spinal cord bleeding and epidural hematoma. Regional analgesia can be done only when laboratory data show a normal blood profile. Von Willebrand's disease presents special problems, in that bleeding can occur even when coagulation studies are within normal limits. Separation of the placenta or severe toxemia can present a picture like disseminated intravascular coagulopathy (DIC). Coagulation studies must be done before attempting regional analgesia. Epidural hematoma can result from these coagulation disorders which produce compression symptoms, with initial motor weakness, loss of sensation, loss of sphincter tone, deep pain, and postural hypotension. Surgical evacuation of the hematoma is required.

Most anesthesiologists avoid region analgesia in patients who have preexisting neurological disease of the spinal cord or peripheral nerves.

Cerebral or abdominal aneurysms are not contraindications. These patients should receive regional analgesia to ease the stress of labor. Straining efforts may endanger their existing conditions.

PARACERVICAL NERVE BLOCK

Paracervical nerve block is performed by obstetricians during the first stage of labor. The needle is injected transvaginally into the submucosa of the vaginal fornix, posterior and lateral to both sides of the cervical rim, at 3 o'clock and 9 o'clock positions or at 4 o'clock and 8 o'clock positions. The procedure blocks Frankenhauser's ganglion with all the sensory nerve fibers that innervate the uterus. This is a highly vascular area and rapid maternal absorption of the local anesthetic can produce sudden elevated and excessive blood concentration. The placental transmission is rapid—about 2 minutes.

The major drawback of this nerve block is the frequent bradycardia and acidosis observed and the reported fetal deaths. The fetal bradycardia is produced by hypoxia due to decreased placental perfusion as a result of uterine arterial vasoconstriction and uterine hypertonicity, which are toxic manifestations of local anesthetics. If fetal bradycardia persists, the result is fetal metabolic acidosis. Fetal acidosis increases the absorption and placental transfer of anesthetic agent, resulting in further local anesthetic toxicity which severely jeopardizes the fetus. Fetal death may occur as a result of medullary and direct myocardial depression. Paracervical block is contraindicated in prematurity, uteroplacental insufficiency, and any compromised fetal environment.

Other complications of paracervical block are intravascular injections, accidental injection into the fetal head, hematoma of the parametrium, and sciatic neuritis.

PUDENDAL BLOCK

Pudendal block is performed by the obstetrician at the second stage of labor. The block is done transvaginally, with injection of local anesthetic into the vaginal mucosa below the tip of the ischial spine, piercing the sacrospinous ligament. This blocks the pudendal nerves supplying the perineum, vagina, and vulva and is sufficient for the use of outlet forceps and repair of episiotomy. For low forceps and low mid-forceps delivery, nitrous oxide may be supplemented in analgesic concentration.

Some complications of pudendal block are inadvertent intravenous injections, hematoma, sciatic nerve block, and puncture of the rectum.

CHOICE OF LOCAL ANESTHETICS IN OBSTETRICAL ANALGESIA (Table 37.1)

Local anesthetics are divided into two groups—the amides and the esters. The most commonly used amides are lidocaine (Xylocaine), mepivacaine (Carbocaine) and bupivacaine (Marcaine). They are metabolized by the liver microsomal enzymes. Their protein-binding capacity is an additional factor that modifies toxicity. The commonly used esters are 2-chloroprocaine (Nesacaine) and tetracaine (Pontocaine). They are hydrolyzed by plasma cholinesterase. This is a more rapid process than liver metabolism. Therefore, they have a lower toxicity than the amides.

Xylocaine and Carbocaine were the local anesthetics that were used for epidural and caudal analgesia in the past. They lost their importance in obstetrical analgesia because they had an adverse effect on the neurobehavioral assessment of newborns.

The two drugs of choice for epidural analgesia at the present time are Nesacaine and Marcaine.

Nesacaine is the least toxic local anesthetic used for obstetrical analgesia, due to its rapid hydrolysis by plasma pseudocholinesterase. Its half life in the mother is 21 seconds; in the fetus the half life is 42 seconds, if it ever enters the fetal blood. It has a rapid onset of action and a high safety index. Its duration of action is 35–45 minutes for a low dose and 45–60 minutes for a larger dose. Cumulative effect does not develop, despite frequent reinforcements during labor. It has no adverse effect on neurobehavioral assessment of the newborn.

Marcaine has a longer duration of action than does Nesacaine—about $1-1\frac{1}{2}$ hours with lower doses used during labor and up to 3 hours with a larger dose such as for cesarean section. Its longer duration means that the need for reinforcement is less frequent. Its protein-binding capacity in the mother is 95%, which makes this drug quite safe for obstetrical analgesia. The half life of Marcaine in the neonate is 2 hours, and it has been found that the newborn can metabolize it into 2, 6 pipecoloxylidide (ppx) besides excreting the drug unchanged in the urine. It is not detected in maternal or neonatal blood after 8 hours, and it is no longer detected in maternal or neonatal urine 24 hours after delivery. Recent neurobehavioral studies of newborns showed no harmful effects.

Table 37.1.   Common Local Anesthetics used in Obstetrics

	Chloroprocaine (Nesacaine)	Bupivacaine (Marcaine)	Tetracaine (Pontocaine)
Type	Ester	Amide	Ester
Onset	Fast	Intermediate	Slow
Duration	Short	Long	Long
Plasma protein-binding capacity	—	95.6%	75.6%
Local infiltration of perineum	0.5%	0.125%	—
Pudendal and paracervical block	1.5%	0.25–0.5%	Seldom used
Spinal block (mg)	—	—	4–10 mg
Epidural block for labor	2%	0.25–0.5%	—
Epidural block for cesarean section	3%	0.75%	—
Maximum initial dose	20 mg/kg	2–3 mg/kg	1.5 mg/kg
Half life	42 seconds in neonate 21 seconds in maternal blood	2 hr in neonate	

Bibliography

1. Albright, G.A. *Anesthesia in Obstetrics: Maternal, Fetal and Neonatal Aspects.* Addison-Wesley Publishing Company, 1978.
2. Bieniarz, J., Corttogini, J.J., Curuchet, E., et al. Aorto-caval compression by the uterus in late human pregnancy: II. An arteriographic study. *Am. J. Obstet. Gynecol. 100 (2):*203–217, 1968.
3. Mendelson, C.L. The aspiration of stomach contents into the lungs during obstetric anesthesia. *Am. J. Obstet. Gynecol. 52:*191–205, 1946.
4. Roberts, R.B., and Shirleys, M.A. The obstetrician role in reducing the risk of aspiration pneumonitis: With particular reference to the use of oral antacids. *Am. J. Obstet. Gynecol. 124:*611–617, 1976.
5. Shnidner, S.M., and Levinson, G. *Anesthesia for Obstetrics.* Williams & Wilkins, Baltimore, 1979.

Operative Delivery

CHAPTER 38

Forceps

RICHARD A. RUSKIN, M.D.

The need of aid for the problems of childbirth is as old as life itself. Invented devices started as instruments of destruction to separate the dead infant from the mother. As time progressed, knowledge increased and techniques were modified so that instruments could successfully aid in the completion of the birth process. The first name associated with the forceps as a conservator of life is that of William Chamberlen, a French Huguenot who emigrated to England in 1569.

Simpson stated that "the best efforts of the forceps were secured when we use them, not as a substitute for the efforts of nature, but as an aid when these are like to fail." This holds true today. The beneficial use of forceps are three in number; extraction, rotation and flexion. Forceps have to be able to achieve the same results that the mechanism of labor produces. Indications for the use of the instruments may be divided into three groups:

A. Maternal: having to do with problems arising from the care of the mother which would necessitate an attempt to shorten labor
   1. Toxemia
   2. Acute disease: pneumonia
   3. Chronic diseases: tuberculosis, cardiac disease, malignancy
   4. Hemorrhage
   5. Exhaustion

B. Fetal distress
   1. Persistent fetal heart irregularities
   2. Meconium
   3. Acidosis

C. Obstetrical (diagnosed by obstetrician)
   1. Progress
      a. Lack of— due to malposition (arrest, etc.), inertia (prolonged labor)
      b. Prolonged second stage
      c. Rigid perineum
   2. Aftercoming head of a breech
   3. Prophylactic— Popularized by Dr. DeLee, in the early 1920s. Prophylactic forceps application to prevent problems of the second stage of labor

Prerequisites for the use of forceps have to be properly understood and fulfilled before the forceps delivery can be successfully accomplished.

I. Cervix—The patient has to be in the second stage of labor before any vaginal delivery can be done.
II. Engagement and station—The vertex must be engaged in the pelvis and its correct station diagnosed. An unengaged head is a definite contraindiction to the use of forceps.

The vertex is situated in the pelvis in a relationship of its biparietal diameter to one of the planes of the pelvis. The planes are four in number, namely, high, mid, low-mid, and low, and are defined as follows (Fig. 38.1):

A. High— The plane of the obstetrical conjugate
B. Mid— symphysis to the junction between the second and third sacral vertebrae
C. Low-mid— symphysis to the sacrococcygeal junction, through the dimensions of the ischial spines
D. Low— symphysis to the sacrococcygeal junction, but through the dimensions of the ischial tuberosities

To enable one to accurately determine station, a bimanual examination is performed with the abdominal hand exerting downward pressure at the same time a labor contraction is started. The internal fingers evaluate the leading bony part of the head in relationship to certain diagnostic factors. This may have to be supplemented with a rectal examination to help determine the relationship of the vertex with the posterior part of the pelvis.

Low station is confirmed when the hollow of the sacrum is filled with the bony part of the vertex. The leading bony part so bulges the perineum that one cannot insert an examining finger between it and the perineum. The vertex is in the A-P diameter (occipitoanterior or occipitoposterior (OA or OP)).

Low-mid station is confirmed when the hollow of the sacrum is filled with the bony part of the head and the leading bony part is one fingerbreadth off the perineum.

Mid station is confirmed when the hollow of the sacrum is only partially filled with the bony part of the head, with the leading bony part reaching just below the spines.

High station is confirmed when the hollow of the sacrum is empty, with the leading bony part just reaching the spines. (Note: This is analogous to engagement.)

Another way of putting this into perspective is to realize the following matching diagnoses, namely,

1. High station = 0 (biparietal diameter through inlet; leading part of vertex at the ischial spines)
2. Mid station = +1 (leading part of vertex is 1 cm beyond the ischial spines)
3. Low-mid station = +2
4. Low station = +3

Any finding of the vertex above high station or 0 is defined as unengaged or is given a minus designation.

The type of forceps operation is defined by the station of the vertex at the time the procedure is started, namely, high forceps operation, mid-forceps operation, low-forceps operation.

III. Position—A forceps procedure has to have 100% cephalic application for a successful outcome, as the instruments are applied to the fetal head and not to the maternal pelvis. One should place most effort on the proper evaluation of the fetal sutures rather than depending on the palpation of a fontanelle. The fontanelle may be misleading because of distortion due to caput formation. The asynclitic attitude of the vertex as it engages in the pelvis may make diagnosis of the position very difficult. Therefore one should take care in tracing the sagittal suture as far as possible to see if there is any curving of the line into a U or inverted U, confirming the diagnosis of asynclitism.

IV. Pelvis—The definition of type of pelvis or passageway is needed to

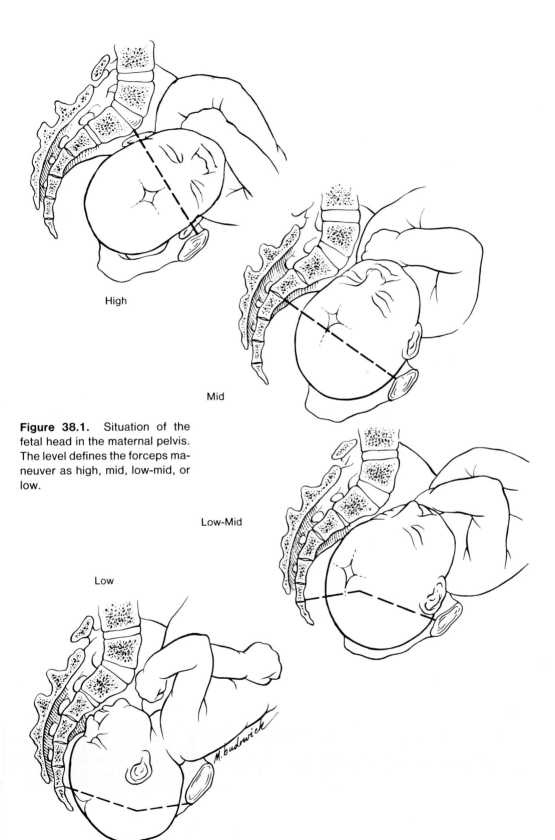

High

Mid

Figure 38.1. Situation of the fetal head in the maternal pelvis. The level defines the forceps maneuver as high, mid, low-mid, or low.

Low-Mid

Low

determine the route that one has to follow with the use of the instrument and to confirm that the diameters are ample for delivery from below.

V. Choice—After complete evaluation of the above prerequisites, one can then proceed to the choice of the correct instrument for the successful outcome of delivery.

A simple classification of forceps based upon uses is:

I. Classical—best used for traction with minimal rotation
  A. Simpson type (separated shanks) —for moulded heads (Fig. 38.2)
  B. Elliot type (overlapping shanks) —for rounded heads
II. Special—for correcting malpositions of the vertex
  A. Kjelland—for correcting asynclitism, rotation of the transverse and posterior positions (Fig. 38.3)
  B. Barton—application and traction in transverse position
  C. Piper—for aftercoming head in a breech delivery (Fig. 38.4)

Classical instruments consist of two parts one of which is a mirror image of the other with the labelling, blade, shank, handle; pelvic curve, cephalic curve; fenestrations or solid blade, anterior lip, posterior lip, toe, heel, finger guard, handles left side, right side, etc. (Fig. 38.2).

Because of its separated shanks the Simpson type has a long tapering cephalic curve which will better fit a moulded head. The Elliot type, because of its overlapping shanks, has to start its curve closer to the shanks, therefore making a wider curve which adapts better to rounded heads.

As stated before, the proper and only application is a cephalic one (Fig. 38.5). This should be biparietal, bimalar and anchored well below the malar eminence. The blades are evenly placed between the lateral borders of the eye and the tragus of the ear so that the pivot point of the head coincides with the point of equilibrium of the forceps. To determine if the forceps is accurately applied, there are three confirmatory examinations:

A. The posterior fontanelle is felt to be one fingerbreadth above the plane of

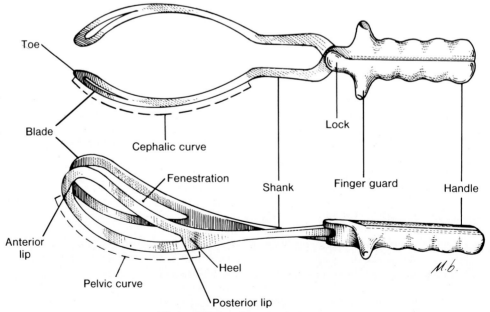

Figure 38.2.   Simpson's forceps.

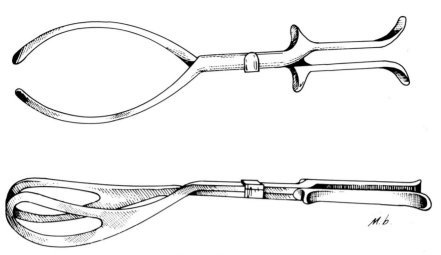

Figure 38.3. Kjelland's forceps.

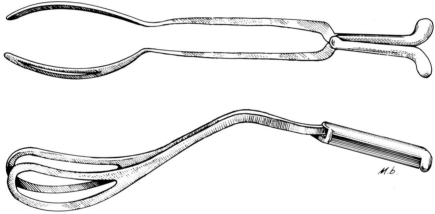

Figure 38.4. Piper's forceps.

the shanks and equidistant between the blades.

B. The sagittal suture is perpendicular to the plane of the shanks throughout its entirety.

C. The fenestrations of the forceps are barely felt, if at all (Fig. 38.6).

Application to moulded heads in anterior positions of the pelvis (namely, right occipitoanterior, occipitoanterior, left occipitoanterior (ROA-OA-LOA)) is best accomplished with a Simpson type instrument. An Elliot type instrument with a shorter curve will not fit evenly, therefore producing a pressure effect, and cannot anchor far enough down.

For an operative vaginal delivery the patient is placed on the delivery table in the lithotomy position, sterilely prepared, and draped, membranes being ruptured. For many years the dictum of catheterization was always carried out. However, the probability of introducing bacteria into the urinary tract outweighs the minimal benefits of the procedure. Therefore, this is done only when the patient presents with a grossly distended bladder. Anesthesia is necessary for a successful procedure. Local infiltration or pudendal block supported by nitrous oxide and oxygen may be used for low stations. However, a more effective anesthetic, such as general, epi-

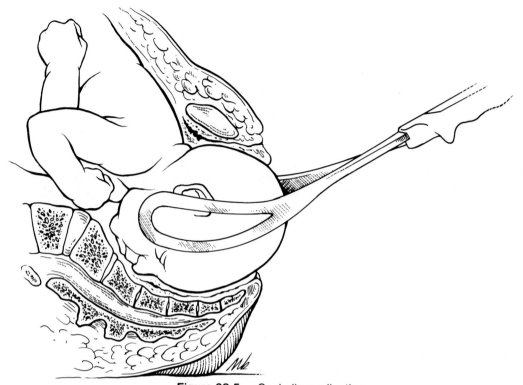

Figure 38.5. Cephalic application.

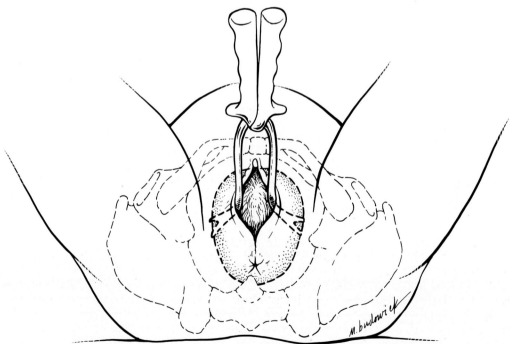

Figure 38.6. Correct application by three confirmatory examinations.

dural or caudal, is necessary for any procedures performed at a higher station.

For application of instruments to a vertex in an anterior position (ROA-OA-LOA), a classical instrument should be used and applied by a posterior blade technique. It should be understood that when the forceps is in position, the left blade is placed on the left side of the baby's head and the right blade on the right side. This means using the blade that splints or holds the head in the position that it has arrived at by its mechanism of labor. If labor started with the vertex engaged in a left-sided position (left occipitoposterior, left occipitotransverse (LOP-LOT)), progress has to be made anteriorly. Therefore in a LOA the vertex has progressed over an arc of 45–90 degrees from its original LOP or LOT position. To enable the head to maintain this position and not to be forced back into a malposition, the operator applies the left blade first as this will go toward the left ear of the baby and help the head maintain its favorable position.

To correctly apply the instruments, the four cardinal points as espoused by Dennen are used; namely, the left blade held in the left hand and facing the left inner thigh of the mother being placed near the left ear of the baby. Conversely, when using the right blade the cardinal points apply as follows: right hand, right blade, right side of pelvis, right ear of the baby. With very few exceptions when forceps are applied correctly, the left blade is applied in front of the baby's left ear and the right blade in front of the baby's right ear. It is easy to diagnose which ear is posterior if the exact position is confirmed. In all left-sided positions of the vertex in the pelvis, the left ear is always posterior; in all right-sided positions of the vertex, the right ear is posterior.

When the forceps is held in both hands with the pelvic curve up, the left hand grasps the left blade and the right hand grasps the right blade. Therefore one automatically picks up the correct blade for insertion. If the vertex is an exact OA, it is always better to insert the left blade first as then there will be no need to cross

handles for locking the instruments in place.

When inserting the forceps, the instrument in the left hand is held perpendicular to the longitudinal axis of the mother; then the tips of the index and middle finger on the right hand are inserted in the vagina alongside the bony part of the baby's head. No more than the tips of the fingers should be inserted, or displacement of the vertex upward will occur, producing a loss of station with a possible loss of anterior rotation and flexion. These fingers help guide the forceps into place, using the thumb alongside the heel of the blade to aid in the procedure. This is done in a gentle maneuver and never requires force. After the initial blade is inserted, the four cardinal principles for the second blade are used and this one is inserted toward the right side at a higher level so that it is not impeded by the brow of the baby's head. The handles are then locked in position and checked as previously noted for 100% cephalic application. When confirmed, the vertex is helped to complete its rotation to an OA. Application is then rechecked before any traction is started.

A similar procedure is done for the vertex in an ROA position. The major problem that occurs in this application is that the forceps handles have to be crossed over (creating some pressure to the baby's head) before they can be locked in position. There have been instruments made for this with a lock on the right blade but they are not universally available. Traction is never accomplished until the vertex is in an OA position with only one exception. Rarely, this may be done with a direct posterior position (if there is a pelvic contraindication to rotation) but the instrument loses an advantage in a less accurate application.

The line of traction one uses should be in a path that encounters minimal resistance. One must visualize the planes of the pelvis as shown in Figure 38.7. With a perpendicular dropped from each plane, this would give a path that is fishhook in appearance from the highest station through the lowest station for delivery.

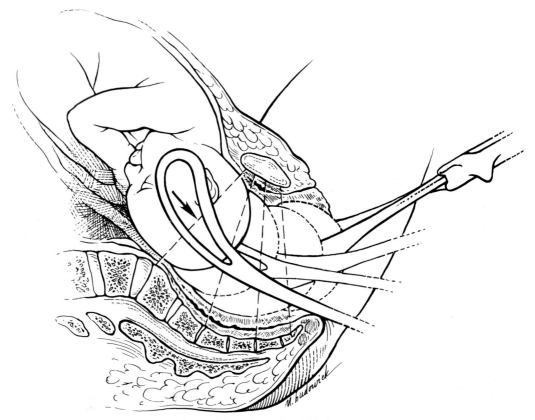

Figure 38.7.   Line of traction with forceps.

This path is midway between the symphysis and the sacrum and is called the *pelvic axis*. When one applies traction along this axis, it is a path of least resistance and the axis-traction principle is fulfilled.

Traction can never be exerted directly outward unless the vertex is in a low station. Therefore to enable one to exert the proper line of force with a head at low-mid, mid or high station, more aid is needed. This can be accomplished by a so-called Pajot or Saxtorph maneuver, which is a manual aid with downward pressure with one hand on the shanks and extraction with the other hand on the handle. This will fulfill the axis-traction principle from the low-mid station (Fig. 38.8). A greater amount of manual aid will be needed for a head that is in a mid or higher station. This is best accomplished by the use of a classical type instrument aided by a traction bar on the handle, attached to the finger guards or a bend in the shanks. These instruments are DeWees (Fig. 38.9), Hawks-Dennen or Bill-Bar attachment for the handle.

The operator sits facing the patient with feet properly balanced on the floor (for a vertex in mid station or a higher station, a lower stool is beneficial) and traction is made in the pelvic axis keeping in mind the changing line of traction as progress continues from one plane to another. This would be roughly downward, outward and upward. Never at any time is undue force exerted. If progress is not made, one should always recheck application, as an error in diagnosis of the position may have been made. Reevaluation of size of the infant and type of pelvis may also be needed.

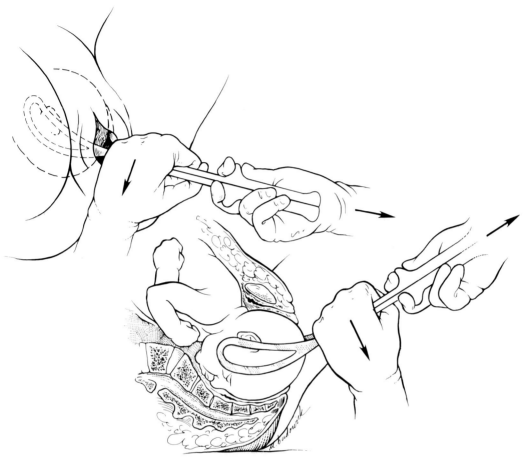

Figure 38.8.   Axis-traction principle: Pajot maneuver.

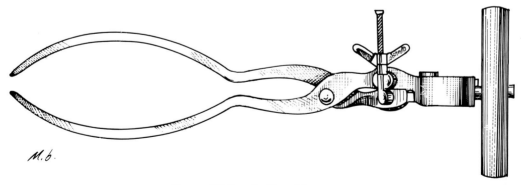

Figure 38.9.   DeWees' forceps.

Traction is continued until the perineum is bulging well (Fig. 38.10); at this time usually an episiotomy is cut. A median or mediolateral incision is made, depending on the anatomy. As the head extends over the perineum, a modified Ritgen maneuver is done; at which time the forceps is removed in a reverse manner to which it

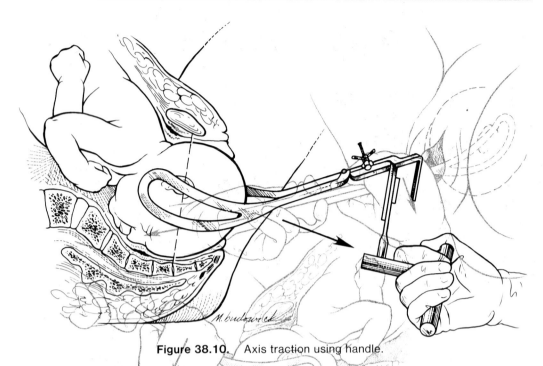

Figure 38.10. Axis traction using handle.

was applied. This is done before completing delivery of the head; a simple maneuver without ever needing force.

A transverse position of the occiput is usually caused by a degree of persistent asynclitism of the head, preventing a flexion and then rotation of the vertex to a more favorable position for progress. Digital rotation, accomplished by using the tips of the index and middle finger against the anterior part of the lambdoidal suture, may be tried at first to help progress. Manual rotation is not usually successful because the operator in placing the hand under the head must lose station, causing further problems for rotation. A classical instrument cannot be applied to the vertex in a transverse position. This is the place for the use of one of the special instruments.

The Kjelland instrument (Fig. 38.3) was developed in 1915 and presented the ability to solve this problem because of its construction. It has a reverse pelvic curve, a sliding lock on the shanks and a beveled inner surface on the cephalic curve. This forceps has a special technique in application known as inversion. The use of right

blade to right ear and left blade to left ear still holds true. However, the posterior blade technique no longer holds true in the application of this instrument. To enable a correct application, the anterior blade is inserted first. It is easy to recognize each blade of this instrument as the lock is attached to the left blade.

Therefore in a LOT position, since the right ear is anterior the right blade is applied first. Conversely in ROT positions, the left ear is anterior and the left blade is applied first. The anterior blade is held in an inverted manner with the inner surface of the cephalic curve facing upward, making the shank about 45 degrees above the horizontal. The middle and index vaginal fingers, placed under the symphysis resting with the fingernails adjacent to the bony part of the baby's head, are used to guide the blade in its progress against the head and under the cervix. As the forceps guides into place, the shanks come below the horizontal. Now the blade has to be turned so that the cephalic curve is adjacent to the skull. Rotation is made by turning the finger guards in a motion away from the occiput and toward the midline.

The posterior blade is always inserted between the anterior one and the mother's right thigh. The vaginal fingers guide this into place in a direct motion, taking care to have the toe of the blade hug the baby's head and making sure that it does not go outside the cervix, which could cause a cul-de-sac perforation. The two handles of the instrument are now brought to a locking position and it may be noticed that one is at a higher level than the other. This is due to an asynclitic attitude of the baby's head and is now correctable by pressure on the finger guards against the sliding lock. As the finger guards equally come into place, a synclitic attitude is accomplished. After the correct cephalic application is confirmed, the head is rotated to its OA position. Because of the reverse pelvic curve of the blades, this is done in a direct arc. After rotation is accomplished, traction is continued using a modified Pajot maneuver for assistance. However, the completion of traction cannot be accomplished by elevating the handles over the horizontal (as one would do with a classical instrument), because the reverse pelvic curve may dig into the sulcus causing tears or may abrade an androidal type arch. Therefore with the aid of fundal pressure, traction is made on the baby's head until the posterior fontanelle comes underneath the symphysis. Then the forceps is disengaged, decreased to 2–3 finger's breadth below the posterior fontanelle and traction made downward, causing the vertex to be extended. A modified Ritgen maneuver is then obtained, and the forceps is removed in a direct manner.

Use of the Kjelland forceps is contraindicated where there is not enough depth in the A-P diameter for the inversion technique and rotation. This occurs in a platypelloid pelvis, with a straightening of the sacrum causing a narrowing of the A-P diameter. Because of this the vertex can only move downward in a transverse position. Therefore this is a situation, mentioned before, in which forceps have to be selected for use to apply traction in the transverse diameter.

The Barton forceps (the instrument to accomplish this) was developed in 1925; it has an anterior blade attached to the shanks by a hinge so that it can be inserted over an arc of 90 degrees. The posterior blade has a deep cephalic curve; the lock again is of the sliding type and there is a traction handle that is applicable. The hinged blade is the anterior blade in all positions. This is applied in a wandering maneuver over the face or occiput; then the posterior blade is inserted between the anterior blade and the mother's right thigh. They are locked in position, and asynclitism is corrected in a similar maneuver as with the Kjelland. Traction is applied using the traction bar until approaching low station. Rotation is then made to the OA. At this time the Barton instrument becomes awkward to use, because the handles point in one direction and the traction bar in another with no definitive maneuver for delivering downward. Each hand therefore is applied, one to the traction bar and one to the handle, and progress is attempted. An episiotomy is cut and a modified Ritgen maneuver is obtained as usual. The forceps is then removed. On occasion if the vertex is rotated at station of application, traction will not be feasible with this instrument. The instrument would have to be removed and a classical type instrument would have to be applied.

For posterior position of the baby's head the Kjelland instrument is usually the instrument of choice. This can be applied by the inversion technique in LOP and ROP cases, but in a vertex in a direct OP this technique obviously cannot be used. To be successful with this position, the station of the head has to be at a low or low-mid station. Any higher station would not allow a correct application. Again one has to always keep in mind the prerequisites, namely the passageway or pelvis. A contraindication could arise which could complicate the successful outcome of the case. Therefore another method would have to be used. If one is dealing with an anthropoid-type pelvis, the pelvis would prevent rotation. A direct posterior delivery would be the method of choice with a Simpson-type instrument. An android type pelvis might contraindicate the use of a Kjelland in rotation, and another method would have to be used. With this direct posterior position the Kjelland forceps is applied upside down. It is inserted from below upward; the right blade being applied first, then the left. The forceps would be locked in position, a cephalic application confirmed and a rotation made over an arc of 180 degrees to the OA. Care is taken to rotate over the side in which the vertex was at the onset of labor. Then when rotation is accomplished, application is rechecked and traction is made as before.

Another technique which had been used long before the introduction of the Kjelland instrument is the Scanzoni maneuver. With this an Elliot type of instrument is used. The forceps is applied in a classical manner, using the technique for a ROA when a true LOP position is present, and the technique for an LOA when a true right occipitoposterior (ROP) position exists. After application the forceps is rotated with the handles over a wide arc, therefore keeping the toes of the blades in a narrow circle. When the OA position is attained the forceps is removed and then reapplied, confirming correct cephalic application before traction is made.

The third special instrument, the Piper, was introduced in 1924 for use in delivering the aftercoming head in a breech. This instrument has the advantage of long shanks with a backward curve, with a special construction giving more spring to the blades therefore permitting less head compression (Fig. 38.4).

After delivery of the breech including the shoulders and arms, examination has to confirm the chin directed toward the posterior segment or the hollow of the pelvis. Then the forceps is directed from below upward in the application. As an assistant holds the baby in a horizontal level, the left blade is inserted first and then the right blade is inserted and locked into position. Traction is applied, after cephalic application is confirmed with the chin midway between both blades and the line of the chin to the nose taking the place of the saggital suture (Fig. 38.11).

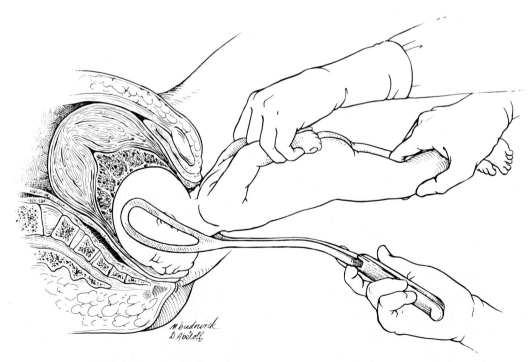

Figure 38.11.   Application of Piper's forceps to aftercoming head.

Other malpositions of the head, namely face and brow, are best handled by cesarean section if any delay occurs. To use instruments for these positions one has to sacrifice a correct application, making vaginal delivery very complicated.

At all times the operator must keep in mind the correct understanding of the prerequisites. This has to be fulfilled in each individual case. Indications have to be completely evaluated; for example, an acute emergency exists or delay can occur to give more time for an improvement in descent or rotation of the head. The correct application of the forceps and the traction-line that is necessary are the basic factors in understanding the effort needed for delivery, so as not to cause trauma to the mother or baby.

Axis-traction may not be neglected. The operator may waste the traction force against the symphysis by not obtaining the correct flexion, even in low stations. One should always keep in mind the need for rechecking when progress is not going as expected. There is no one universal forceps that will solve all problems. Therefore the choice of instrument in each situation is important.

Most cases in which forceps are used are those in which the hollow of the sacrum is filled by the bony parts of the fetal head, the perineum is bulging, and the vertex is in the direct occipitoanterior position: fulfilling all the criteria for low forceps. Higher stations of the head in the pelvis (mid, including low-mid, and high) should be reevaluated, with the guidelines being the force of the indications—the more difficult the situation, the more one would lean to cesarean section.

Bibliography

1. Dennen, E.H. *Forceps Deliveries.* F.A. Davis, Philadelphia, 1955.

CHAPTER 39

Vacuum Extraction

LARS L. CEDERQVIST, M.D.

An attempt to assist the delivery of a baby by the application of vacuum to its head was reported more than 275 years ago. However, it was not until Malmström in 1953 introduced his vacuum extractor (VE) that this type of delivery became popular. It has now almost completely replaced the obstetrical forceps in most European countries. The vacuum extraction is an extremely physiological method of delivery as the head can rotate freely during its movement through the birth canal. In addition, the VE does not encroach on the space of the fetal head in the pelvis. Our experience is that the VE should serve as a useful complement to rather than replacement of the forceps.

The VE is a traction instrument with a suction cup which can be attached to the fetal head. It mainly serves as an aid to the maternal expulsive efforts and the tractions must be synchronous with the uterine contractions. The various sizes of the cups allow the obstetrician to attach the VE without having to wait for full dilatation. The vacuum should be increased slowly by 0.1–0.2 kp/cm^2 at 2-minute intervals up to 0.6–0.7 kp/cm^2. The vacuum can then be increased temporarily to 0.8 kp/cm^2 during traction. The suction cup is applied as close to the posterior fontanelle as possible in order to promote flexion and to achieve the most favorable attitude of the head. The intracranial tension created by the VE under the least favorable circumstances is only one twentieth of that created by the forceps under the most favorable conditions.

The main indications for vacuum extraction are 1) prolonged first or second stage, 2) secondary uterine inertia, 3) malrotations, 4) fetal distress and 5) inability to apply forceps correctly.

A firm but gentle traction with the VE will usually result in reestablishment of uterine activity by stimulation of the paracervical plexus if there are no contractions as a result of uterine inertia. An occipital application of the VE and traction will often lead to increased flexion followed by forward rotation when the occiput is in a lateral or posterior position. In some cases, a forced rotation of the fetal head may be needed and is carried out with one hand rotating the cup as the other hand is used simultaneously for traction. A vacuum extraction should, however, not be done when the head is above the level of the ischial spines; the only exception to this rule is application of the VE to the head of a second twin. If a delivery is not completed in 20–30 minutes, it is highly probable that the VE will fail.

Contraindications for the use of the VE are uncorrected face or brow presentations, breech delivery and relatively severe cephalopelvic disproportion. We also consider premature birth with its increased risk for intracranial hemorrhage as a contradiction for vacuum extraction, although some studies failed to demonstrate an increased risk for the premature baby delivered by the VE.

The most common complication in the use of a VE delivery is detachment of the suction cup, usually caused by an incorrect direction of the traction. There is no increased risk to the mother associated with the use of a VE over the risk of the use of forceps. Vaginal rupture is less frequent with vacuum extraction than with forceps extraction, while the incidence of cervical tears is about the same. The artificial caput succedaneum on the baby's head disappears quickly and as a rule the baby leaves the hospital without any scalp marks. Small abrasions or ulcers on the scalp can be seen if too high a vacuum is used or if the extraction time is too long. The incidence of cephalhematoma is higher in babies delivered by the VE than in those delivered by forceps; it is not, however, of any serious clinical importance although it has been associated with hyperbilirubinemia. Prospective studies have shown that VE delivery in full-term babies is associated with no increased risk of serious cerebral sequelae.

Several new models of the VE have recently been introduced. The metal cup of Malmström's instrument has been replaced by cups of softer material. These new cups can be firmly attached to the fetal head without the need to first develop an artificial caput succedaneum. Thus, a more rapid delivery can be accomplished with less damage to the fetal scalp. There is an important limitation associated with the new instruments: forced rotation of the fetal head to correct certain malpositions cannot be done. It is too early to predict if the new modifications of the VE will lead to an increased use of vacuum extraction in the United States.

References

1. Malmström, T. The vacuum extractor, an obstetrical instrument, and the parturiometer, a tokographic device. *Acta Obstet. Gynecol. Scand. (Suppl.)* 36:7–50, 1957.
2. Plauché, W.C. Vacuum extraction: Use in a community hospital setting. *Obstet. Gynecol.* 52:289, 1978.

CHAPTER 40

Cesarean Section

RONALD M. CAPLAN, M.D.

The incidence of cesarean section in North America has been rising.[3] In years past, much attention was given to improving perinatal and maternal mortality rates. With the realization that the quality of the newborn infant and its long-term intellectual functioning could be adversely affected by traumatic delivery and asphyxia, cesarean section has become the preferred mode of delivery[4] in many situations (Tables 40.1 and 40.2).[1]

It can be seen (Table 40.1) that relative cephalopelvic disproportion, fetal distress, lack of progress, and breech presentation are some of the most frequent causes of primary cesarean section. Diabetic patients have a high rate of cesarean section, as do patients with twins.

A study of the incidence of forceps deliveries at the New York Hospital—Cornell University Medical Center revealed a significant decline in this mode of delivery. This bears an inverse relationship to the rise in the cesarean section rate, so that the percentage of all patients delivered by operative means remains relatively constant. Neonatal outcome was found to be significantly improved in both the forceps delivered group in the later years and the combined forceps and cesarean section group and in the total delivered population.

It is important to adequately assess the status of mother, fetus, and labor prior to performing a cesarean section for suspected dystocia. This includes assessing fetal well-being by adequate monitoring (see Chapter 36: "Fetal Monitoring in La-

bor") and by appropriate measurement of uterine contractility (see Chapter 33: "Uterine Contractility"), with due consideration given to the usage of oxytocin.

Cesarean section is an abdominal surgical procedure in which the peritoneal cavity is entered, with all the attendant risks to the mother. General or epidural anesthesia may be utilized. With the former, it

Table 40.1. Major Indications for Cesarean Section, New York Hospital, 1980

Indication	Percentage
Cephalopelvic disproportion	18.9
Repeat cesarean section	26.4
Breech presentation, term	10.3
Fetal distress	13.0
Lack of progress	6.8
Premature breech	2.9
Premature separation of the placenta	1.5
Placenta previa	1.8
Previous myomectomy	1.8
Failed induction	2.9
Cesarean section rate—twins (uncorrected)*	67.9
Cesarean section rate—diabetic pregnancies (uncorrected)*	49.2

* Twins and diabetics are included in the specific indication.

is important that all preparations for the procedure are carried out prior to induction of anesthesia so that the baby is removed from the uterus quickly after induction. This lessens the possibility of severe respiratory depression in the neonate. The use of epidural anesthesia allows the mother to be awake and see her newborn infant.

Table 40.2. Other Indications for Cesarean Section, New York Hospital, 1980

Failed forceps
Preeclampsia moderate, unfavorable cervix
Prolapsed cord
Multiple myomata
Postmature, falling estriols
Poor obstetrical history
Obstructing myoma
Previous repair of a prolapsed rectum
Eclampsia
Condylomata
Failed vacuum extraction
Large myoma
Uterus didelphys
Known omphalocele
Erythroblastosis
Achondroplastic dwarf
Abnormal N.S.T.
Positive C.S.T.
Placental insufficiency
Carcinoma of cervix
Compound presentation
Polyhydramnios hydrocephalic

* Twins and diabetics are included in the specific indication.

LOW SEGMENT CESAREAN SECTION

Currently, this is the more commonly performed type of the procedure. After the peritoneal cavity is entered, the peritoneum over the anterior aspect of the uterus is incised and reflected downward exposing the lower uterine segment, which at term and during labor is generally thinned. The urinary bladder is mobilized downward, and usually a transverse, but sometimes longitudinal, incision is made in the lower uterine segment. If the membranes have already ruptured, amniotic fluid will come from the incision. If the membranes are intact, they will bulge into the incision and can be ruptured at this point. The surgeon introduces a hand into the incision and with gentle traction on the presenting part, aided by a surgical assistant exerting downward pressure transabdominally on the uterine fundus, delivers the baby. The umbilical cord is doubly clamped and cut, and the baby is handed to a waiting member of the pediatric team.

Subsequently, the placenta is removed, and the uterine cavity is manually ex-plored to ensure that no fragments of placenta or membranes remain. The cervical os is checked without contamination to ensure that it is open, so that proper postpartum drainage of lochia may occur.

The uterine incision is then closed in two layers, the second imbricating the first. The peritoneal incision over the uterus is then closed, and the abdomen is closed in layers.

CLASSICAL CESAREAN SECTION

This procedure is reserved for cases such as the transverse lie or twins with abnormal lies or placenta previa with the placenta lying over the anterior lower uterine segment, where delivery through a lower segment incision could be difficult and traumatic. Occasionally, a preterm delivery, where there is effectively no developed lower uterine segment, can be effected less traumatically through a classical incision, especially with the baby in breech presentation. The classical section involves a vertical incision being made in the anterior wall of the uterus. The musculature here is thick and vascular, and the procedure usually results in more blood loss then does a low segment section. The resultant scar leaves an area of weakness in the anterior uterine wall.

DELIVERY IN SUBSEQUENT PREGNANCIES

If a cesarean section had to be done because of a significant degree of cephalopelvic disproportion or if a classical cesarean section had been done, all further pregnancies must be delivered by cesarean section.

However, in many instances, cesarean section was undertaken because of an abnormal presentation of the fetus, such as breech presentation, or because a condition such as placenta previa, that in a given case did not necessitate a classical section, existed. In these cases, it is possible to allow the patient who spontaneously commences labor to undergo a normal vaginal delivery,[2] provided that careful monitoring is utilized, always mindful that rupture of the previous low segment scar is possible, although not probable in the normal course of events.

References

1. Hawks, G.G., and Varnis, C. Annual Report of the Department of Obstetrics, New York Hospital—Cornell Medical Center, 1980.

2. Lavin, J.P., Stevens, R.J., et al. Vaginal delivery in patients with a prior cesarean section. *Obstet. Gynecol. 59:* 135, 1982.

3. Rosen, M.G., Alper, M.H., et al. (The Cesarean Birth Task Force) NIH consensus development statement on cesarean childbirth. *Obstet. Gynecol. 57:*537, 1981.

4. Williams, R.L., and Chen, P.M. Identifying the sources of the recent decline in perinatal mortality rates in California. *N. Engl. J. Med. 306:*207, 1982.

Section 4
Postpartum

CHAPTER 41

Postpartum Complications

RONALD M. CAPLAN, M.D.

The puerperium is defined as the 6-week period following delivery of the fetus during which the maternal reproductive organs return to their nonpregnant state.

Maternal hemorrhage and infection are significant possibilities during this period, and toxemia remains a danger in the early postpartum period.

HEMORRHAGE

Postpartum hemorrhage may occur almost immediately following the birth of the baby or may be delayed. Uterine atony, lacerations in the birth canal, and retained placenta are the important causative factors.

Long, exhausting labors and induced labors may be associated with uterine atony postpartum. The "latticework" of muscle fibers in the uterus, through which the uterine vessels pass, do not contract adequately, and bleeding occurs from the raw placental site. Retained placental fragments may also prevent adequate uterine contraction, resulting in persistent bleeding postpartum. Lacerations may occur in the vulva, vagina, cervix or even the lower uterine segment. Prolonged or hypertonic labor may result in uterine rupture in the lower uterine segment. A previous cesarean section scar, or myomectomy scar, may rupture.

Immediately after delivery of the placenta, many consider it to be good obstetrical practice, with proper sterile technique, to manually explore the uterus, ensuring that no placental fragments are left behind. The placenta itself should always be inspected for signs of missing cotyledons.

The cervix is then inspected around its circumference to ensure that it is intact. The vagina is totally inspected, from the vaginal introitus to the fornices, to ensure that no lacerations are present. If an episiotomy has been made to prevent tearing of the introitus, it is important to begin the vaginal suture above the apex of the incision and to ensure that hemostasis is secured while suturing each successive layer of the incision.

Pitocin is generally given by intravenous infusion postpartum, especially in cases where induction of labor has been employed.

The patient who hemorrhages is a prime candidate for postpartum infection, and, conversely, the patient with a postpartum endometritis typically has a subinvoluted uterus and thus may continue to bleed. Moreover, retained fragments of placenta not only can cause hemorrhage but also are prime sites for infection.

Treatment of hemorrhage consists of identifying the source of bleeding, by sterile examination under anesthesia if necessary. Retained placental fragments are removed, and lacerations are sutured. Pitocin and ergotrate may be given to combat uterine atony. Blood transfusions are given. The patient is closely monitored for signs of shock or developing coagulopathy.

In extreme cases, such as laceration of a uterine artery, abdominal operative intervention may be necessary to ligate the vessel, or to perform a hysterectomy. Ligation of the internal iliac vessels is rarely required.

HEMATOMAS

Not all postpartum hemorrhage is obvious, with blood issuing from the vagina. If a blood vessel is torn by manipulation or tears spontaneously, hematoma formation—an occult accumulation of blood—may occur. Most commonly, this is seen at the site of the episiotomy or where vulvar and vaginal lacerations have occurred. In such cases, bleeding vessels, often at the apex of the wound, are the causative factor. Blood accumulates in the wound and may track into the ischiorectal fossa. Bleeding from cervical lacerations is generally obvious, but damage to the lower uterine segment or to the uterine vessels laterally (which can occur spontaneously in uterine rupture, during intrauterine manipulations, with forceps application, or with extension of a cesarean section scar) can result in retroperitoneal accumulations of blood that can track laterally through the broad ligaments to the lateral pelvic sidewalls, compressing the ureters. If the peritoneum is opened or torn, direct bleeding into the peritoneal cavity can result.

Prevention of these complications involves careful suturing of the episiotomy, beginning above the apex of the wound. Careful sterile examination of the postpartum patient to check the integrity of the uterus, cervix, and vagina should be done, followed by suturing of any lacerations. In spite of the most careful observance of these techniques, however, hematoma formation still can arise.

If the hematoma occurs in the episiotomy or in a vulvar laceration, the patient will experience pain at the site. Swelling and bluish discoloration of the overlying skin are obvious. The incision may later break down, due to the tension or to infection. A risk of infection in a hematoma, with subsequent abscess formation, exists.

A retroperitoneal hematoma can result in lower abdominal pain; if appreciable blood loss has occurred, a mass may be in evidence on abdominal, pelvic, or rectal examination. The patient will manifest a dropping hematocrit and, ultimately, shock, characterized by weakness, dizzi-

ness, rapid pulse, falling blood pressure (especially when standing), and a decreased urinary output. Pelvic ultrasonography or computerized axial tomography may be used to delineate the hematoma.

If the hematoma stabilizes and bleeding does not persist, supportive treatment to prevent shock and careful observation may be all that is necessary. Blood transfusions may be required. If bleeding persists, reoperation with identification of and suturing of bleeding points may become necessary.

INFECTION

The natural defenses of the female reproductive tract are diminished postpartum, and the new mother is a prime target for ascending infection. The episiotomy may become infected and "break down"— that is, the sutures may open, leading to hemorrhage from that site and necessitating resuturing. Endometritis may occur, manifested by subinvolution of the uterus, uterine tenderness, pelvic pain, increased "lochia" or postpartum blood flow which might or might not be purulent or have a foul odor, and fever. Further progression might lead to salpingitis, pelvic peritonitis, and generalized peritonitis.

Aerobic and anaerobic cultures of the uterine cavity and blood cultures must be taken in these cases, and appropriate intravenous antibiotics must be instituted. (See Chapter 25: "Infectious Diseases.")

The nursing mother may develop mastitis, infection usually introduced through "cracks" around the nipple. The mother develops a painful, tender erythematous area in the breast and fever. Cultures of the milk are taken, and appropriate antibiotics are given. If the mother continues to nurse, care must be taken in the choice of antibiotics, as they pass in the breast milk to the fetus.

TOXEMIA

The preeclamptic patient is not free of the danger of progression to eclampsia until significant diuresis occurs postpartum. Therefore careful monitoring, including frequent vital signs, intake and output, and daily weights, is employed until the patient has stabilized. (See Chapter 20: "Hypertensive Disorders of Pregnancy.")

THROMBOPHLEBITIS

Thrombophlebitis occurs more often in the puerperium than during the pregnancy itself. It more commonly occurs in the lower extremities, either superficially or deep, but pelvic vein thrombophlebitis may be associated with postpartum pelvic infection. Pulmonary embolism is a possibility.

Early ambulation is a preventative measure advocated in the postpartum patient. If superficial phlebitis does occur below the knee, elevation of the leg, warm packs, and bed rest may be sufficient treatment. If deep vein phlebitis occurs, anticoagulation is employed, with attention being paid to the possibility of increased uterine bleeding.

AMNIOTIC FLUID EMBOLISM

This rare complication in the immediate postpartum period frequently is fatal. However, definitive diagnosis is difficult without demonstrating fetal material in the maternal lungs by biopsy, so some surviving cases may go undiagnosed. The examination of blood from a maternal central venous pressure catheter and the examination of maternal sputum for fetal squames are alternatives. A lung scan can be helpful.

The condition is more likely to occur in the older multigravida or in the gravida who experiences a tumultuous labor. Uterine stimulants have been implicated. Cesarean section, retained placenta, and placenta accreta all increase the possibility of amniotic fluid embolism. The relatively innocuous acts of rupturing membranes or placement of an intrauterine pressure catheter may have some slight influence on the incidence.

The patient develops respiratory distress, cyanosis, cardiovascular collapse with hypotension out of proportion to the blood loss, and coma.

The particulate matter in the amniotic fluid causes pulmonary vascular obstruction, leading to a decrease in left atrial pressure and decreased cardiac output which causes the hypotension. The perfusion defect leads to anoxia, and pulmonary hypertension occurs. The circulating amniotic fluid leads to disseminated intravascular coagulation, with resultant consumption of fibrinogen and an increase in fibrinolytic activity.

Therapy consists of cardiopulmonary resuscitative measures and treatment of the coagulopathy. Blood and fibrinogen are replaced. Hydrocortisone is employed. In some cases, heparinization may be warranted.

SHOCK

The most common cause of shock in the postpartum patient is blood loss. The patient will display the symptoms and signs alluded to in the discussion of hemorrhage and hematoma. The treatment is essentially twofold—prompt blood transfusion and careful monitoring of vital signs. Hourly urinary output is monitored with an indwelling Foley catheter. A central venous pressure catheter is utilized, and in extreme situations a Swan-Ganz catheter is used to monitor pulmonary capillary bed pressures.

The coagulation profile and hematocrit are monitored. Equally important, prompt attention is paid to stopping the bleeding, by measures outlined in the previous discussion.

Infection may lead to shock, secondary to release of endotoxins. In these cases, the blood pressure may stay in the low normal range, while urinary output drops significantly. Intravascular coagulation occurs, and clotting defects ensue. The treatment includes the monitoring previously discussed, aggressive use of antibiotics, whole blood transfusion monitored by placement of a central venous pressure line or a Swan-Ganz catheter, and, if necessary, steroids.

Surgery may rarely become necessary to remove the grossly infected uterus.

Pulmonary embolism and amniotic fluid

embolism can result in shock, as previously described. In the former condition, anticoagulation with intravenous heparin is utilized, as well as cardiopulmonary resuscitative measures.

Rare cases of acute myocardial infarction with subsequent cardiogenic shock have been described in older women, in the second stage of labor or postpartum.

Inversion of the uterus is a rare complication that leads to immediate profound shock. In this condition, after delivery, traction on the umbilical cord of a placenta attached to the uterine fundus leads to the uterus turning "inside out." The patient becomes comatose, with unobtainable blood pressure. Treatment consists of immediate sterile manual conversion of the uterus to its normal state, following which manual removal of the placenta can be done. The danger of hemorrhage after this event is significant. The condition is largely preventable: traction on the umbilical cord should not be used as a means to remove the placenta.

PITUITARY

Very rarely, severe postpartum hemorrhage and shock results in anterior pituitary infarction and amenorrhea: Sheehan's syndrome.

The Chiari-Frommel syndrome refers to the postpartum appearance and persistence of amenorrhea and galactorrhea: that is, the constant leakage of milk in the non-nursing mother.

DEPRESSION

Postpartum depression is a well-recognized phenomenon. It is usually self-limited in nature and generally does not last for more than 10 days. Episodic emotional lability, with mood swings and crying spells, is in evidence. Less commonly, the depression may be severe.

Bibliography

1. Lumley, J., Owen, R., and Morgan, M. Amniotic fluid embolism: A report of three cases. *Anaesthesia* 34:33, 1979.
2. Melges, F.T., and DeMaso, D.R. Postpartum psychiatric reactions. In *Psychological Aspects of Gynecology and Obstetrics*, edited by Wolman, B.B. Medical Economics, Oradell, NJ, 1978, p. 201.
3. Morgan, M. Amniotic fluid embolism. *Anaesthesia* 34:20, 1979.
4. Wasser, W.G., Tessler, S., et al. Nonfatal amniotic fluid embolism: A case report of postpartum respiratory distress with histopathologic studies. *Mt. Sinai J. Med.* 46:388–391, 1979.

Index